Current Topics in Pathology
84/1

E. Grundmann and E. Vollmer (Eds.)

Reaction Patterns of the Lymph Node

Part 1 Cell Types and Functions

Contributors
C. Bélisle · S. Bödewadt-Radzun · B. Brado
A. Castenholz · Y. Cho · P.P.H. de Bruyn
J. Delabie · C. de Wolf-Peeters · F. Facchetti
S. Fossum · M.-L. Hansmann · E.C.M. Hoefsmit
E.W.A. Kamperdijk · F.G.M. Kroese · P. Möller
P. Nieuwenhuis · M.R. Parwaresch · F.S. Peng
H.J. Radzun · G. Sainte-Marie · W. Timens
J.J. van den Oord · E.B.J. van Nieuwkerk
M.A.M. Verdaasdonk · H.-H. Wacker

Springer-Verlag
Berlin Heidelberg New York
London Paris Tokyo
Hong Kong Barcelona

E. GRUNDMANN, Professor Dr.
E. VOLLMER, Dr. Dr.

Gerhard-Domagk-Institut für Pathologie
der Universität Münster, Domagkstr. 17
4400 Münster, Federal Republic of Germany

C.L. BERRY, Professor, M.D., Ph.D., F.R.C. Path.

Department of Morbid Anatomy, The London Hospital,
London E1 1BB, United Kingdom

With 102 Figures and 11 Tables

ISBN-13:978-3-642-75521-7 e-ISBN-13:978-3-642-75519-4
DOI: 10.1007978-3-642-75519-4

Softcover reprint of the hardcover 1st edition 1990

2113/3130-543210 – Printed on acid-free paper

List of Contributors

Bélisle, C., Dr.	Département d'Anatomie, Université de Montréal, CP 6128 Succ. A, Montréal, Québec, H3C 3J7, Canada
Bödewadt-Radzun, S., Dr.	Pathologisches Institut der Universität Kiel, Michaelisstraße 11, D-2300 Kiel
Brado, B., Dr.	Pathologisches Institut der Universität Heidelberg, Im Neuenheimer Feld 220, D-6900 Heidelberg
Castenholz, A., Prof. Dr.	Gesamthochschule Kassel, Institut für Humanbiologie, Universität Kassel, Heinrich-Plett-Straße 40, D-3500 Kassel
Cho, Y., Dr.	Department of Surgery, University of Illinois, Chicago, IL 60612, USA
de Bruyn, P. P. H., Dr.	Department of Organismal Biology and Anatomy and Committee on Immunology, The University of Chicago, 1025 E. 57th Street Chicago, IL 60637, USA
Delabie, J., Dr.	Department of Pathology II, Laboratory of Histo- and Cytochemistry, University Hospital St. Rafael, Catholic University of Leuven, B-3000 Leuven, Belgium

DE WOLF-PEETERS, C., Prof. Dr.
Department of Pathology II,
Laboratory of Histo- and Cytochemistry,
University Hospital St. Rafael,
Catholic University of Leuven,
B-3000 Leuven, Belgium

FACCHETTI, F., Dr.
Department of Pathology II,
Laboratory of Histo- and Cytochemistry,
University Hospital St. Rafael,
Catholic University of Leuven,
B-3000 Leuven, Belgium

FOSSUM, S., Dr.
Anatomical Institute,
University of Oslo,
Karl Johansgate 47,
N-0162 Oslo 1, Norway

HANSMANN, M.-L. Prof. Dr.
Pathologisches Institut
der Universität Kiel,
Michaelisstraße 11,
D-2300 Kiel

HOEFSMIT, E. C. M. Prof. Dr.
Department of Cell Biology,
Division of Electron Microscopy
Medical Faculty, Vrije Universiteit,
Van der Boechorststraat 7,
NL-1081 BT Amsterdam, The Netherlands

KAMPERDIJK, E. W. A., Dr.
Department of Cell Biology,
Division of Electron Microscopy,
Medical Faculty, Vrije Universiteit,
Van der Boechorststraat 7,
NL-1081 BT Amsterdam, The Netherlands

KROESE, F. G. M., Dr.
Department of Histology and Cell Biology,
Immunology Section,
University of Groningen,
Oostersingel 69/1,
NL-9713 EZ Groningen, The Netherlands

MÖLLER, P., PD, Dr.
Pathologisches Institut
der Universität Heidelberg,
Im Neuenheimer Feld 220,
D-6900 Heidelberg

NIEUWENHUIS, P., Prof. Dr.	Department of Histology and Cell Biology, Immunology Section, University of Groningen, Oostersingel 69/1, NL-9713 EZ Groningen, The Netherlands
PARWARESCH, M. R., Prof. Dr.	Pathologisches Institut der Universität Kiel, Michaelisstraße 11, D-2300 Kiel
PENG, F. S., Dr.	Département d'Anatomie, Université de Montréal, CP 6128 Succ. A., Montréal, Québec, H3C 3J7, Canada
RADZUN, H. J., Prof. Dr.	Pathologisches Institut der Universität Kiel, Michaelisstraße 11, D-2300 Kiel
SAINTE-MARIE, G., Dr.	Département d'Anatomie, Université de Montréal, CP 6128 Succ. A., Montréal, Québec, H3C 3J7, Canada
TIMENS, W., Dr.	Department of Pathology, University of Groningen, Oostersingel 69/1, NL-9713 EZ Groningen, The Netherlands
VAN DEN OORD, J. J., Dr.	Department of Pathology II, Laboratory of Histo- and Cytochemistry, University Hospital St. Rafael, Catholic University of Leuven, B-3000 Leuven, Belgium
VAN NIEUWKERK, E. B. J., Dr.	Department of Cell Biology, Division of Electron Microscopy, Medical Faculty, Vrije Universiteit, Van der Boechorststraat 7, NL-1081 BT Amsterdam, The Netherlands

Verdaasdonk, M.A.M., Dr. — Department of Cell Biology, Division of Electron Microscopy, Medical Faculty, Vrije Universiteit, Van der Boechorststraat 7, NL-1081 BT Amsterdam, The Netherlands

Wacker, H.-H., Dr. — Pathologisches Institut der Universität Kiel, Michaelisstraße 11, D-2300 Kiel

Preface

Due to the topology and structure of the lymph nodes, their role in the pathogenesis and development of diseases is a very special one. Each organ and even each organ-related region of the body has its own group of lymph nodes, specific topological reactions, such as in circumscribed inflammation or in the metastatic spread of malignant tumors. On the other hand, all the lymph nodes of an organism join in a uniform function effected by highly differentiated structures.

Volume 84 of *Current Topics in Pathology* presents our current knowledge about the structure and reaction patterns of this "secondary" lymphoid organ. Despite our original intention to publish all the contributions in one book, it became necessary to divide them: Part 1 focuses on the involved nodal compartments, cell types, and functions, while Part 2 describes their reactions in inflammatory, neoplastic, and immune-deficient diseases. Even with the cooperation of more than 30 authors, the coverage cannot be exhaustive. The scope of both parts is limited to those reactions that can be described by direct and indirect morphological methods, including modern techniques such as immune electron microscopy.

The opening chapter of Part 1 centers around the basic structures and the cellular multiformity of lymph nodes in their respective functional contexts. In lymphoid tissue, cellular reactions cannot be fully understood unless their basic architecture is also taken into consideration, as it is here. A valuable tool for this purpose is the three-dimensional respresentation of tissue at lower and higher magnifications in combination with the corrosion cast technique. Insight into the nodal architecture also improves our understanding of the intranodal passage of blood and lymphoid cells. Each compartment of the lymph node is linked to this flow of blood and lymphoid cells and equipped with a specific reactivity, for example in the different strata of the cortex and medulla.

One chapter is devoted to the deep cortex, and its functional units describing their specific reactions to antigenic stimulation. The correlation of structure and function is particularly evident in a comparative study of lymph nodes in nude and euthymic rats.

Of particular significance regarding the passage of lymphocytes through the nodes are the high endothelia of postcapillary venules, since the attachment of lymphocytes to these endothelia represents the first phase of transmural lymphocyte passage, followed by their eventual penetration. There is an obvious lymphocyte-endothelial interaction that is of considerable importance under normal conditions and exhibits specific reactions to pathologic changes.

The functional structure of lymph nodes corresponds with a specific disposition of immunoactive cells. Germinal centers are the chief site of B cells and the B cell immune reaction. One chapter presents the other cell types within that zone, such as germinal center T cells, dendritic reticulum cells, and macrophages. Pathologic conditions evoke typical germinal center reactions of varying specificity.

T lymphocytes, in contrast, are not subject to such strict local confinement. Though their preferred site is the paracortex, they are also found in immune-stimulated areas and, during the immune response proper, in other compartments of the node, where they may form T nodules or special organoid structures depending on the actual stage of the response. A cell type particular to the T zones of human lymphoid tissue is known as the plasmacytoid T cells or plasmacytoid monocytes. Although their function is largely unclear, they are known to express CD4 antigen in the absence of B cell antigens.

In rodent and human lymph nodes professional "accessory cells" have the capacity to stimulate specific T or B cell responses following antigen pulsing. Most of them have a tree-like appearance, and the term "dendritic cells" is widely used. Corresponding to the bimodal differentiation of lymphocytes, there seem to be two types of dendritic accessory cells: those involved in cellular immunity (T accessory cells) and those involved in humoral immunity (B accessory cells). The functional activities of these cells is comprehensively presented for the first time.

Two chapters are devoted to the role of macrophages in the structural and functional system of the lymph node. The first describes the characteristic types of macrophages attributed to the different compartments of the node, including the Langerhans' cells of the skin. These may pick up and transport antigen as "veiled cells" by way of the afferent lymphatics and subcapsular sinus into the outer cortex of the node. Also, Langerhans' cells are known to share Fc receptors and CR1 with the macrophages and to express macrophage-specific markers. The second describes the different phenotypic features of macrophages, using a set of fairly specific reagents. Reference is also made to classification and to certain other features distinguishing between professional phagocytes and non phagocytic dentritic cells that are specialized for the processing and the presenting of antigens. Here, too, a bimodal differentiation of cells reflects their functional engagement in either cellular or humoral immunity.

Immune electron microscopy is of great assistance in the ultrastructural localization of target antigens. The value of this approach is exemplified in the distinction of B and T cells and of the macrophage subtypes, the interdigitating and dendritic cells, and the sinus-lining cells. Further consideration is given to the problems of tissue preservation and of the predictability of required electron density of various structures, especially in the nuclear cell compartments.

Part 1 of this volume attempts to survey the relevant structural and functional relationships between the different compartments of the lymph node, with particular emphasis on the different cell components involved, thereby providing the base for Part 2, which reviews the specific reaction patterns of the nodes in neoplastic and immune-deficient disease.

Münster, June 1990

EKKEHARD GRUNDMANN
EKKEHARD VOLLMER

Contents

Indexed in ISR

Architecture of the Lymph Node with Regard to Its Function

A. Castenholz

1 Introduction

Together with the spleen, the tonsils, and the gut-associated structures (GALT), the lymph nodes represent secondary lymphoid organs. The main task of all these organs consists in enabling lymphoid cells, most of which originate from the primary lymphoid organs (thymus and bone marrow), to react with antigens and so to initiate immune responses. As integrated parts of the lymph vascular system, the lymph nodes carry out further functions by filtering lymph.

This chapter will be concerned with the basic morphology of the mammalian lymph node and will demonstrate its functions as far as they are reflected in morphological findings. For this purpose *scanning electron microscopy* is preferable to light microscopy; it provides pictures with a three-dimensional representation of the tissue at both low and high magnification and thus is very effective in elucidating the special architectural conditions in different parts of the node. In combination with the corrosion cast technique, scanning electron microscopy can visualize interstitial spaces as well as lymphatic vascular structures and the intranodal lymph spaces (Kobayashi et al. 1976; Kurokawa and Ogata 1980; Castenholz 1983c, 1985a, b, 1989a). It should be pointed out that lymph nodes of different species may exhibit structural and functional features which differ to a greater or lesser extent from those outlined here. Moreover, depending on the particular antigenic and metabolic situation, the morphology of the node tissue quickly alters even within individuals, and the transition from a state to be regarded as normal to a reactive pattern that can be assessed as pathological is fluid (in this context, see Chap. 4 by FOSSUM in this volume).

2 General Arrangement

Lymph nodes are bean-shaped organs located throughout the body (Fig. 1). They are interposed as links in the lymph-conducting vascular system. Between the finest roots of this system in the tissue, the initial lymphatics, and the large lymph stems joining the blood circulation at the level of the jugular veins, a number of lymph nodes are inserted as special controlling stations for the lymph. The tributary lymph nodes of an organ are arranged in groups and are found in typical locations under the skin or in the bowels. Aggregates of lymph nodes exist along the superficial and deeper cervical pathways, in the axillary,

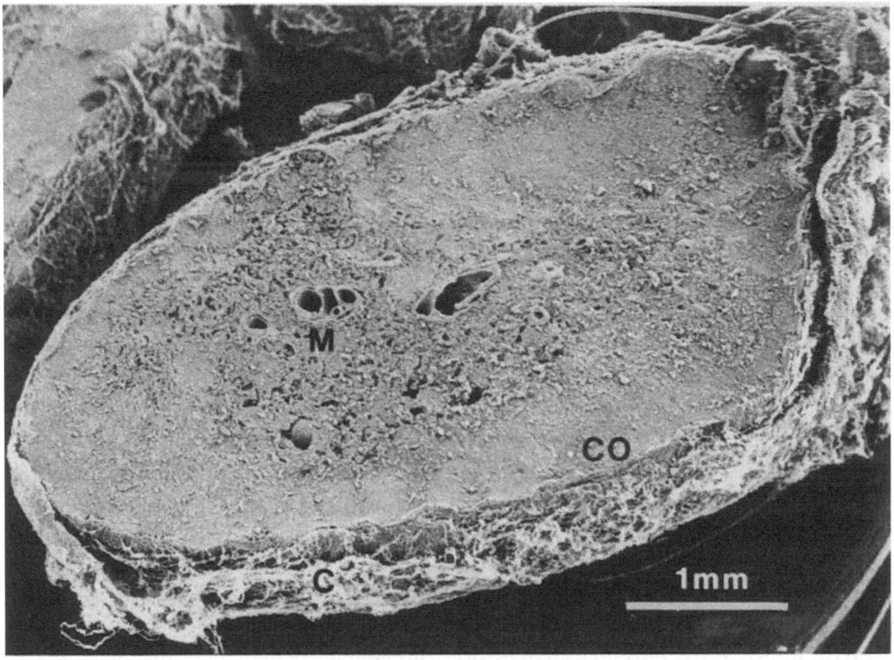

Fig. 1. Scanning electron micrograph of a cat lymph node. The small capsule (*c*) is covered by fine strands of loose fibrous connective tissue, which anchors the node in the surrounding body region. The cut plane shows the dense area of the cortex (*CO*) and the sponge-like zone of the medulla (*M*) with some vascular structures

supraclavicular, and infraclavicular fossae, in the groin, and along the iliac and mesenteric arteries.

Lymphoid tissue in connection with a lymph-draining system first appears in birds. In the higher vertebrates it reaches a high degree of complexity, comprising diffuse lymphoid tissue as well as highly organized solitary lymph nodes. With the progress of phylogeny, the number of lymph nodes also increases. The dog possesses about 60 nodes, the pig 190, cattle 300, and man 500–1000, while in the horse up to 8000 nodes have been counted (BAUM and TRAUTMANN 1933; EHRLICH 1946).

The lymphatic vascular system consists of different kinds of vessels exhibiting special structural and functional features. The initial lymphatics are thin-walled tubes comparable to the blood sinusoids and arranged in a plexus-like manner in many organs. The functional morphology of these vessels, which forms the base for our knowledge of the lymph-forming process, has been described in previous papers (CASTENHOLZ 1984, 1985a, 1987a, 1989b). The lymph flows from the initial lymphatics into the precollector channels and from there into the collecting vessels proper with the lymph node stations. Precollectors and collectors are richly equipped with valvular structures. The valves appear in collectors at regular distances, so creating characteristic circular constrictions of the outer vascular contour. Thus, single vascular units, the lymph angions, are formed in course of a collector (MISLIN 1983). Owing to the contractile properties of each lymph angion, the prenodal and postnodal lymph is actively propelled.

The prenodal lymph enters the lymph node via several afferent lymphatics and leaves it mostly only via one afferent vessel. By the grouping of lymph nodes associated with a tributary lymphatic pathway system, either at the same level or in a chain-like system of connected nodes, two effective principles are realized. One is the convergence of many peripheral lymphatic pathways upon one node or only a few nodes; the other is the repeated flow passage of the lymph through nodal tissue.

Although it has been observed that the lymph never reaches the blood circulation without passing at least one lymph node (and more frequently a series of lymph nodes) (DRINKER et al. 1934; YOFFEY and COURTICE 1970), it has been reported that in rats testicular lymph is drained without entering a lymph node (ENGESET 1959). It remains to be ascertained to what extent this observation represents an exception related to a certain species and a special organ.

3 Architecture

Lymph nodes are solitary structures endowed with a capsule of dense fibrous tissue. They are embedded in the surrounding loose connective tissue by fine strands of collagenous fibers. The capsule consists of a firm layer of collagenous fibers and fibrocytes, fine elastic fibers, and a few smooth muscle fibers,

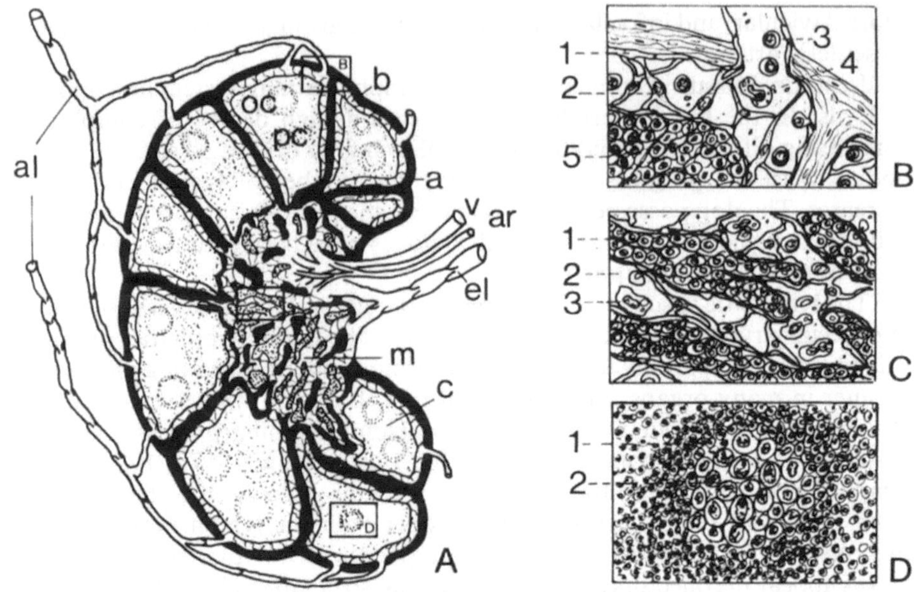

Fig. 2. **A** Basic architecture of the human lymph node. The framework of the capsule and trabeculae (*a*) surrounds compartments, with the parenchyma consisting of the sinuses (*b*) and the reticular tissue (*c*). The interior of the lymph node contains three zones: outer cortex with nodules (*oc*), paracortex (*pc*), and medulla (*m*). Afferent lymphatics (*al*) enter the node at points over the entire circumference, while one efferent lymphatic (*el*) leaves it at the hilus. There are also the supporting blood vessels, artery (*ar*) and vein (*v*). **B** Enlargement of area similar to *rectangle* indicated in **A**. The marginal sinus is represented. *1*, littoral cell; *2*, reticulum cell; *3*, lymphocyte; *4*, macrophage; *5*, B cell population of the reticular tissue of the outer cortex. **C** Enlargement of corresponding area in **A**. *1*, medullary cords with columns of plasma cells and other lymphoid cells; *2*, medullary sinuses; *3*, macrophage. **D** Enlargement of the nodular zone corresponding to *rectangle* in **A**. *1*, small lymphocytes of the peripheral corona; *2*, germinal center with large lymphocytes (immunoblasts)

and from its inner surface *trabecular structures* of similar composition branch off to cross the interior of the node. The capsule and the trabecular structures form the framework responsible for the constancy of the nodes' shape (Fig. 2A). Most trabeculae have a radial orientation and so converge toward the inner zone of the node. Some compose small tissue formations with broad fenestrations and numerous interconnections to each other.

The capsule is pierced by several *afferent lymphatics* with their twigs, while commonly only one *efferent lymphatic* leaves the node at the *hilus* (Fig. 3a, b). In this particular area the outer contour of the node shows a slight indentation. The hilus is also the place where the supporting blood vessels pass. The spaces between the compact collagenous tissue of the capsule and the trabeculae, which together form the *stroma*, contain a meshwork of fine collagenous and reticular fibrils occupied by a large number of lymphoid cells. A very dense accumulation of lymphocytes exists in the outer region of the node, the *cortex*. In young and adult individuals this zone possesses spherical structures with a

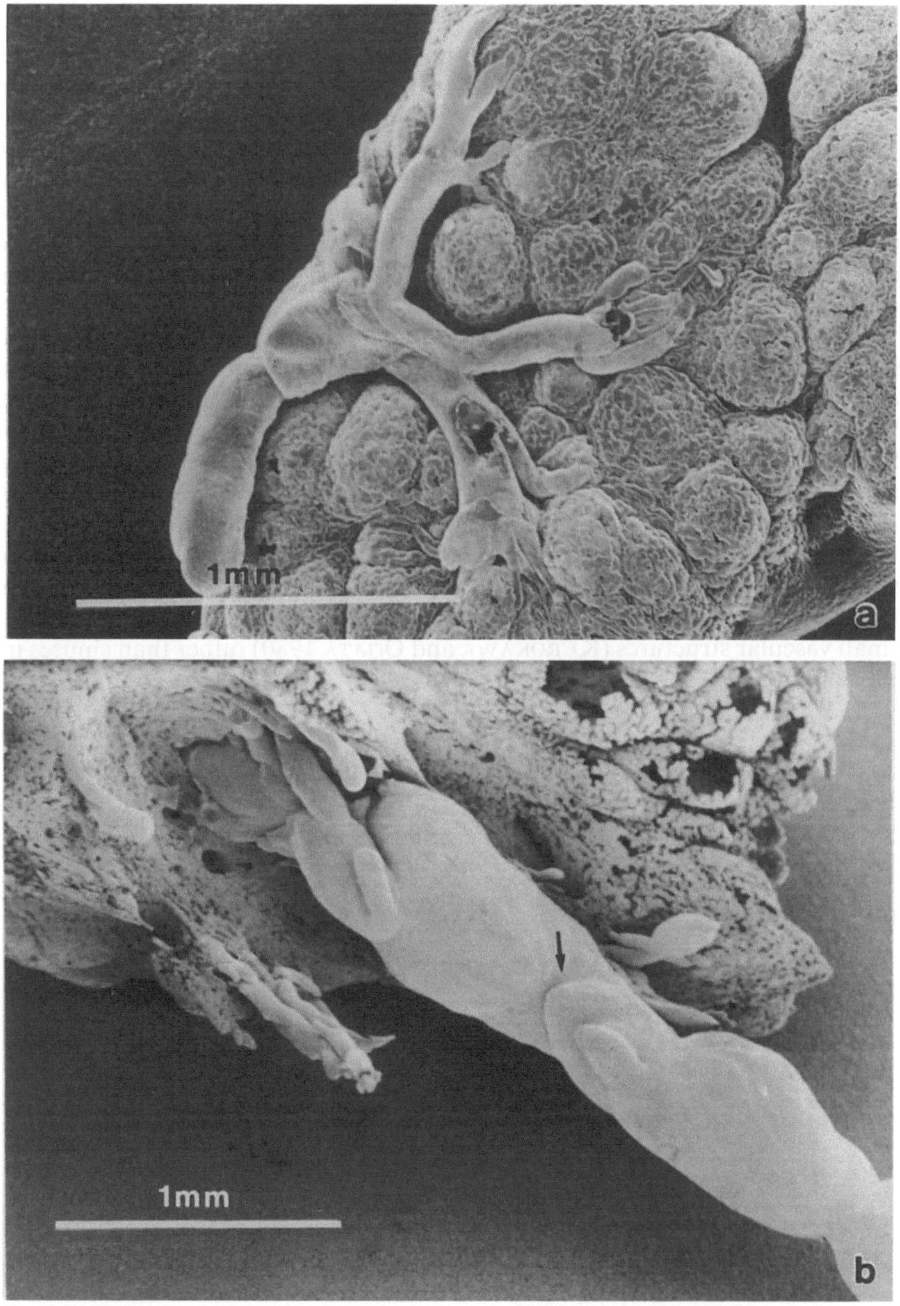

Fig. 3 a, b. In these scanning micrographs of a corrosion cast of a rabbit mesenteric lymph node the afferent lymphatics (**a**) and the efferent lymphatic (**b**) are represented as resin casts. The valves of the vessels have been imprinted as sharp indentations (*arrow*). In **a** the marginal sinus has been filled by the resin, too

special cellular pattern, termed *primary* and *secondary nodules* (Fig. 2D). Together with the reticular tissue of other nodal regions, these structures form the *parenchyma*. The nodules are unstable structures which undergo changes in size, composition, and dimension in accordance with age and state of health.

The tissue of the central part of the node, the *medulla*, has a looser character. Although the cellular elements of the medulla do not essentially differ from those of the cortex, the lymphoid cells are arranged toward the hilus in irregular strands, *medullary cords*, which interlace to form a coarse plexiform system (Fig. 2C). The intermediate zone between the outer cortex and the medulla is called the *paracortex*.

A system of small and broader continuous and interconnected ducts and spaces, the *sinuses*, constitutes a further element of the lymph node. The system of sinuses, which is filled with lymph, can be regarded as an intranodal link between the afferent and efferent lymphatic pathways. According to their location, different kinds of sinuses – subcapsular (marginal) sinus, penetrating (trabecular, intermediate) sinus, and medullary sinus – can be distinguished (Fig. 4). The space upon which all medullary sinuses converge and which joins the efferent lymphatic is termed the *terminal sinus*. The sinuses commonly form wide, irregular spaces and channels crowded by cells (Figs. 2B, 5). Deviating from such a sinus type, fine *tubular sinuses* have been observed which resemble small vascular structures (KUROKAWA and OGATA 1980) rather than sinuses in the common sense.

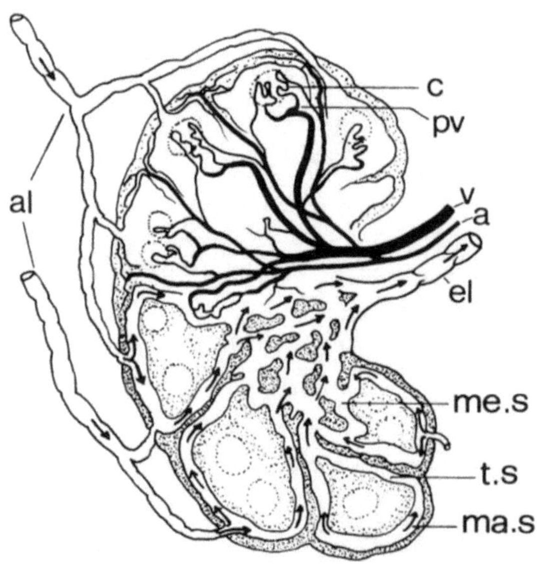

Fig. 4. Blood vascular system (*upper half*) and sinus system (*lower half*) of a rat lymph node. *a*, nodal artery; *v*, nodal vein; *c*, capillaries in nodular area; *pv*, postcapillary venules; *al*, afferent lymphatics; *el*, efferent lymphatic; *ma.s*, marginal sinus; *t.s*, trabecular sinus; *me.s*, medullary sinus. *Arrows* indicate the direction of the main lymph stream through the sinus system. Percolation of lymph through the reticular tissue has not been considered in this diagram

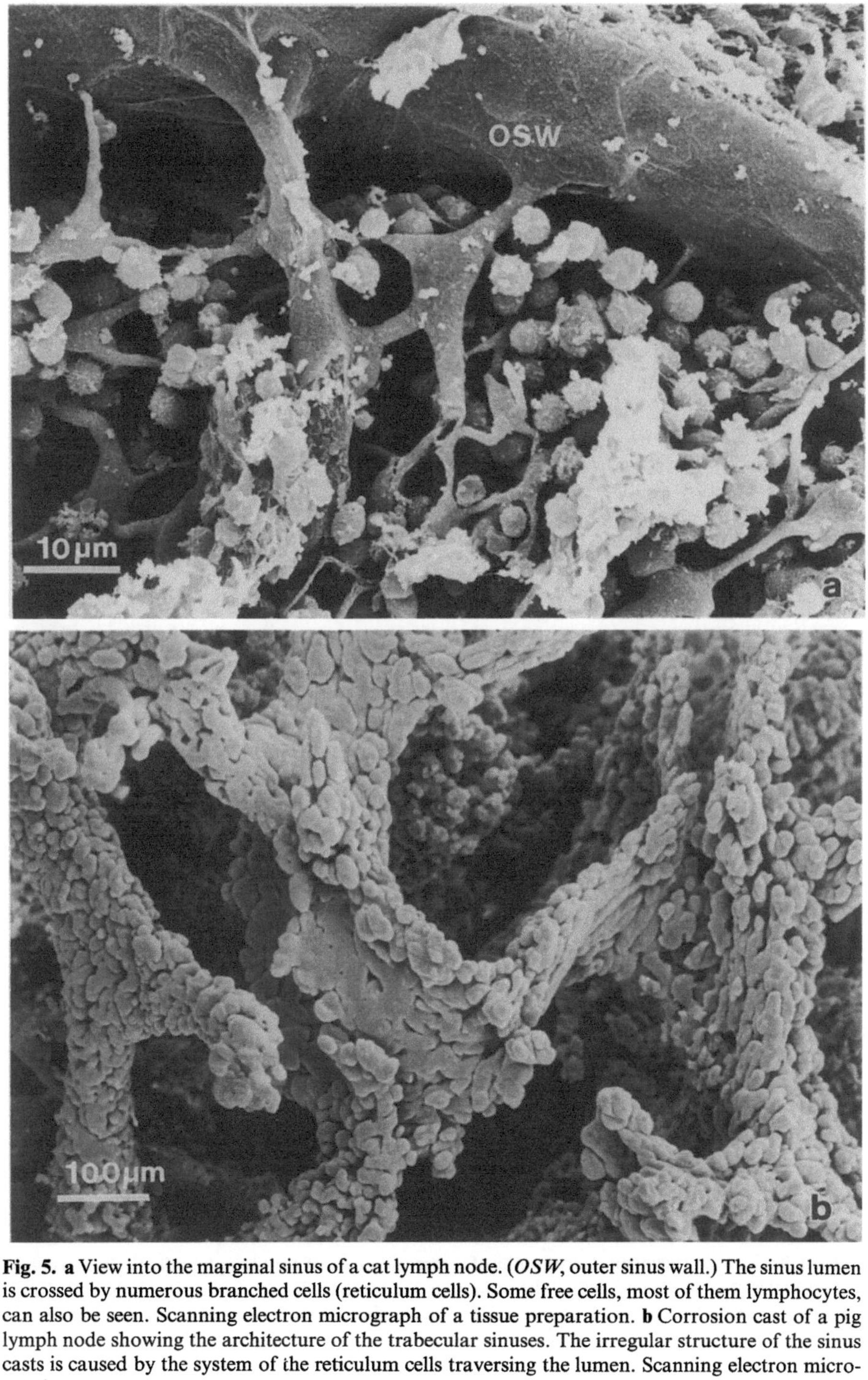

Fig. 5. a View into the marginal sinus of a cat lymph node. (*OSW*, outer sinus wall.) The sinus lumen is crossed by numerous branched cells (reticulum cells). Some free cells, most of them lymphocytes, can also be seen. Scanning electron micrograph of a tissue preparation. **b** Corrosion cast of a pig lymph node showing the architecture of the trabecular sinuses. The irregular structure of the sinus casts is caused by the system of the reticulum cells traversing the lumen. Scanning electron micrograph

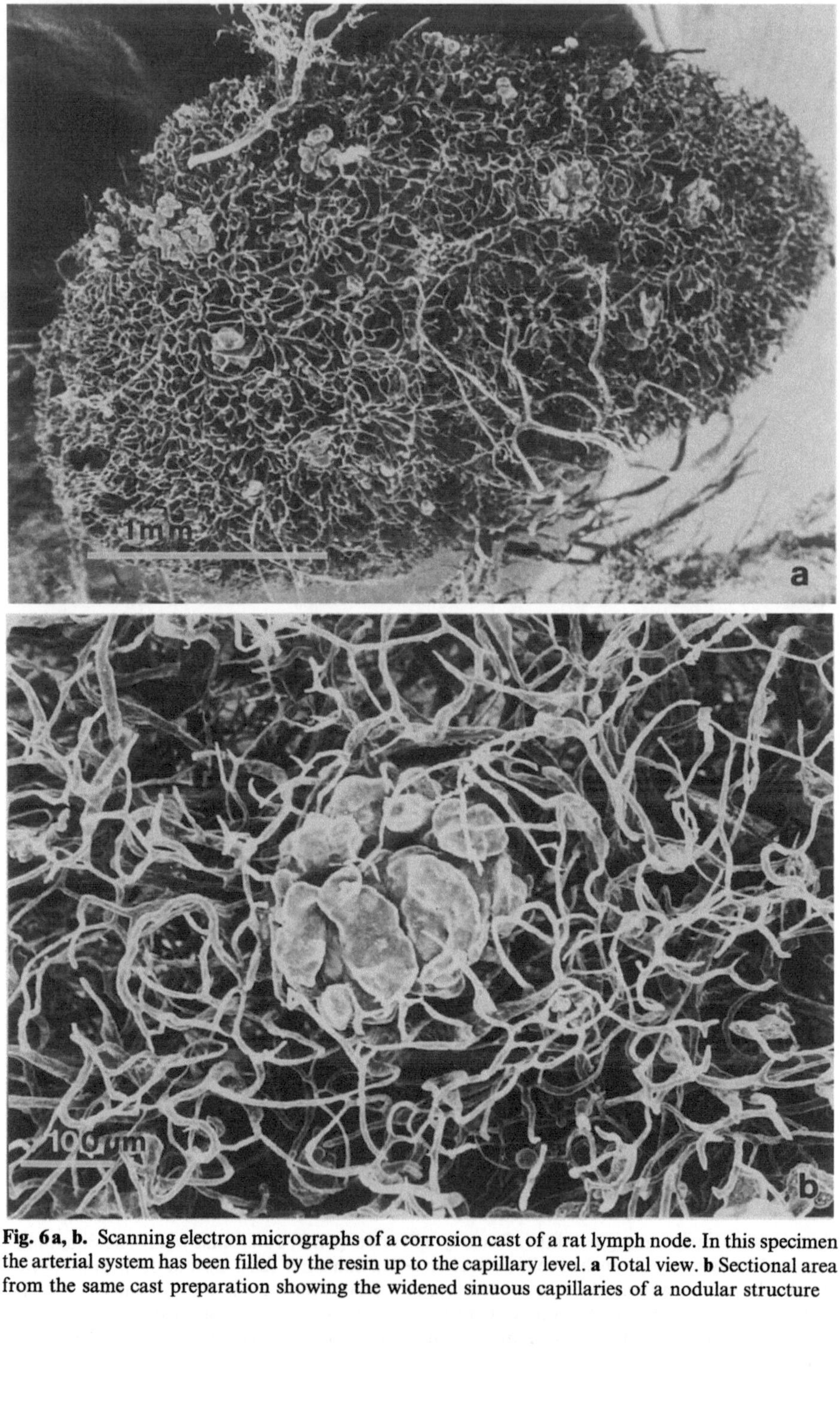

Fig. 6 a, b. Scanning electron micrographs of a corrosion cast of a rat lymph node. In this specimen the arterial system has been filled by the resin up to the capillary level. **a** Total view. **b** Sectional area from the same cast preparation showing the widened sinuous capillaries of a nodular structure

The lymph node is everywhere permeated by *blood vessels,* whose arrangement corresponds to a certain vasoarchitectural principle (Figs. 4, 6): The nodal artery enters the node at the hilus, where it gives off some twigs to the capsule. Within the node the artery leads into several smaller arteries and arterioles, which follow the trabeculae. Within the medulla, twigs spread into the medullary cords, forming a capillary network that supplies the related area and the cortex. A special arteriolar vessel enters primary or secondary nodules and there branches off into several sinuous capillaries. Single arterioles reach the capsule via trabecular structures at many sites and so anastomose with branches coming from the hilus.

The venous system, consisting of postcapillary venules, muscular venules, and small veins, generally uses similar routes to the hilus, where the main vein leaves the node accompanied by the efferent lymphatic. The vascular system nowhere communicates with that of the sinuses. Such a situation only exists in *hemal nodes,* which are seldom found in humans. Most of the postcapillary venules are situated in the paracortex, where they represent a special site for cellular traffic between blood and lymph system (see below). Further details concerning the basic morphology of the lymph node have been reported in previous papers (Castenholz 1983 a, b).

4 Fine Structure

4.1 Reticular Tissue

The compartments between the capsule and the trabeculae are filled by a three-dimensional network of *reticulum cells* and fine fibrils. The reticulum cells are branched elements with an extremely irregular surface and a shape varying from stellate to spindle-shaped. With their long processes neighboring cells have firm contact to each other and so form a syncytium with small and wide meshes.

The cytoplasm of the reticulum cells contains numerous lysosomes, mitochondria, small vesicles, and phagosomes. A granular endoplasmic reticulum and free ribosomes are also found at certain sites. The *fibrils,* as far as they are reticular fibrils, show a positive reaction in silver-impregnated specimens under light microscopy (agyrophil fibers). Other fibers are regarded as special delicate modifications of the collagenous fibers. Most of the fine fibrils are in an extracellular position but some are in close connection to the cellular surface of reticulum cells. In the sinuses the fibrils are enwrapped by the cytoplasm of the long extensions of these cells traversing the lumen. Thus, nowhere does direct contact exist between the fibrils and the lymph.

The structural organization of the reticular tissue in lymph nodes and other lymphatic organs can be well demonstrated by scanning electron microscopy in organs washed out by a physiological saline solution and so cleared of the free cells normally occupying the spaces between the reticulum cells (Fig. 7).

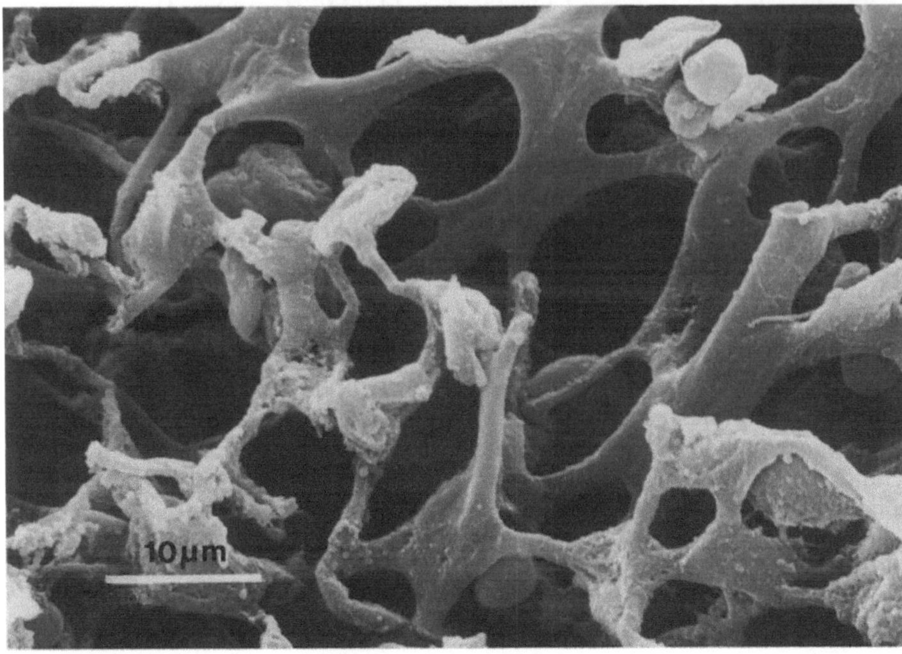

Fig. 7. Reticular tissue of a rat mesenteric lymph node, represented as a continuous framework after removing the free cells by washing out the node tissue before fixation. Scanning electron micrograph

Otherwise, in untreated nodes, the whole reticular tissue within the framework of the capsule and the trabeculae is masked by the accumulation of lymphoid cells.

4.2 Nodules

Many parts of the outer cortex show a special differentiation in the form of concentric structures: the nodules or follicles. Each nodular area is characterized by a special arrangement of the lymphoid cells. The cells are embedded in a fine stroma of reticular cells and reticular fibrils. The central part of secondary nodules, the *germinal center,* is composed of medium-sized and large

Fig. 8. **a** Mesenteric node of a simian (*Cebus apella*). This light micrograph of a semithin section shows the cortical area with a secondary nodule. The germinal center (*GC*) and the surrounding dense mantle zone or corona (*C*) consisting of small lymphocytes are well visible. **b** Nodular area of a rat lymph node as revealed by scanning electron microscopy. The node has been washed out with physiological saline solution prior to the fixation. Thus, the reticular tissue surrounding the nodule has been almost fully cleared of free cells. The cell population of the nodular area, however, has not been removed by the procedure ▶

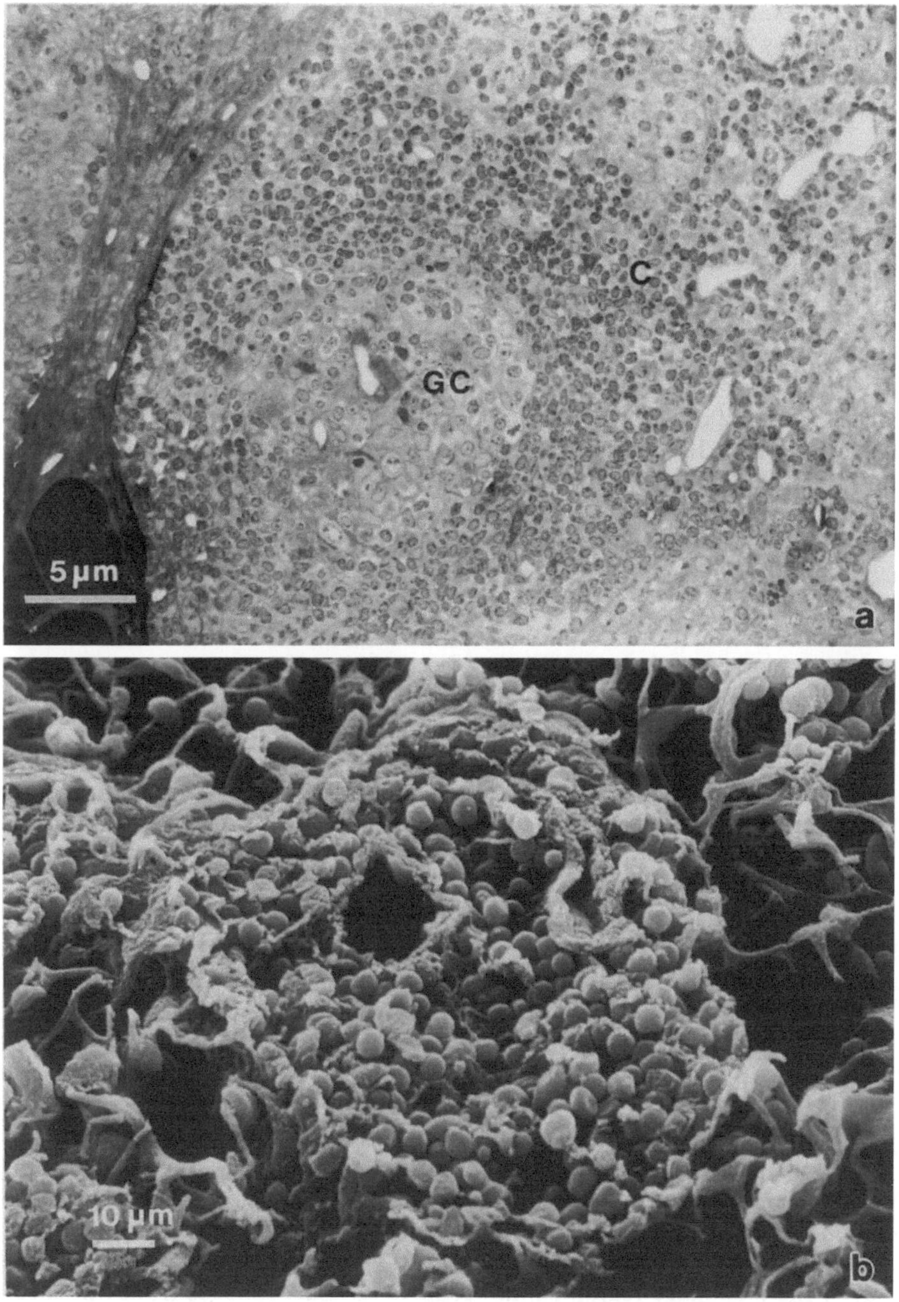
C
GC
5 µm
a
10 µm
b

cells (immunoblasts). It appears in light micrographs as a bright zone surrounded by a dark mantle (corona), in which a great number of small lymphocytes are located (Fig. 8a). Only the nuclei of these cells can be distinguished light microscopically when common stains are employed.

The nodal area also exhibits a special vascularization. There are several sinuous capillaries whose lumina distinctly exceed the width of the capillaries in other parts of the node. In some specimens the sinuous capillaries form glomerular structures, which become very obvious in cast preparations (Fig. 6). As regards the fine structural differentiation and the functional significance of the nodal blood vessels, no further details are known as yet.

Lymphoid cells of the follicular region cannot be removed by washing out lymph nodes prior to fixation (Fig. 8b). In semithin sections of light microscopy (Fig. 9a) or in ultrathin sections of transmission electron microscopy the various types of cells within and around a germinal center can be easily identified (see below). In scanning electron micrographs most of the cells are spherical. They have a smooth surface or possess only a small number of fine microvilli. The differences in size between the lymphoid cells are very great (Fig. 9b). It is impossible to classify them solely on the basis of their scanning electron microscopic appearance.

4.3 Medullary Structures

The medulla of the lymph node is composed of three structural elements, medullary trabeculae, medullary sinuses, and medullary cords. The reticular tissue forms the structural base for two of these elements, the medullary cords and the medullary sinuses, which according to current knowledge, can be regarded as a morphological unit.

The *medullary cords* contain numerous lymphoid cells, most of them plasma cells and small lymphocytes, arranged in parallel columns (Fig. 10a). Many macrophages are also present, preferentially located in the outer zone of each cord. The reticular tissue is little developed. Most cords form longish or irregular tissue formations which are surrounded by the medullary sinuses (Fig. 10b). In most parts of the medulla the spatial ratio between the two systems is about 1:1.

The *medullary sinus* and the neighboring medullary cords are separated by the littoral cells. The sinus lumen is crossed by the reticulum cells at many points (Fig. 11a). In the wide sinus spaces a large number of macrophages and lymphocytes can be found. Some of the macrophages are attached to the sinus wall by means of small cellular extensions, which is the reason why washing out of the medullary region cannot remove all macrophages from our specimens. Due to their different states of activity the macrophages of the medullary sinuses exhibit a great variety in shape, ranging from a nearly smooth surface to a totally irregular profile consisting of extended bleb-like protrusions (Fig. 11b).

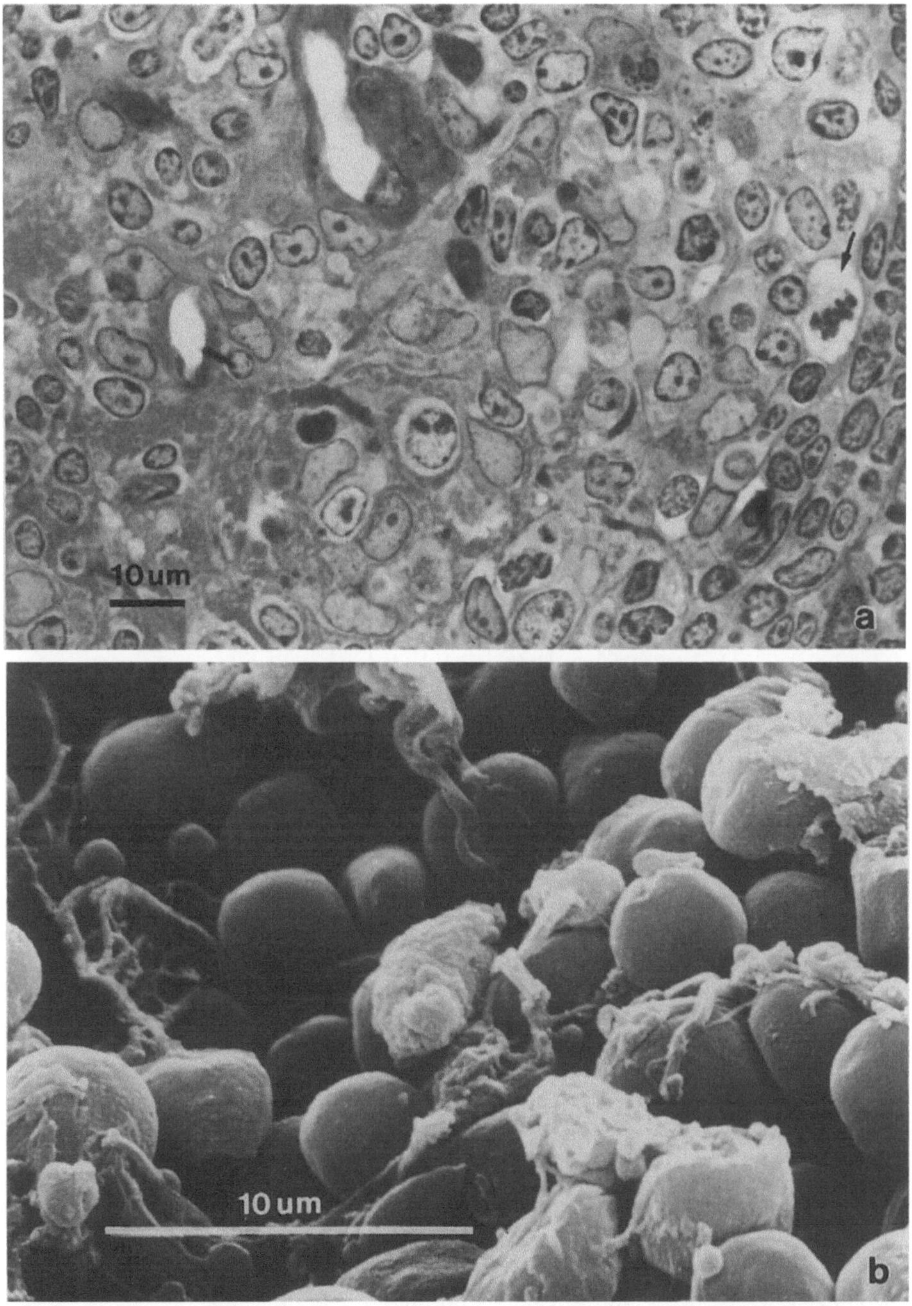

Fig. 9. **a** Enlargement area from Fig. 8 a. Large and medium-sized lymphoid cells, some in a state of division (*arrow*), appear as elements of the lymphopoietic activity of the germinal center (*middle part of the figure*). The small lymphocytes of the mantle zone are found at the periphery (*bottom, right*). **b** Cells of the nodular zone of the rat lymph node shown in Fig. 8 b at high magnification. Most cells are spherical and smooth-surfaced

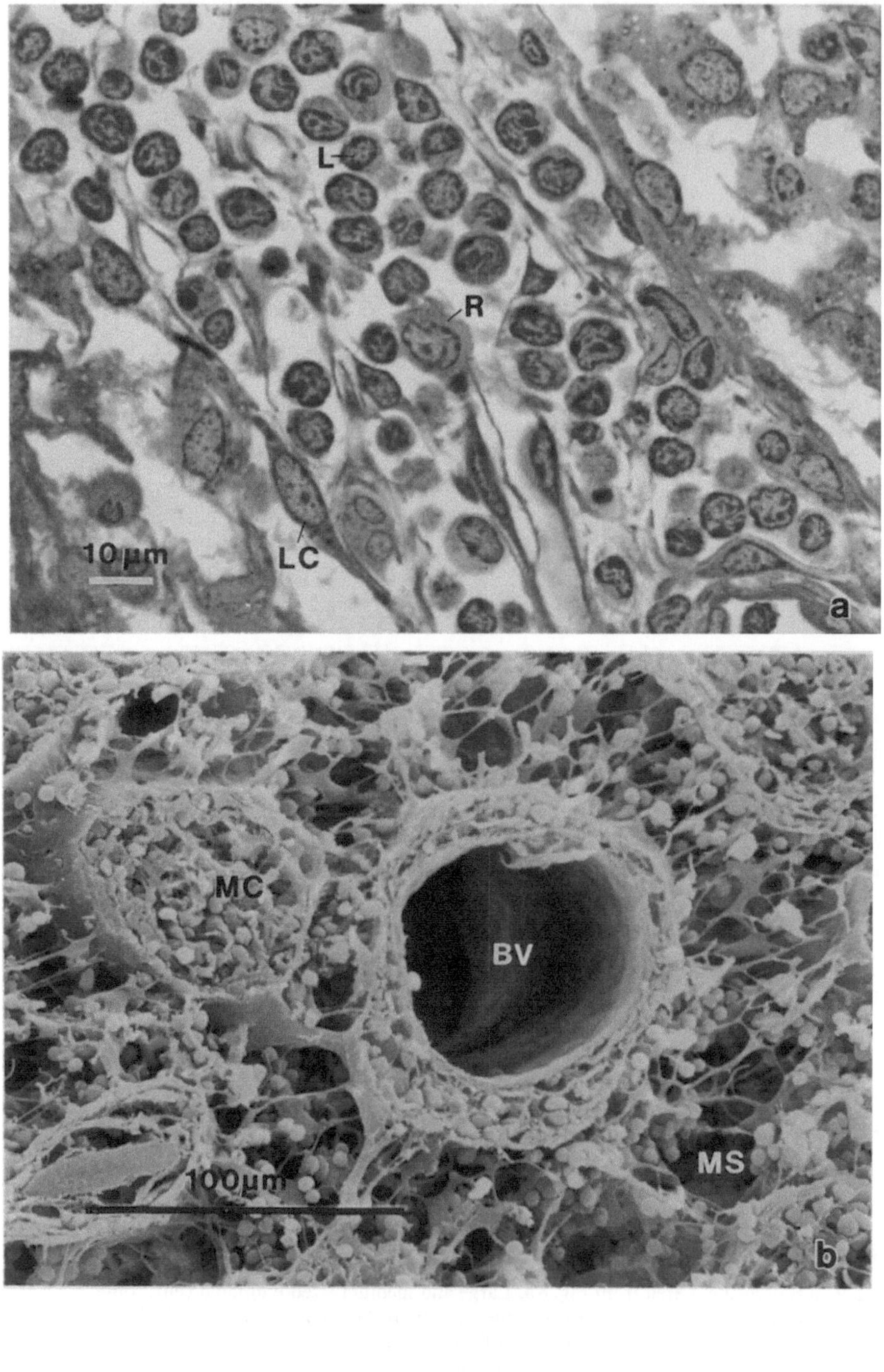
L
R
10 µm
LC
a
MC
BV
MS
100µm
b

The *trabeculae* of the medulla are composed of dense connective tissue, so providing guide structures for blood vessels and nerves. There are also trabeculae which form a small zone of loose connective tissue around blood vessels. The tissue area is also richly occupied by free lymphoid cells.

4.4 Sinuses

The different sinuses of the lymph node are lined by a layer of flat cells of endothelial nature, the *littoral cells*. These cells, regarded as special kind of reticulum cell, do not form a continuous layer. Thus, at many sites, broad intercellular gaps exist in the sinus wall through which the meshes of the reticular tissue are in direct communication with the sinus lumen. The fine structural features of the different sinuses of a lymph node vary somewhat. While the composition of the marginal sinuses appears relatively simple, that of the intermediate medullary sinus is much more complex. A basement membrane underlying the littoral cells only exists on the capsular side of the marginal sinus. Such a structural element is missing in the inner wall of that sinus and also in the wall of the other sinuses. A few reticular fibers cover the outer sinus wall everywhere.

The sinus lumen is crossed by *reticulum cells*, as already mentioned, which interlace to form a cellular network (Figs. 2B, 5a, 10b, 11a). Strands of enwrapped reticular fibers accompany the extensions of these cells. Neighboring littoral cells are united by desmosomes. A smooth endoplasmic reticulum, several mitochondria, and a great number of pinocytotic vesicles are characteristic elements of the cytoplasm. Further structures like a rough endoplasmic reticulum, a few lysosomes and vacuoles, and fine filamentous elements are especially prominent in lining cells of the inner marginal, the intermediate, and the medullary sinus. These organelles quantitatively increase if the node is stimulated by various factors.

The well-developed basement membrane covering the littoral cells on the capsular side of the marginal sinus and the trabecular side of other sinuses consists of an amorphous or filamentous material. Only sparse filamentous material and a small amount of amorphous matter can be occasionally observed with the electron microscope at the outer surface of the sinus wall facing the lymphoid reticular tissue. No clear distinction can be made between the fine structural differentiation of littoral cells and that of the reticulum cells traversing the sinus lumen. Consequently, both types of sinus cell are classed

◀ **Fig. 10. a** Semithin section of the medullary region of a mesenteric lymph node of a simian (*Cebus apella*). A medullary cord with accumulations of plasma cells, small lymphocytes, and macrophages is seen in the *middle part of the figure*. On both sides (*top right, bottom left*) the medullary sinuses are separated from the cord area by littoral cells (*LC*). The sinus' lumen is filled by reticulum cells (*R*) and lymphocytes (*L*). **b** Scanning electron micrograph of a guinea pig lymph node showing medullary cords (*MC*), the medullary sinus (*MS*), and a cord structure with a big blood vessel (*BV*). Note the numerous free cells within the sinus spaces and the well-developed system of reticulum cells crossing the sinus lumen

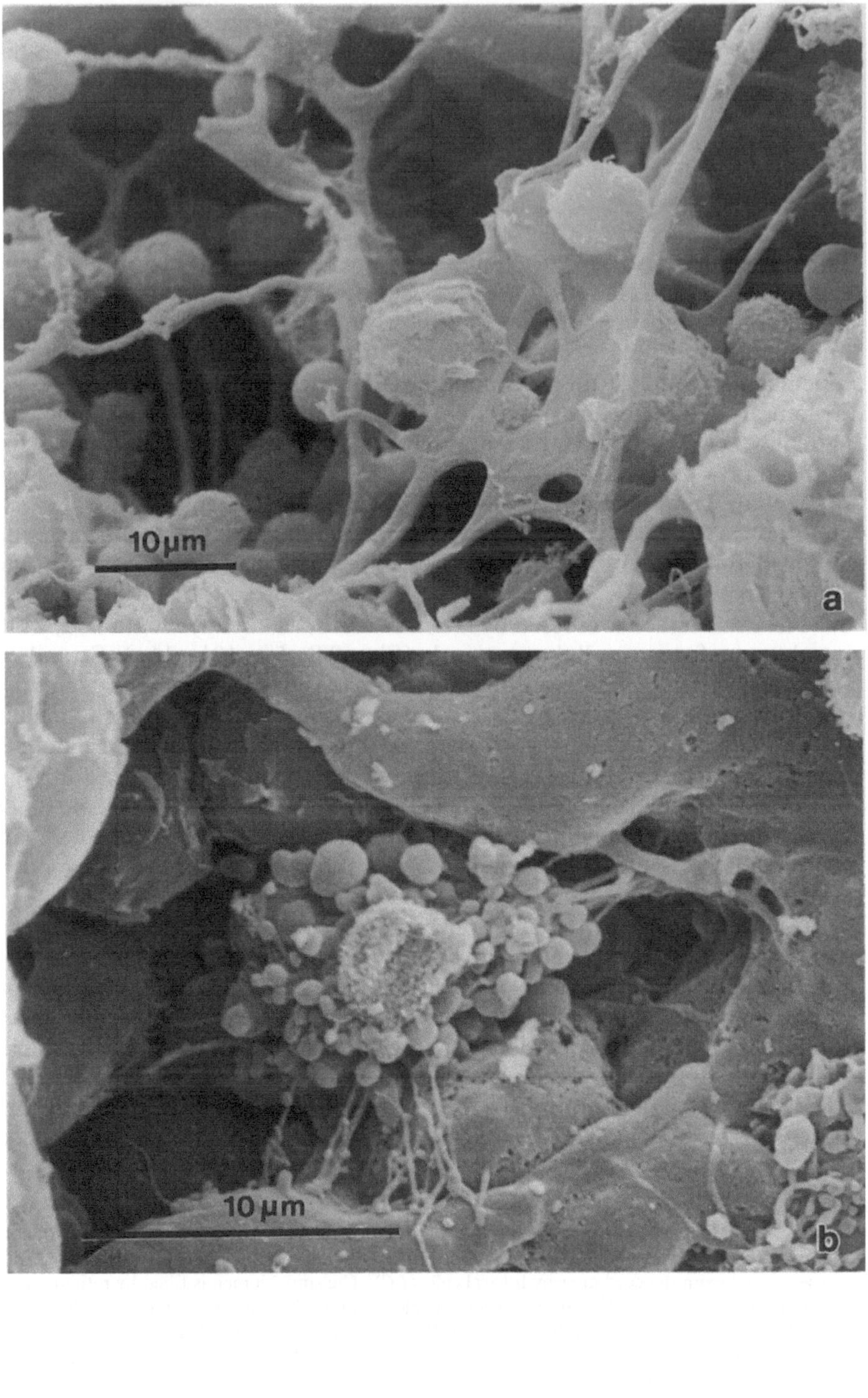
10 µm
a
10 µm
b

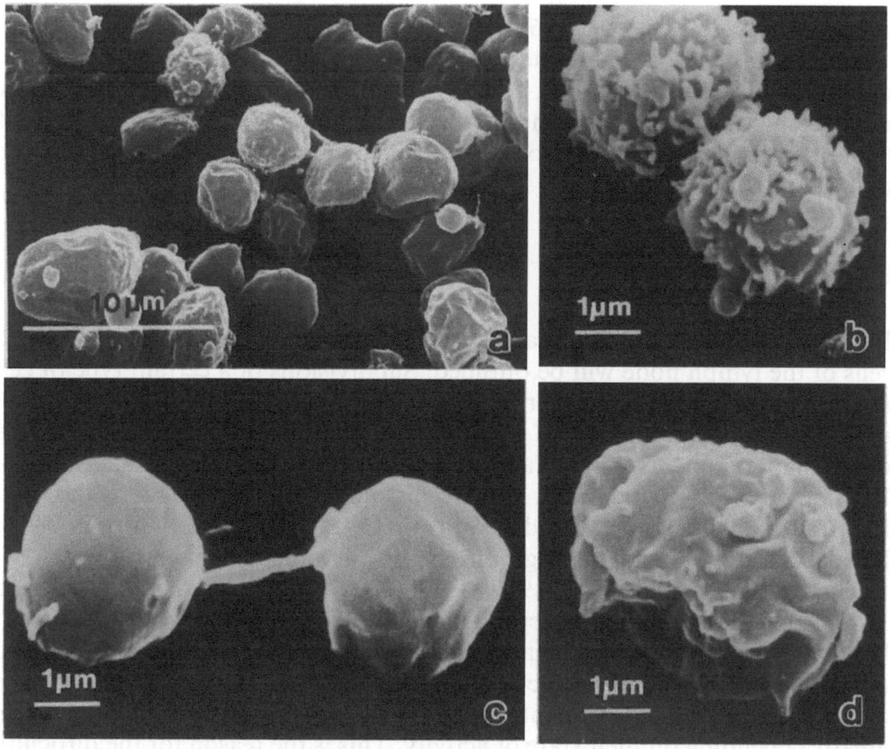

Fig. 12 a–d. This series of scanning electron micrographs depicts free cells which have been isolated from a fresh rat lymph node by perfusion with physiological saline solution. **a** Survey of the cells concentrated by centrifuging the rinsed sample several times. Note the great differences in shape and dimensions among the cells. Some of them, such as small lymphocytes and macrophages, can be recognized by the typical surface pattern. **b** Two *lymphocytes* exhibiting many small microvilli and a few bleb-like protrusions. **c** Two smooth-surfaced *lymphocytes* touching via a filopodial extension of one cell. **d** *Macrophage* with an undulating surface profile and some bleb-like protuberances

◀ **Fig. 11.** **a** Enlarged view into the lumen of a medullary sinus (same preparation as shown in Fig. 10b). In the foreground a reticular cellular element appears with several slender processes spanning the lumen. Supporting reticular fibrils run together with the cellular processes. However, these structures are not visible in this figure because they are covered by the cytoplasm of the reticulum cell. **b** Scanning electron micrograph with a view of the wall of the medullary sinus. A macrophage is recognizable attached to the littoral cells with the help of filopodial extensions. A large number of bleb-like protrusions appears on the cell surface as signs of phagocytotic activity as *retothelial cells* (LENNERT 1961). As freely moving cellular elements there are lymphocytes, macrophages, and occasionally plasma cells and monocytes in the lumen of the sinuses (Figs. 2B, 5a, 10b, 11). Most of them can be easily removed by washing out the sinuses and so examined in smear preparations of light or scanning electron microscopy independent of their environment in the node (Fig. 12).

4.5 Free Cells

In this chapter only the essential structural features of the most characteristic cells of the lymph node will be outlined. Subdivisions of a certain type of cell are not considered. For further details on the cytological differentiation, the light microscopic appearance, and the modifications of lymphoid cells, see other chapters in this volume and textbooks of immunology (KELLER 1977; REYNOLDS 1982; ROITT et al. 1985), histology and cytology (MORI and LENNERT 1969; JUNQUEIRA and CARNEIRO 1971; WEISS 1972; RHODIN 1974; BARGMANN 1977), and monographs on the lymphatic system (HELLMANN 1943; RUSZNYAK et al. 1957, 1969; KAMPMEIER 1969; YOFFEY and COURTICE 1956, 1970). It should also be kept in mind that the morphology of the different lymphoid cells is subject to many factors such as development, species and organ specificity, and antigenic stimulation, and that their structural features and dimensions can consequently alter. The surface profile of the cells varies greatly depending on their state of activity. This is the reason for the difficulty in recognizing and classifying certain lymphoid cells and for at least some of the controversy on this matter in the literature.

The *lymphocytes* are spherical or ovoid cells whose diameters are smaller than 8 μm. The roundish nucleus occupies a large area of the cell. Sometimes the nucleus is slightly indented. The chromatin is concentrated as dense mass near the nuclear membrane and in the nuclear center. In the small cytoplasmic zone around the nucleus a few mitochondria, lysosomes, and free ribosomes as well as elements of smooth- and rough-surfaced endoplasmic reticulum occur. In the scanning electron microscope the cellular surface appears covered with a pattern of small knot-like or finger-like microvilli (Fig. 12). Although the differentiation of T lymphocytes and B lymphocytes is very difficult on the basis of their structural features alone, some investigators have been able to distinguish them employing scanning electron microscopic criteria (LIN et al. 1973). According to these authors, a surface furnished with many fine microvilli is typical for the B cells, whereas a surface with only a few microvilli is a characteristic sign for T cells.

Germinocytes with an ovoid or irregular shape have a somewhat larger diameter, ranging up to 10 μm. These specialized lymphocytes are found only in the germinal center of the secondary follicles (Fig. 9 a). Their ovoid nucleus is slightly indented and exhibits pocket-like structures. The chromatin forms a small zone along the nuclear border. One or two large nucleoli are characteristic elements of the nucleus. Several mitochondria are scattered in the cytoplasmic zone but no endoplasmic reticulum – either smooth or rough – can be detected. *Germinoblasts* are cells with diameters up to 12–14 µm, which as a rule exhibit prominent nuclear pockets and in the cytoplasm a few lysosomes, ribosomes, and a well-developed Golgi apparatus.

The *plasma cells* measure about 10 µm in diameter. The roundish nucleus is eccentrically located in the cell. Due to the concentration of the chromatin substance at the nuclear periphery, the nucleus displays as a characteristic sign a wheel-like structure. The granular endoplasmic reticulum of plasma cells, containing sac-like and enlarged tubular sections, is very prominent. There are also large mitochondria and a well-developed Golgi zone. The surface morphology is similar to that of the lymphocytes.

Free *macrophages* are large cells of about 20 µm or more in diameter. Their surface is very irregular and changes its appearance in accordance with the phagocytotic activity. Thus, extended bleb-like or long finger-like pseudopodia, but also small microvilli and flat or wavy portions, are found in this cell type (Figs. 11b, 12d, 16). The nucleus appears oval and has several indentations. It contains one or two nucleoli and a large amount of chromatin. The cytoplasm exhibits free ribosomes, structures of a granular reticulum, a few mitochondria, and a very prominent Golgi zone. There are also pinocytotic invaginations of the cellular surface and pinocytotic vesicles of the smooth and coated type in the cytoplasm. As special characteristics most macrophages have several phagosomes (vacuoles with engulfed matter, Fig. 16a), lysosomes, and residual bodies.

The *monocytes* vary in diameter between 12 and 20 µm and have a typical kidney-shaped large nucleus in an eccentric position. The chromatin is less densely packed than in lymphocytes. Knob-like microvilli and filopodial protrusions occur on their cellular surface. Beside structures of the endoplasmic reticulum and a great number of ribosomes, the cytoplasm contains many small vesicles, a few mitochondria, and some fine filaments.

4.6 Postcapillary Venules

While the fine structural properties of most nodal blood vessels – arteries, arterioles, capillaries, and veins – are not especially conspicuous and so do not differ from the morphology of corresponding vessels in other organs like muscle or skin, the postcapillary venules of the paracortex are a distinct exception. The endothelium of these vessels, inserted between the capillaries and the muscular venules, can be regarded as unique in regard to both cytological differentiation and functional significance. It is appropriate for the structural features of this vessel type to be briefly characterized here, inasmuch as this is necessary for a comprehensive understanding of certain nodal functions. Detailed information on the morphology and function of the postcapillary venules is given in Chap. 5 by De Bruyn and Cho in this volume.

The *endothelium* of postcapillary venules, commonly called high endothelial venules (HEVs), is composed of cuboidal and squamous cells whose surface strongly bulges into the lumen (Figs. 13, 14). Their cytoplasm is provided with a well-developed granular endoplasmic reticulum, a large Golgi zone, and a great number of cytoplasmic filaments. Single lymphocytes adhere at the luminal endothelial surface at many sites. This phenomenon is very obvious in nodes which have been treated by perfusion with physiological saline solution from the arterial or venous side and have been fixed in the same way (Fig. 13b). The adherent cells exhibit different stages of diapedesis. Most of them apparently use the interendothelial gaps for their transmural passage, but it has also been suggested that the cells can choose the intraendothelial passage (CHO and DE BRUYN 1979, 1981; YAMAGUCHI and SHOEFL 1983a, b).

With the help of the corrosion cast technique the rough surface profile of the HEVs is replicated in the hardened resin. Deep hole-like indentations reaching diameters of about 10 μm presumably are created by the adherent lymphocytes. The zones of high endothelium are sharply marked against the area of flat, nondifferentiated endothelium lining the subsequent muscular venule (Fig. 14b).

5 Functions

It is a well-known fact that the lymph nodes and the spleen are the sites most endowed with the ability to produce antibodies (YOFFEY and COURTICE 1970). Keeping this in mind, it is consistent to understand processes like filtration of lymph, lymphocytopoiesis, and phagocytosis as events subserving this major task. It must be pointed out, however, that only a few of the great number of cellular and humoral reactions permanently occurring in the node can be represented and assessed by conventional morphological methods. Many immune biological reactions are not expressed in morphological findings as dealt with in this chapter; rather, special immunohistochemical or other differentiated methods are required (see Chap. 3 by HANSMANN and WACKER in this volume). The morphological techniques of today are also incapable of providing exhaustive information on lymphocytopoiesis or cellular differentiation. Thus, in the following functional-morphological approach it is mainly the general architecture of the node and some cytological phenomena that are outlined.

Fig. 13. a Semithin section of a simian lymph node (*Cebus apella*). The light micrograph demonstrates a sectional area from the paracortical zone. Two postcapillary venules (high endothelial venules, HEVs) are represented. Note the high endothelial lining of these vessels. From the luminal side single lymphoid cells attach to this layer (*arrows*). Accumulations of small lymphocytes, mostly T lymphocytes, are found in the reticular tissue around the vessels. **b** This scanning electron micrograph offers a view into a postcapillary venule from the paracortex of a perfused rat lymph node. An assembly of recirculating lymphocytes is recognizable. The cells have firm contact to the prominent endothelial layer, some of them being in a state of diapedesis ▶

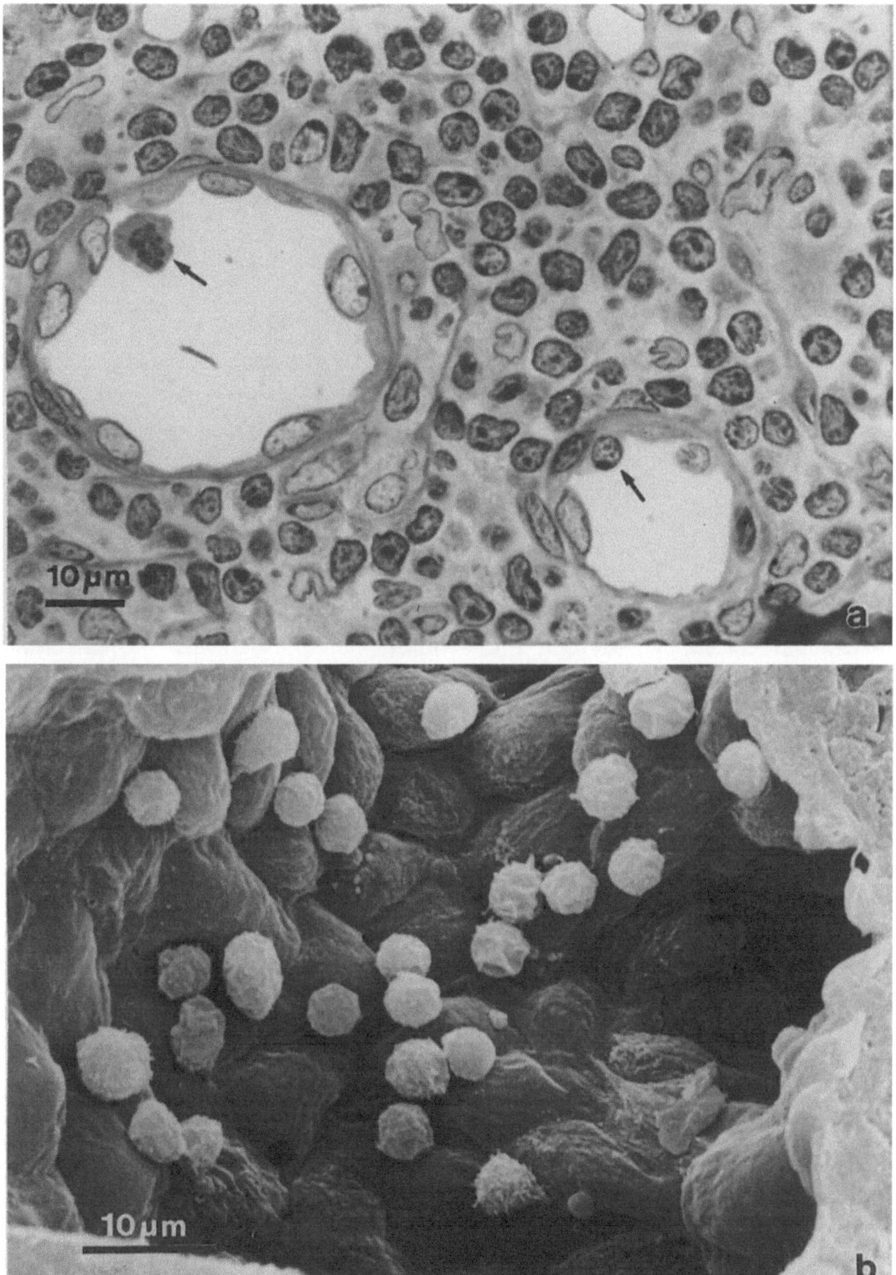
10 µm
a
10 µm
b

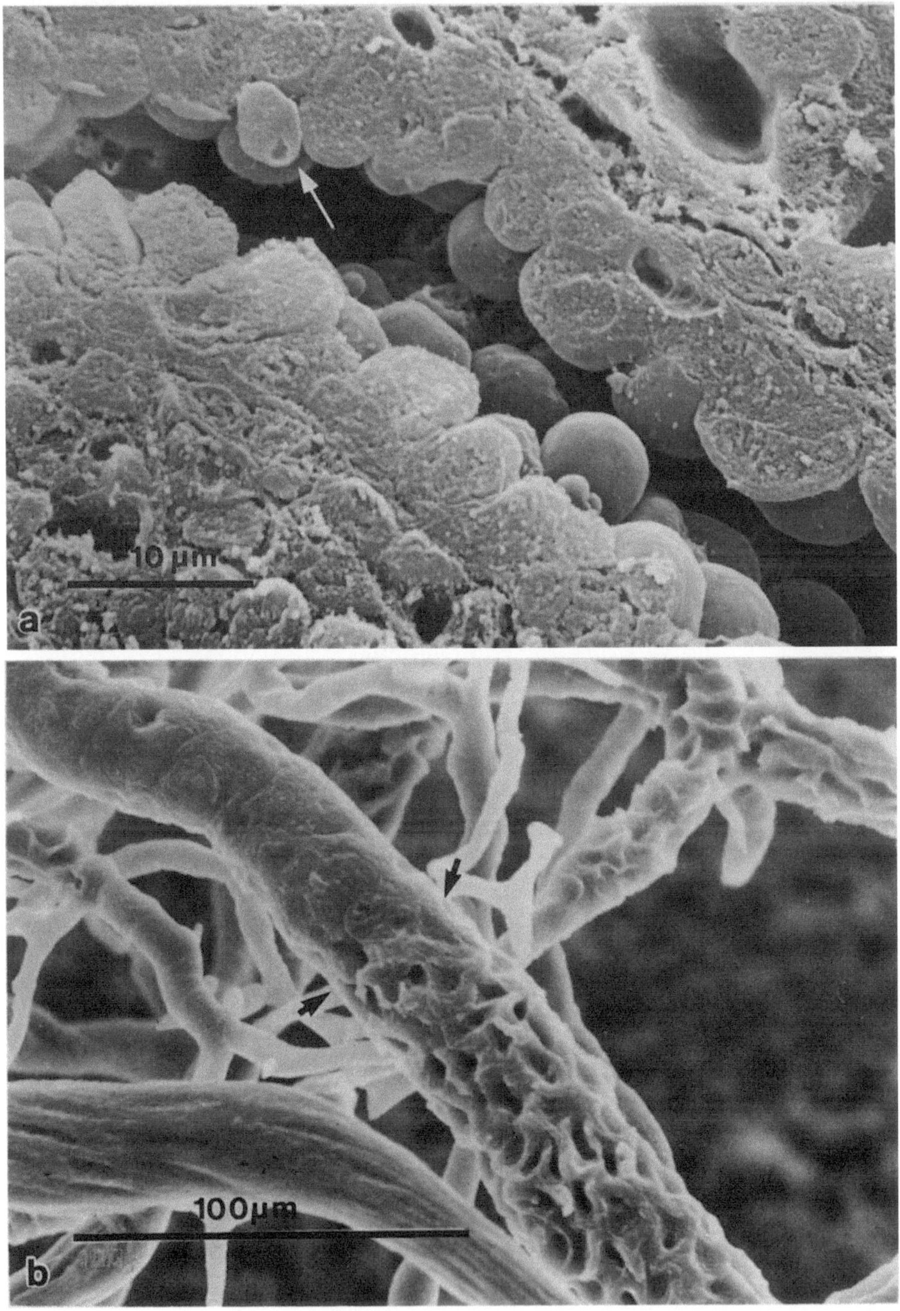
10 µm
a
100µm
b

5.1 Filtration of Lymph

The general organization of the lymph node, consisting of the external rigid capsule, the framework of trabeculae, the widely branched system of sinuses, and the sponge-like reticular tissue, provides an ideal *filter station* for the lymph. Interconnected as a special unit between afferent and efferent lymphatic vessels, the node receives lymph from a broad entrance zone and delivers it to a smaller output area, similar to the way a funnel functions. The interior of the node is provided with a structure like a weir, represented by the coarse plexus-like structure of the sinuses and the finer network of the reticular tissue. The main flow of the lymph percolates through the preformed pathways of the sinuses, while only 1% of the lymph is assumed to pass the reticular tissue.

After entering the node via the afferent lymphatics, the lymph first spreads in the extended marginal sinus, which embraces nearly the whole circumference of the node. From here, the lymph reaches the system of medullary sinuses in the center of the node via the numerous intermediate sinuses. As stated by NORDMANN as long ago as 1928, there are three routes by which lymph traverses the node (Fig. 4). One is around the marginal sinus without entering other sinuses. The second route follows the intermediate sinuses through the interior of the node. A third possibility involves the drifting of small amounts of lymph from the marginal sinus over the reticular tissue of the cortex into the intermediate and medullary sinuses.

Thus, the principle of lymph flow is based on a system of low resistance pathways realized by the different sinuses of the node enabling rapid distribution of the lymph within the entire node. On the other hand, the spatial system of the reticular tissue can be regarded as a system of high resistance pathways which slows the exchange of lymph due to the dense accumulation of cells and narrow passageways but enables intense contact of cells with the antigen for a long period.

The filtering capacity of the lymph node does not concern only the mechanical filtration of lymph; it also influences important biological reactions such as the formation of antibodies and cell-mediated immune responses. It seems probable that the antibody production in a lymph node depends upon factors like the complete retention of antigen and its fastening to special cells, predominantly reticulum cells.

During its passage through the complex narrow and traversed intranodal sinuses and tissue spaces, the *lymph* with its cells, bacteria, and foreign material is forced to come into contact with lymphocytes, littoral cells, macrophages,

◀ **Fig. 14. a** This scanning electron micrograph shows a postcapillary venule of the paracortex of a rat lymph node. The cut plane runs longitudinally through the vessel in this specimen; thus, the extraordinary thickness of the endothelial layer is very obvious. The *arrow* indicates a part of a sticking lymphocyte (from CASTENHOLZ 1989a). **b** In corrosion casts the postcapillary venules exhibit a rough surface with deep imprints and high crests. This striking profile corresponds to the morphological differentiation of this vessel type. The transition from the postcapillary venule to the subsequent nondifferentiated venule is sharply distinguished (*arrows*)

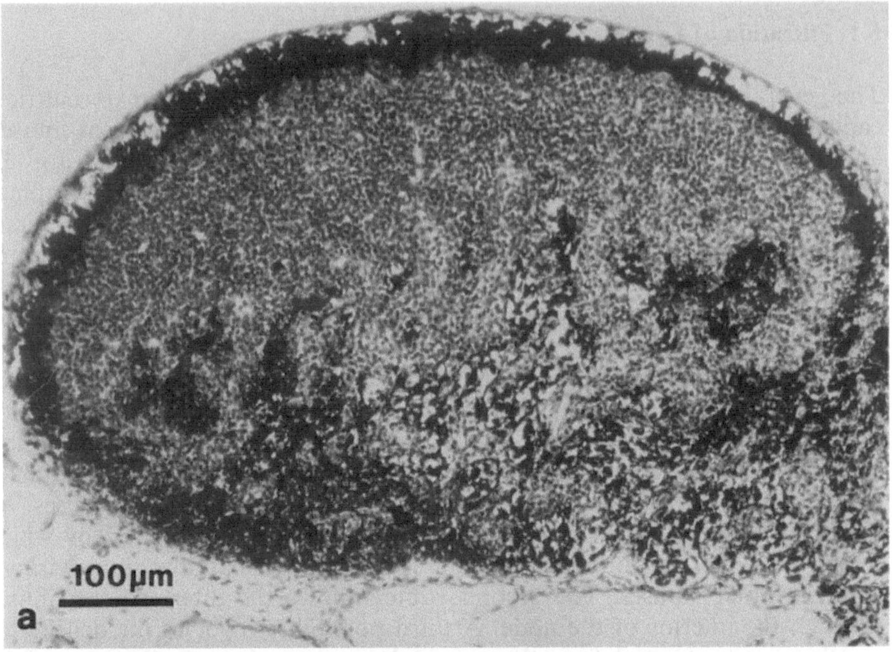
100µm
a

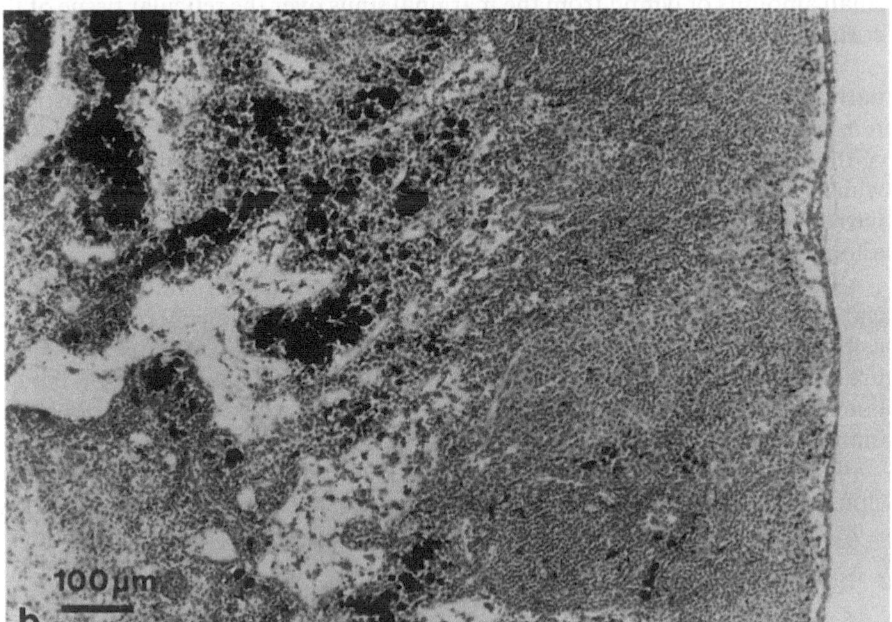
100µm
b

monocytes, and reticulum cells. Different cellular interactions are thus initiated. The antigenic front is directed from the medulla to the paracortex and the cortex. The sinus wall obviously does not represent a noteworthy hindrance for amoeboid cells such as monocytes and for small lymphocytes. Large cells such as macrophages and cell clusters, however, are scarcely able to leave the sinuses and may be arrested at narrow sites.

After interstitial injection of Indian ink or other particulate substances it can be observed that the marginal sinus first becomes blackened while the intermediate and medullary sinuses are distinctly less affected (Fig. 15a). The amount of ink penetrating the reticular tissue is very small. At a later stage of the experiment the carbon is stored in macrophages spread over all areas of node tissue, including germinal centers (Fig. 15b). The fact that cell-independent carbon does not easily enter the parenchyma is not primarily due to an impermeable sinus wall; rather it is chiefly the result of dense packing of lymphoid cells in the reticular meshwork of the parenchyma.

The filtration process must clear the lymph of foreign material, of bacteria, and in part of host cells before it is discharged into the blood circulation. When the node becomes overloaded by these elements, its spatial capacity and immuno-biological efficiency would soon be exhausted. Two kinds of body defense mechanism operate during the filtering of the lymph. One is *phagocytosis*, the other, a different mode of *interaction of lymphoid cells* with each other or with antigenic substances.

5.2 Phagocytosis and Peripolesis

The cells primarily engaged in phagocytosis are the freely movable *macrophages* (true wandering cells) and *reticulum cells* (fixed macrophages, resting wandering cells). Although the two types of cells are different in shape, they exert their function according to the same principle: material such as particulate matter, tissue debris, and effete cells (e.g., erythrocytes, lymphocytes, and other lympoid cells) is taken up by an invagination of the cell membrane and so engulfed into the cytoplasm in the form of smooth-walled vacuoles (phagosomes). Here, the material is digested and rendered harmless by enzymes of the primary lysosomes, which fuse with the phagosomes to secondary lysosomes.

Undigestible matter such as dust or carbon particles is stored in the fixed macrophages over long periods and so is kept inert. The initial stage of phagocytosis can be recognized by scanning electron microscopy. Characteristic signs

◀ **Fig. 15.** **a** Micrograph of a submandibular lymph node of a young rat which has been dissected 2 h after interstitial injection of a carbon deposit into the tongue. The carbon masses fill the whole marginal sinus and in part the medullary sinuses. No carbon has penetrated the area of the reticular tissue in this acute phase of the experiment. **b** Section of a submandibular lymph node of a young rat 6 weeks after interstitial injection of carbon into the tongue. The carbon particles have now been picked up by the macrophages of the medullary region. There are also single carbon-loaded macrophages in the paracortical and corticales areas

are bleb-like protrusions on the surface of the macrophages by which parts of foreign cells or other material are trapped (Figs. 11 b, 15). Phagocytosis is very prominent in the macrophages of the sinuses; to some extent it also occurs in the littoral cells and reticulum cells of the reticular tissue.

Beside acting as "scavenger cells," removing foreign matter or effete cellular elements, macrophages provide specific information to the antibody-forming cells. This important role is due to their content of various antigens picked up by phagocytosis and to the ability to interact with other cells without destroying them. It is a known fact that lymphocytes can come into close contact with one another (Fig. 12c) and also with reticulum cells and macrophages (KLEIN 1958a, b; SHELTON and RICE 1959; SUNDBERG and DOWNEY 1955; SUNDBERG 1960). Groups of lymphocytes often surround a macrophage, attaching it intimately (SHELTON 1962). This phenomenon has been described as *"peripolesis"* in lymph nodes and spleen (SHARP and BURWELL 1960). A corresponding situation but with entry of lymphocytes into the surrounded cell (megakaryocyte) had already been designated *"emperipolesis"* by HUMBLE et al. (1956). We have been able to recognize similar phenomena in lymph nodes of rats after application of carbon (Fig. 16b) (CASTENHOLZ 1988).

"Peripolesis" and "emperipolesis" obviously represent a process of close functional interrelationship of lymphocytes and macrophages, which is based on the very high active surfaces of these cells (see YOFFEY and COURTICE 1970). (Other authors use the term "emperipolesis" for the phenomenon of the migration of lymphocytes through the wall of postcapillary venules (SANDRITTER and BENEKE 1974)). Thus, it can be suggested that in touching or fusing of cellular membranes a very intensive exchange of information occurs that is necessary for a specific defense response in the immune system. Such an act of cellular interaction probably achieves its highest degree of efficiency with temporary fusion of interacting cells, when lymphocytes enter the cytoplasm of the macrophages and circulate in them. However, after exchange of immunological reactions the incorporated cells are released without any damage and so can participate in further cellular interactions.

Fig. 16. **a** Scanning electron micrograph of a submandibular rat lymph node showing a group of cells consisting of carbon-containing macrophages (*M*) and some lymphocytes (*L*) within the reticular tissue. The node was dissected 4 days after interstitial injection of carbon into the tributary tissue area of the tongue. Due to the carbon uptake the macrophages have assumed a roundish shape. At one site the surface of one macrophage was partly removed during preparation of the specimen; thus, many phagosomes are recognizable in the cytoplasm (*arrows*). **b** Scanning electron micrograph of a submandibular lymph node of a rat which was loaded with carbon particles after interstitial injection of a carbon deposit into the tongue 30 days before the lymph node was dissected. A strongly distended macrophage (*M*) of the medullary sinus is represented. A group of lymphocytes (*L*) is attached to its surface. This phenomenon can be interpreted as sign of an exchange of information between both types of cell (peripolesis). *LC*, littoral cell; *RC*, reticulum cell ▶

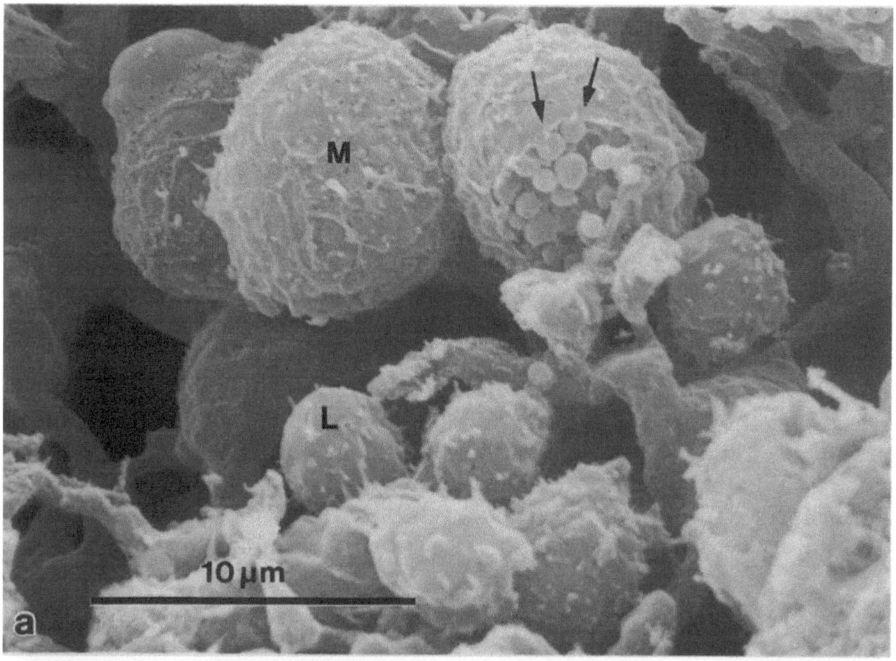
M
L
10 µm
a

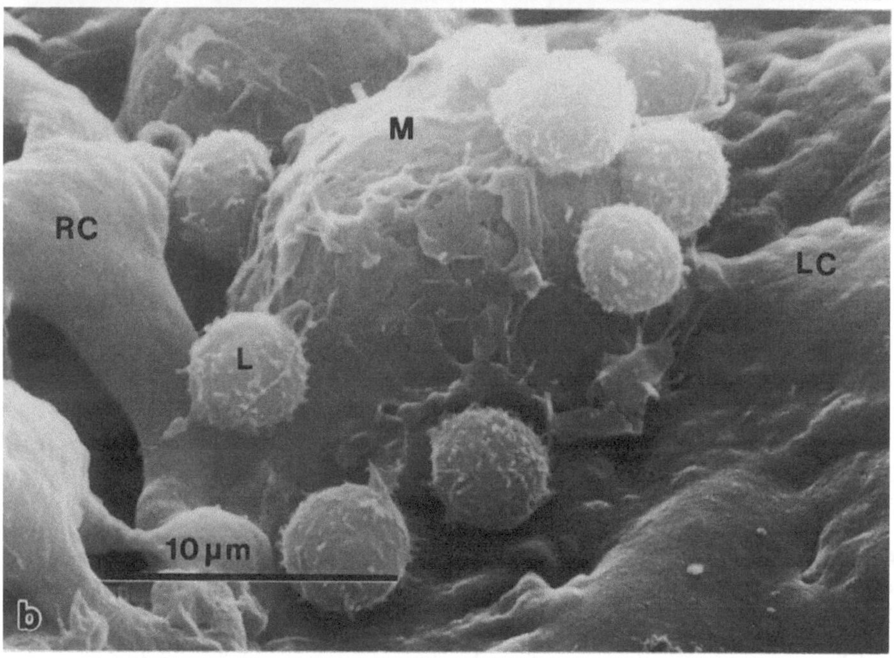
M
RC
LC
L
10 µm
b

5.3 Dynamic Cell Populations

As already stated, lymph nodes contain a large number of free cells which permanently move through the loose framework of the reticular tissue and the sinus system. These organs thus exhibit *dynamic structures*. Nevertheless, the architecture of lymph nodes from all regions of the body seems to be organized according to a uniform structural conception, if one ignores the fact that there are some relevant distinctions between nodes of young and old animals and also among different species. It should, however, be kept in mind that the appearance of histological specimens only characterizes a single phase of a constantly changing dynamic process: cells are constantly moved in the lymph stream, cells move through the labyrinth of the spaces of the reticular tissue, and cells wander between the blood circulation and the lymphatic system (Fig. 17). In the course of these events, sites of accumulation and reduction of lymphoid cells develop in the lymph node which contribute essentially to the histological nature of the node. To some extent even fixed reticulum cells can be transformed into moving cells so that the basic structure of the parenchyma is subject to dynamic changes, too.

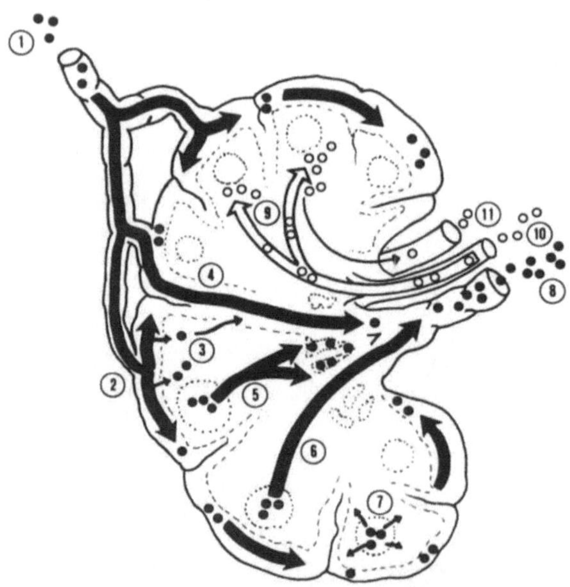

Fig. 17. Routes of intranodal passage of lymphoid cells. Cells using the lymph system are indicated as *black spots*, those transported by a blood vessels as *small circles*. *1*, Input of cells from initial lymphatics preset to the lymph node; *2*, distribution of cells along the marginal sinus; *3*, entering of the reticular tissue by cells penetrating the sinus wall; *4*, transnodal passage along trabecular and medullary sinuses; *5*, migration of cells from the germinal center to medullary cords; *6*, passage of cells from the germinal center into trabecular and medullary sinuses; *7*, spreading of cells from the nodular area into the surrounding cortex; *8*, cells escaping the node via efferent lymphatic; *9*, returning of cells from the blood vessel (HEV) into the parenchyma of the paracortex; *10*, nodal artery with returning lymphoid cells; *11*, escape of cells from the node via nodal vein

The *follicular structures* with their characteristic zones develop when the node has been sufficiently exposed to antigens. Hence, primary follicles with a uniform distribution of lymphocytes and a missing marginal zone are only found in newborns and animals kept in an antigen-free environment. After antigen exposure, the differentiation to secondary follicles occurs, with two clearly distinguishable zones, the germinal center and the perifollicular zone. At the periphery of each germinal center the reticular tissue is densely packed with small lymphocytes. The more loosely structured germinal center, which appears in stained sections as a bright zone, is composed of cells of the reticulum cell type as well as of immunoreactive *B lymphocytes* (immunoblasts). This area becomes especially prominent in a state of high antigen stimulation.

The peculiar cellular organization of the follicular zone of the cortex and other parts of the lymph node becomes better understandable when the process of lymphocytopoiesis and lymphocyte transformation is considered. According to LUKES and COLLINS (1975), B lymphocytes migrate when stimulated by antigens from the perifollicular zone into the germinal center, where they first transform over several steps, involving small and large cleaved and noncleaved cells, into large *immunoblasts*. In contrast, LENNERT et al. (1975) have claimed that the process of transformation of the lymphocytes is initiated by stem cells (immunoblasts) of the germinal center, and that from here the B lymphocytes proceed in the opposite direction to the perifollicular zone (LENNERT et al. 1975).

Plasma cells are a further product of the process of lymphocyte transformation in the lymph node, probably deriving from special medium-sized lymphocytes (plasmablasts) of the follicles. It is also believed that there is another means of plasma cell development, based on the conception that immunologically competent small lymphocytes proliferate and differentiate to medium-sized lymphocytes and finally transform to plasma cells everywhere in the parenchyma.

The transformed cells migrate into the cortical and medullary zone. While most of the plasma cells remain in the lymph node, many of the small lymphocytes reach the blood circulation together with the lymph. Thus, there is a constant movement of lymphoid cells from the reticular area to the marginal sinus and the intermediate sinuses. But another orientation of cells is also possible, from the follicular area to the medullary cords, either via the sinus system or directly through the reticular tissue. The latter route is discussed as being a response to a demand for high antibody formation.

The functional significance of the *medullary cords* is mainly based on the fact that in this node area a very close association exists between small lymphocytes or plasma cells and macrophages of the medullary zone. The arrangement of the lymphoid cells in small columns ensures a broad base of contact to the surrounding sinuses containing a great number of antigen-loaded macrophages. Although the cell population of the medullary cords is considered a static one, it seems likely that single cells continuously change their position in order to form new combinations for cellular interactions. Some cells may also drift with the lymph stream to merge into the blood pool.

The *paracortex* represents a special transitional zone for lymphocyte migration. Characteristic elements of this area are the dense population of *T-lymphocytes* and the postcapillary venules (HEVs) mentioned above. This is the site where the lymphocytes, once discharged into the blood circulation, return to the node tissue to encounter lymphoid cells again and to be available for a new immune response.

The recirculating lymphocytes reenter the lymphatic reticulum via the high endothelium of the postcapillary venules, as mentioned. This layer is especially enlarged when an active response to antigens occurs. The differentiated endothelial cells, obviously by virtue of receptor abilities, recognize the lymphocytes, both B and T cells, and force them to adhere at the luminal surface and subsequently to migrate through the endothelium. The intricate mechanism involved in this transmural passage will not be examined here (see Chap. 5 by DE BRUYN and CHO in this volume). While the T cells stay in the paracortal zone, the B cells proceed to the outer cortical area, where they form compact conglomerates within primary follicles and corresponding structures in the perifollicular zone of secondary follicles.

Due to its structural differentiation and the dynamic behavior of special lymphoid cells, the lymph node contains several *compartments,* each with a special immunological function. Thus, the germinal center of the secondary follicles is responsible for the generation of immunocompetent B cells. The marginal cortex and the medullary cords are responsible for a humoral response by plasma cells and the paracortex for the cell-mediated immunity provided by the T cells. The importance of the sinuses relates to an equal division of antigens in all these compartments and to the carrying of the products created in them. But there are also tissue zones in the lymph node which exert many more functions than such a simple model indicates. The fact that there exists a permanent fluctuation of cells and that many cells are able to transform into other cells with a new functional significance makes it impossible to subordinate a distinct region of lymph nodes only to a single function. It must also be taken into account that a lymph node from a certain region in the body represents only a small unit among the widely scattered lymphatic system, which also comprises organs like the spleen, thymus, and bone marrow. Thus, it is only provided with a limited immunological efficiency. Although the lymph node reacts very sensitively to all antigen influences originating from the body area of its narrower destination, it is also subject to general rules that govern the immune system as a whole.

References

Bargmann W (1977) Histologie und mikroskopische Anatomie des Menschen. Thieme, Stuttgart

Castenholz A (1983a) Der menschliche Lymphknoten aus funktionsmorphologischer Sicht. Z Lymphol VII/2:57–72

Castenholz A (1983b) Morphologie und Funktion des menschlichen Lymphknotens. Z Lymphol VII/2:137

Castenholz A (1983c) Neue Erkenntnisse über das Lymphgefäßsystem: REM-Darstellungen von Lymphbahnen in Zunge und Lymphknoten. Z Lymphol VII/2:143
Castenholz A (1984) Morphological characteristics of initial lymphatics in the tongue as shown by scanning electron microscopy. Scan Electron Microsc II:1343–1352
Castenholz A (1985a) The demonstration of lymphatics in casts and fixed tissue with the scanning electron microscope. In: Bollinger A, Partsch H, Wolfe JHW (eds) The initial lymphatics. New methods and findings. Thieme/Thieme-Stratton, Stuttgart New York, pp 75–83
Castenholz A (1985b) REM-Darstellung von interstitiellen Raumsystemen und Lymphbahnen mit der Kunststoffinjektion. GIT Verlag [Suppl] 2:16–21
Castenholz A (1986) Corrosion cast technique applied in lymphatic pathways. Scan Electron Microsc II:599–605
Castenholz A (1987a) Structural and functional properties of initial lymphatics in the rat tongue: scanning electron microscopic findings. Lymphology 20:112–125
Castenholz A (1987b) Die Rasterelektronenmikroskopie in der mikroangiologischen Forschung. Beitr Elektronenmikroskop Direktabb Oberfl 20:187–194
Castenholz A (1988) Rasterelektronenmikroskopische Beobachtungen an den feinsten Venen (Venulen) unter besonderer Berücksichtigung ihrer Beziehungen zur Lymphbahn. Phlebol Proktol 17:38–47
Castenholz A (1989a) Interpretation of structural patterns appearing on corrosion casts of small blood and initial lymphatic vessels. Scan Electron Microsc III:315–325
Castenholz A (1989b) Structure of initial and collecting lymphatics. In: Olszweski WL (ed) Lymph stasis – pathophysiology, diagnosis and treatment. CRC Press, Boca Raton
Cho Y, De Bruyn PPH (1979) The endothelial structure of the postcapillary venules of the lymph node and the passage of lymphocytes across the venule wall. J Ultrastruct Res 69:13–21
Cho Y, De Bruyn PPH (1981) Transcellular migration of lymphocytes through the walls of the smooth-surfaced squamous endothelial venules in the lymph node: evidence for the direct entry of lymphocytes into the blood circulation of the lymph node. J Ultrastruct Res 74:259–266
Drinker CK, Field ME, Ward HK (1934) The filtering capacity of lymph nodes. J Exp Med 59:393–405
Ehrlich WE (1946) The role of the lymphocyte in the circulation of the lymph. Ann NY Acad Sci 46:823–845
Engeset A (1959) The route of peripheral lymph to the blood stream. J Anat 93:96–100
Hellman T (1943) Lymphgefäße, Lymphknötchen und Lymphknoten. In: Möllendorf W v (ed) Handbuch der mikroskopischen Anatomie des Menschen, vol VI/1, pp 233–396, vol VI/4, pp 173–254. Springer, Berlin Heidelberg New York
Humble JG, Jayne WHW, Pulvertaft RJV (1956) Biological interaction between lymphocytes and other cells. Br J Haematol 2:283–294
Junqueira LC, Carneiro J (1971) Basic histology. Lange Medical, Los Albatros, USA
Kampmeier OF (1969) Evolution and comparative morphology of the lymphatic system. CC Thomas, Springfield, Ill
Keller R (1977) Immunologie und Immunpathologie. Thieme, Stuttgart
Klein R (1958a) Etudes des fonctions lymphocytaires par la cinématographie en contraste de phase de cultures de tissus humains foetaux. CR Soc Biol (Paris) 152:265–269
Klein R (1958b) Etude, par la cinématographie en contraste de phase, des cultures de tissu thymique humain foetal. CR Hebd Seanc Acad Sci (Paris) 246:644–647
Kobayashi S, Osatake H, Kashima Y (1976) Corrosion casts of lymphatics. Arch Histol Jpn 39:177–181
Kurokawa T, Ogata T (1980) A scanning electron microscopic study on the lymphatic microcirculation of the rabbit mesenteric lymph node. A corrosion cast study. Acta Anat (Basel) 107:439–466
Lennert K (1961) Lymphknoten. Cytologie und Lymphadenitis. In: Lubarsch O, Henke F, Rössle R, Ühlinger E (ed) Handbuch der speziellen pathologischen Anatomie und Histologie, vol I/3A. Springer, Berlin Heidelberg New York, pp 1–605
Lennert K, Müller-Hermelink HK (1974) Lymphozyten und immunologische Bedeutung. Verh Anat Ges, Kiel

Lennert K, Stein H, Kaiserling E (1975) Cytological and functional criteria for the classification of malignant lymphoma. Br J Cancer 31[Suppl II]: 29–43
Lin SP, Cooper AG, Wortis HH (1973) Scanning electron microscopy of human T-cell and B-cell rosettes. N Engl J Med 289: 548–562
Lukes RJ, Collins RD (1975) New approaches to the classification of the lymphomata. Br J Cancer 31[Suppl II]: 1–28
Mislin H (1983) The lymphangion. In: Földi M, Casley-Smith JR (eds) Lymphangiology. Schattauer, Stuttgart, pp 165–173
Mori Y, Lennert K (1969) Electron microscopic atlas of lymph node cytology and pathology. Springer, Berlin Heidelberg New York
Nordmann M (1928) Studien an Lymphknoten bei akuten und chronischen Allgemeininfektionen. Virchows Arch [A] 267: 158–203
Reynolds GJ (1982) Lymphoid tissue. Wright PSG, Bristol
Rhodin JAG (1974) Histology. A text atlas. Oxford University Press, New York
Roitt JM, Brostoff J, Male DK (1985) Immunology. Gower Medical, London
Rusznyak J, Földi M, Szabo G (1957) Physiologie und Pathologie des Lymphkreislaufes. Fischer, Jena
Rusznyak J, Földi M, Szabo G (1969) Lymphologie, Physiologie und Pathologie der Lymphgefäße und des Lymphkreislaufes. Gustav Fischer, Stuttgart
Sandritter W, Beneke G (1974) Allgemeine Pathologie. Lehrbuch für Studierende und Ärzte. Schattauer Verlag, Stuttgart/New York
Sharp JA, Burwell RG (1960) Interaction ("peripolesis") of macrophages and lymphocytes after skin homografting or challenge with soluble antigens. Nature 188: 474–475
Shelton E (1962) Prolonged survival of rabbit thoracic duct lymphocytes in a diffusion chamber. J Cell Biol 12: 652–655
Shelton E, Rice ME (1959) Growth of normal peritoneal cells in diffusion chambers: a study in cell modulation. Am J Anat 105: 281–342
Sundberg RD (1960) Lymphocytes: origin, structure and interrelationships. In: Rebuck JW (ed) The lymphocyte and lymphocytic tissue. Hoeber, New York, pp 1–21
Sundberg RD, Downey H (1955) Lymphocytes and plasma cells. Ann NY Acad Sci 59: 671–684
Weidenreich F, Baum H, Trautmann A (1933) Das Lymphgefäßsystem der Säugetiere. In: Bolck L, Göppert E, Kallius E, Lubosch W (eds) Handbuch der Vergleichenden Anatomie der Wirbeltiere. Bd. VI, Urban & Schwarzenberg, Berlin Wien, 745–854
Weiss L (1972) The cells and tissues of the immune system. Structure, functions and interactions. Prentice-Hall, Englewood Cliffs, NJ
Yamaguchi K, Shoefl GI (1983a) Blood vessels of the Peyer's patch in the mouse: I. Topographic studies. Anat Rec 206: 391–401
Yamaguchi K, Shoefl GI (1983b) Blood vessels of the Peyer's patch in the mouse: III. High-endothelium venules. Anat Rec 206: 419–438
Yoffey JM, Courtice FC (1956) Lymphatics, lymph and lymphoid tissue. Edward Arnold, London
Yoffey JM, Courtice FC (1970) Lymphatics, lymph and the lymphomyeloid complex. Academic, London

The Deep Cortex of the Lymph Node: Morphological Variations and Functional Aspects

G. SAINTE-MARIE, C. BÉLISLE, and F.S. PENG

1 Introduction

1.1 The Deep Cortex

The lymph node has long been known to comprise a medulla radiating from its hilus and a cortex located along most of its periphery. This "peripheral cortex" contains folliculonodules, each consisting of a follicle and a nodule (or germinal center), separated by an extrafollicular zone (SAINTE-MARIE and SIN 1970). The node is also known to comprise a third main component which, for about the past two decades, has frequently been referred to as the "paracortex" and commonly illustrated as a rather uniform layer underlying the entire peripheral cortex (GUTMAN and WEISSMAN 1972; GOLDSCHNEIDER and MC-

Table 1. Terms used to designate elements of the lymph node corresponding to the deep cortex

Nodule-like elements	
Pseudo-secondary nodule	EHRICH, W. 1929
Tertiary nodule	EHRICH, W. E. 1946
Primary cortical nodule	RINGERTZ and ADAMSON 1950
Primary lymphoid nodule	WAKSMAN et al. 1962
Follicular paracortical area	OORT and TURK 1965
Pseudo-follicle	SAINTE-MARIE and SIN 1970
Paracortical nodule	NOSSAL and ADA 1971
T nodule	REE and FANGER 1975
Ill-defined elements	
Diffuse lymphocyte-rich area	RINGERTZ and ADAMSON 1950
Primary lymphoid mass	WAKSMAN et al. 1962
Mid and deep cortex	GOWANS and KNIGHT 1964
Lymphocyte-filled cortex	OSOBA and MILLER 1964
Paracortical area	OORT and TURK 1965
Thymus-dependent area	PARROTT et al. 1966
Diffuse cortex	WEISSMAN 1967
Diffuse lymphocyte field	GOLDSCHNEIDER and MCGREGOR 1968
Diffuse cortical tissue	NOSSAL and ADA 1971
Parafollicular cortex	GUTMAN and WEISSMAN 1972
Paracortex	GOLDSCHNEIDER and MCGREGOR 1973

GREGOR 1973; COTTIER et al. 1973; KEARNEY 1974; GREAVES et al. 1974; WEISSMAN et al. 1978). However, such a topographical concept of the third component is inconsistent with earlier observations which instead reported the component to comprise elements with diverse appearances. A review of the literature led us to distinguish these elements into two types: nodule-like and ill-defined elements (Table 1). Obviously, the varied terminology used to designate these elements reflected great variations in the histology of the third nodal component and/or an inadequate knowledge of its histology. Therefore, we undertook a detailed study aiming to clarify the histology of this component, which, for reasons presented below, we will refer to as the "deep cortex" by contrast to the peripheral cortex containing the folliculonodules and the extrafollicular zone. The findings summarized here demonstrate that the deep cortex is actually formed of basic structures, which we have now come to term "deep cortex units" or more simply "units," after having used the term "pseudofollicle" for a while (Table 1).

1.2 The Compartmentation of the Lymph Node

It is necessary first to introduce the notion of the compartmentation of the node, since it relates to the pattern of lymph flow in the organ which ultimately influences the topography of the deep cortex. In past literature, the predominant view on the pattern of lymph flow was as follows: The lymph, entering a node by any of its afferent lymphatic vessels, would spread through the entire subcapsular sinus underlying the capsule (DRINKER et al. 1933; HERMAN et al. 1968). Some of the lymph would then enter vaguely described sinuses which cross the cortex and open into medullary sinuses adjoining the efferent lymphatic vessel(s) at the hilus (DENZ 1947). Finally, lymph would also find its way into medullary sinuses at the perihilar margin of the subcapsular sinus (NORDMAN 1928; YOFFEY and COURTICE 1970). Hence, lymph from any afferent lymphatic of a node was presumed to flow into all of its sinuses. Consequently, a node was considered to be a physiological entity, responding as a whole to stimulation by an immunogenic element carried by any of its afferent lymphatics. However, a few authors observed that the distribution of a locally injected tracer could be restricted to a portion of a draining node (HOBBS and DAVIDSON 1976; KETT et al. 1978).

A tridimensional study of the architecture of the rat node, and of the pattern of lymph flow in it, revealed that the node is morphologically and functionally compartmented (SAINTE-MARIE et al. 1982). Each "compartment" of a node is related to an afferent lymphatic vessel, a node having as many compartments as such vessels. Accordingly, a locally injected small dose of a tracer is distributed only in the portion of subcapsular sinus which overlies the compartment related to the given afferent lymphatic via which the tracer enters a draining node. A compartment comprises: the opening of an afferent lymphatic in the subcapsular sinus, the portion of subcapsular sinus which receives the lymph entering from this vessel, the corresponding portion of underlying peripheral cortex, a deep cortex unit, and the medullary cords contiguous to these cortical elements. Here and there at the margin of a compartment, narrow to wide gaps occurring in the subcapsular sinus and the peripheral cortex allow the lymph from the related afferent lymphatic to enter medullary sinuses. These gaps represent outward extensions of one or a few medullary sinuses across the peripheral cortex, which connect directly with the subcapsular sinus. Figure 1a illustrates a "compartment," and defines the terms used throughout this review. Figure 1b schematizes the pattern of lymph flow in a compartment, and the route followed by a circulating lymphocyte, from the afferent lymph or the blood, to reach the structure of the compartment where the immunological process in which it is to be involved will occur.

The morphological variations of structures of the same type possibly observed among compartments of the same node can be explained by the fact that the node's various afferent lymphatics carry lymph from neighboring anatomical sites which can host different immunogenic elements (SAINTE-MARIE et al. 1982). While our study focused on the rat, this conclusion applies also to large species but with a difference. In large species like the sheep, ox, or dog, an afferent lymphatic yields many branches as it reaches a node, and each such "prenodal branch" relates to a compartment (BÉLISLE and SAINTE-MARIE 1981e; HEATH and BRANDON 1983; AIJIMA et al. 1986). A group of neighboring compartments is thus similarly stimulated by the same afferent lymph, so that morphological variations occur mainly among groups of compartments instead of among single compartments.

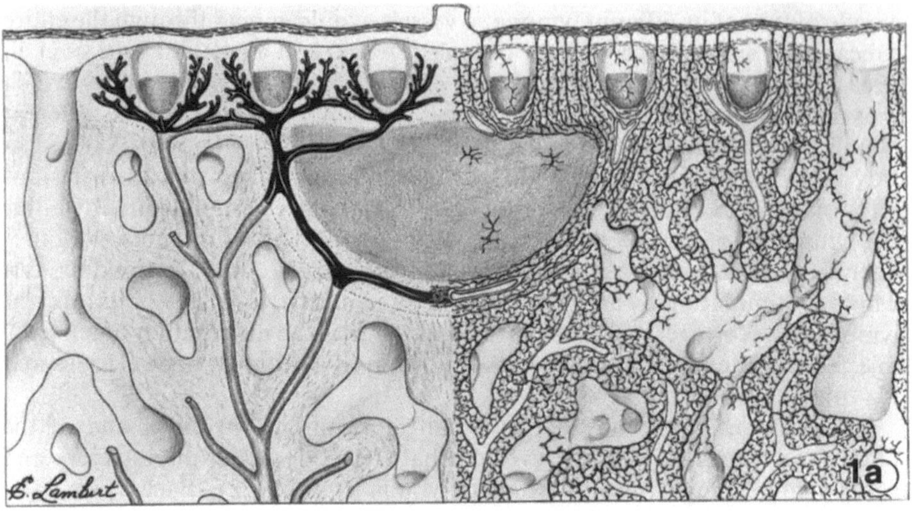

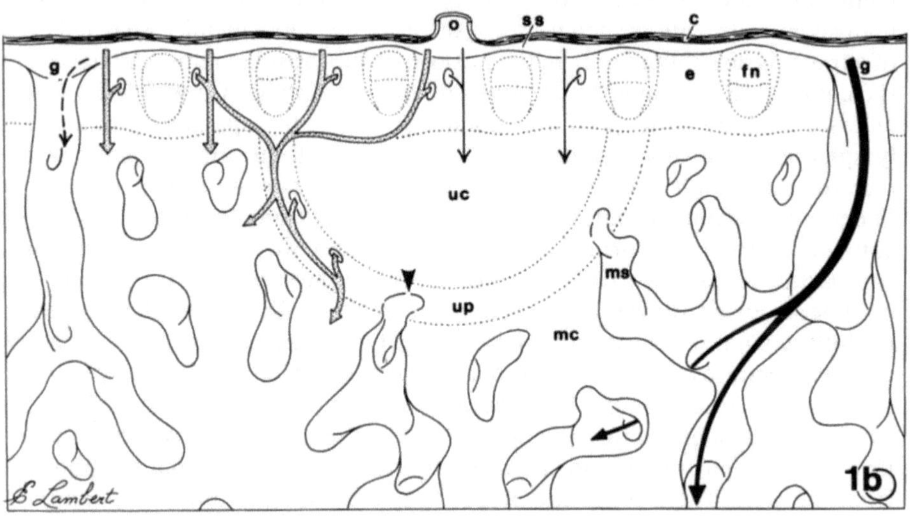

2 Constitution of the Deep Cortex of the Rat Node

2.1 Topography of the Deep Cortex

To elucidate the tridimensional organization of the deep cortex, a histological analysis of 112 serially sectioned nodes of diverse anatomical locations from normal young rats was carried out (BÉLISLE and SAINTE-MARIE 1981 a). The sections were silver impregnated with a variant of the technique of Bielchowsky, and counterstained lightly with Kernechtrot for cell nuclei. The

◀ **Fig. 1 a, b.** Different aspects of a "compartment" of the rat lymph node. The compartment is centered on the opening (*o*) of the related afferent lymphatic vessel into the subcapsular sinus (*ss*) underlying the capsule (*c*). Corresponding portions of subcapsular sinus and of peripheral cortex are delimited, on either side, by a gap (*g*) where subcapsular sinus connects directly with medullary sinuses. The peripheral cortex has an extrafollicular zone (*e*) and folliculonodules (*fn*), i.e., follicles with a nodule (germinal center) comprising an outer pale and an inner dark zone. The compartment includes a deep cortex "unit" with a center (*uc*) and a periphery (*up*). The *arrowhead* points to a "unit sinus" arising as a cul-desac in the unit periphery. Note that the peripheral cortex may extend for variable distances beyond the unit. The compartment also comprises medullary cords (*mc*) and sinuses (*ms*). In **a**, high endothelial venules (*shaded*) run in the extrafollicular zone and the periphery of the unit. At the corticomedullary junction, they transform into the regular venules (*unshaded*) of the medullary cords. Numerous reticular fibers arise from the capsule and extend parallel across the subcapsular sinus, the extrafollicular zone, and the periphery of the unit. As they reach the medullary cords, the fibers acquire a different pattern. In **b**, the *heavy arrows* indicate the pathway of lymph flow; their thickness is proportional to the importance of flow at a given site. Lymph enters indirectly, via anatomoses, the medullary sinuses present under the cortex, flow being minimal in segments beneath the unit. Other *arrows* schematize the routes of migration of incoming circulating lymphocytes. From the subcapsular sinus or the high endothelial venules of the extrafollicular zone above the center of the unit, lymphocytes involved in cellular immune responses (*single full arrows*) migrate toward the unit center; cells involved in humoral immune responses (*dotted arrows*) migrate toward medullary cords. Noninvolved cells (*broken arrow*) enter the medullary sinuses directly

silver blackens the reticular fibers, as well as the nuclear chromatin present at a distance greater than about 4 μm from a fiber; the chromatin closer to a fiber is lightly stained by the Kernechtrot. As a result, the bulk of the deep cortex as well as the folliculonodules, both containing few fibers, have a very dark background since most of their densely packed lymphoid nuclei are blackened. These components hence contrast with the nearby extrafollicular zone or medullary cords, in which the abundant fibers inhibit the blackening of virtually all nuclei.

The analysis revealed the presence of deep cortex units in all nodes, a unit being a component of each node compartment. The smallest nodes contain a single compartment and thus have a single unit. The units are semispherical to semiovoid in shape; they are contiguous to the peripheral cortex and bulge into the medulla (Figs. 2, 3). The apparent shape of a unit in single sections differs greatly according to the angle as well as the level of cutting. Figure 4 schematizes some such variations. Typically, a transverse cut shows the unit as a round structure totally surrounded by medulla. Note that the peripheral cortex of a compartment most often extends for varying distances beyond its unit, where it overlies medulla directly (Fig. 1). Due to this fact, to the cutting incidence, and to the relatively small size of units in some nodes, single sections of a node can exhibit solely peripheral cortex and medulla, even though the node actually has several units.

On the whole, the semispherical units outnumber the wider semiovoid units, which are more frequent in the large mesenteric and cervical nodes (Table 2). The absolute width of a unit reaches a maximum of about 1.6 mm; the absolute thickness ranges from 0.2 to 1.5 mm. Translated into histological terms, as observed in single median longitudinal sections of a compartment, a unit is overlaid by an area of peripheral cortex containing two to six follicu-

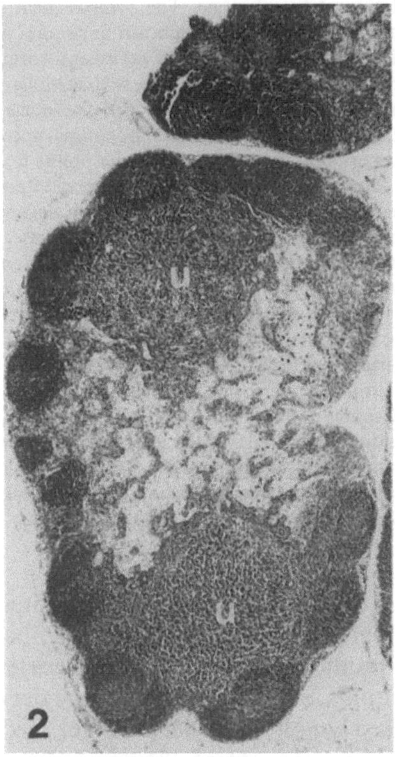

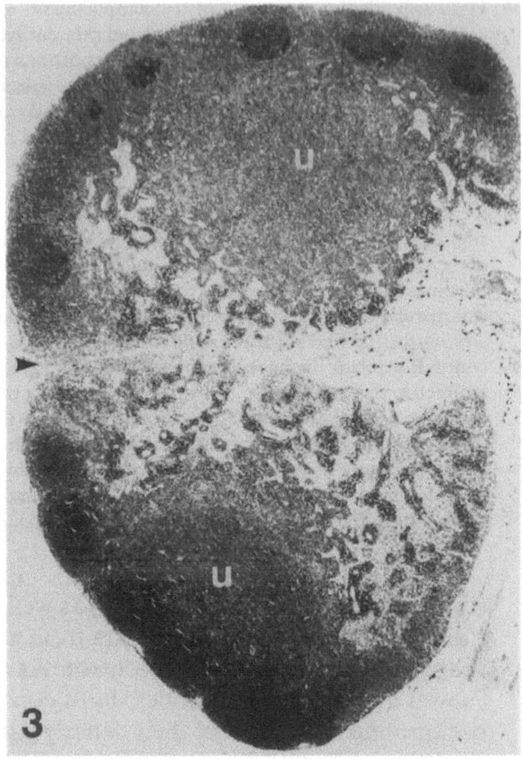

Fig. 2. Mesenteric lymph node from a 10-week-old normal rat. Large and outwardly protruding folliculonodules occur above two deep cortex units (*u*), which are similarly stained because they are equally populated by lymphocytes. The peripheries of the units are not very distinct from the also lymphocytic contiguous medullary cords. Dominici stain, ×23

Fig. 3. Same as Fig. 2, but cervical lymph node. The *arrowhead* indicates a gap at the margin of the two compartments, each showing its deep cortex unit (*u*). The lower unit is stained darker than the upper one, due to a denser concentration of lymphocytes mostly in its center, which is hence also darker than the periphery of same unit. Most medullary cords contiguous to the unit peripheries are distinguishable from the latter, being darker stained because they are plasmacytic. The dark zones of the nodules (germinal centers) above the upper unit are obvious, unlike those related to the lower unit, where lymphocyte concentration is denser around them. Dominici stain, ×23

lonodules depending on its absolute width. The apparent size of a unit in single sections also varies greatly with the incidence of cutting, as is the case for shape. For instance, a unit cut through its edge, or transversely across its bottom, appears much smaller than it is in reality (Fig. 4).

The number and size of units in a node vary to some extent with its location. Nodes of a given location tend to be of a similar size, and their main constituents tend to account for a comparable relative volume of the node (MEYER et al. 1979). This is because, under normal conditions, nodes of the same site are similarly stimulated. On the other hand, the main constituent can account for very different relative volumes, in nodes of different locations in

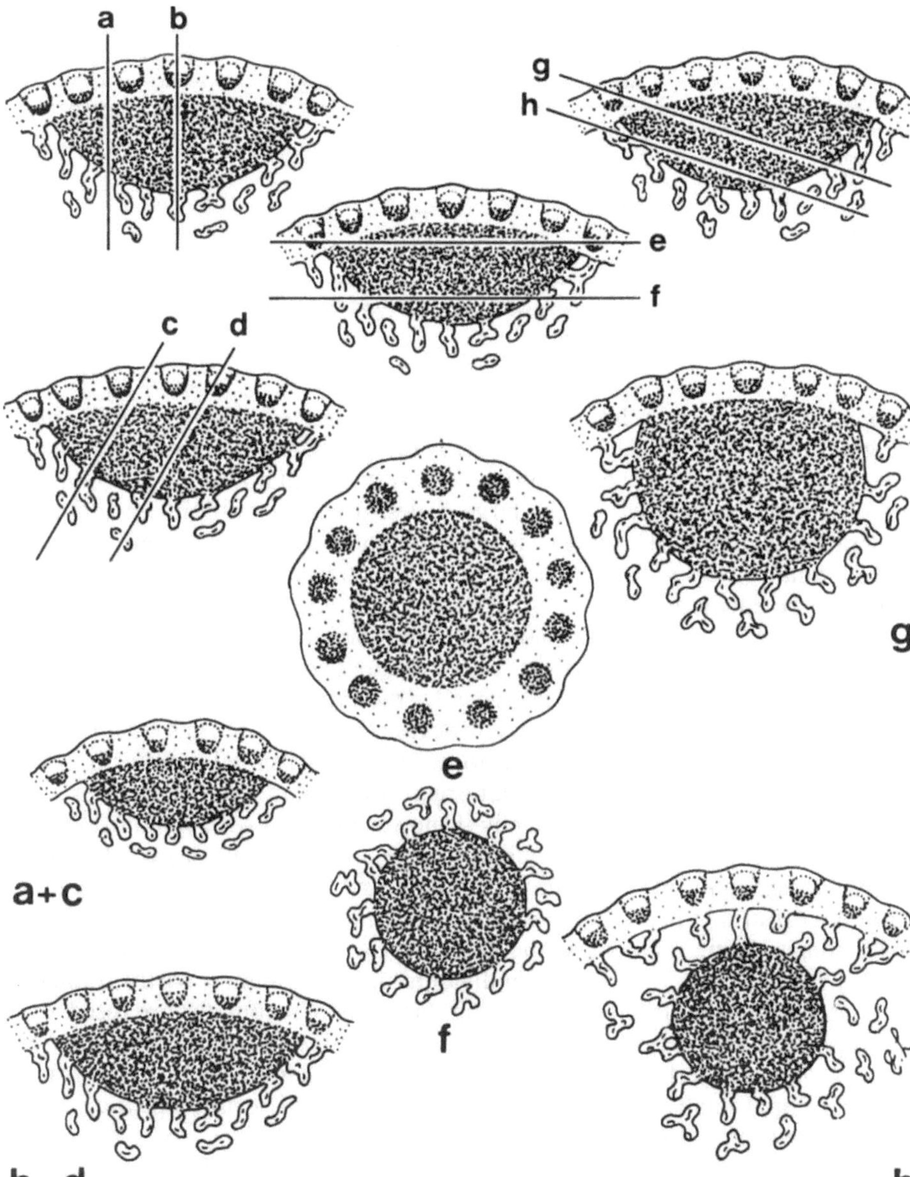

Fig. 4a–h. The variations in shape and size of a deep cortex unit according to the angle and/or level of cutting. The *upper diagrams* indicate, by a letter, the incidence of cutting shown in the diagram below designated by the corresponding letter. The *left column* shows variations in appearance with longitudinal (**a, b**) and longitudinal like (**c, d**) cutting incidences, units exhibiting a semispherical to semiovoid shape. The *central column* demonstrates variations in appearance in transversely cut units. Units are then round and surrounded by cortical (**e**) or medullary (**f**) structures. The *right column* illustrates variations in appearance of obliquely cut units. Here, units vary from semispherical or semiovoid (**g**) to spherical or ovoid (**h**). In the latter conditions, units are totally surrounded by medulla, as in transverse sections (**f**)

Table 2. Deep cortex units in lymph nodes of various sites from eight normal rats

Sites	Number of nodes analyzed	Number of units recorded	Ratio of semispherical to semiovoid units
Brachial	16[a]	95	4.0
Popliteal	14	44	3.7
Inguinal	14[a]	92	3.6
Parathymic	34	65	3.4
Mesenteric	8[a]	60	2.3
Cervical	26	89	2.1

[a] Underestimated figures since, in these cases, the analyzed tissues were often chains of nodes including a few hardly definable organs

particular. Hence, the relative volume of a node occupied by its deep cortex ranges from 10% to 70%, that occupied by the medulla varying approximately inversely. The small units occur most often in the small nodes. The large units are observed almost solely in the large nodes, predominantly in cervical and mesenteric locations. However, departures from this general trend are observed. Small nodes with a large unit(s) and, at times, large nodes with small units can be encountered.

About half of the units are isolated. The remaining units are variably but incompletely fused to one another, thus forming deep cortex "complexes." A complex has two to six units and, usually, the more units in a complex, the more intricate its pattern. The most intricate complexes are thus encountered in the large cervical and mesenteric nodes. A tridimensional analysis is often necessary to understand the particular organization of individual complexes as observed in single sections, especially if they are stained with standard methods. Indeed, differences in the number, the size, the shape, the degree of fusion, the relative orientation of the individual units, and the incidence of cutting lead to great variations in the appearance of complexes in single node sections. With some cutting incidences, the pattern of a complex can be understood readily in single sections, for the individual units show their partly rounded outline. But at other levels of sectioning, the units of a complex are fused and a complex can misleadingly appear as a large ill-defined structure or as a rather uniform layer underlying a broad portion of peripheral cortex. In this case, tridimensional analysis will reveal, on other levels of sectioning, the partly rounded outline of the constituent units.

It was hence established that the deep cortex is made up of units which can form complexes. It is the numerous variations in the above-cited parameters related to units and complexes that give rise to the diverse appearances of the deep cortex in single sections. Further variations result from differences in the particular architecture of a node and in the incidence of cutting of the organ, while variably cut units, or complexes, can occur simultaneously in the same section. One can understand how the great magnitude of resulting variations in the appearance of structures of the deep cortex in single sections gave rise to correspondingly varied terminology. Hence, the many terms used in the past reflected variations in the appearance of basic structures rather than different structures. The nodule-like elements of the literature correspond to transversely cut units, whereas the ill-defined elements correspond to variably cut complexes (Table 1). Among the many terms used previously, we decided to retain "deep cortex." First, it is a topographical term properly applying to this component. Second, it has no functional implication, which was preferable since the function of this component was insufficiently known. Third, the term paracortex was discarded for it implies that this component is not part of the cortex, which is not so, as will be seen later.

2.2 Relation of the Deep Cortex Units to the Afferent Lymphatic Vessels

Certain observations had led to the suspicion that a unit is topographically related to an afferent lymphatic vessel (SAINTE-MARIE and SIN 1970; SIN 1972; KELLY 1975). This hypothesis was tested by a study of rat nodes prefixed by perfusion to prevent the collapse of the afferent lymphatics. The perinodal adipose tissue was furthermore left in place to preserve these lymphatics. This method made it possible to follow, on consecutive sections, the afferent lymphatics from the outline of the adipose tissue to a node's capsule. The tridimensional analysis of the serial sections from 41 nodes revealed that each unit is centered on the opening of an afferent lymphatic and that, conversely, each such opening is underlaid by a unit (BÉLISLE and SAINTE-MARIE 1981 b). The analysis also showed that an afferent lymphatic generally abuts on a subcapsular sinus by way of a single opening. In many instances, however, a lymphatic undergoes a "terminal division" just before entering a node's capsule; this gives rise to two openings and, at times, to more than two openings. The study further revealed the existence of a relationship between the pattern of the opening(s) of an afferent lymphatic and the shape of the related unit. Of the 98 analyzed units, 63 were semispherical and associated with an afferent lymphatic having a single opening (Fig. 5 a). Nine units were semispherical and related to a lymphatic whose terminal division gave rise to two neighboring openings (Fig. 5 b). Twenty-one units which exhibited a broader semiovoid shape were associated with a double-branched lymphatic with more distant openings (Fig. 5 c). The remaining five units, with even broader semiovoid shapes, were related to a vessel whose terminal division gave rise to more than two openings (Fig. 5 d). Furthermore a relationship was observed between the isolation of units, or the partial fusion of neighboring units into complexes, and the distance separating the openings of the related afferent lymphatics. Where two neighboring units were isolated (Fig. 5 e), the distance between the openings of the two related lymphatics was greater than where the units were fused one to another (Fig. 5 f). As to the complexes, they were associated with a number of afferent lymphatics equal to that of the constituent units, the shape of the complexes correlating with the topography of the lymphatic openings. Our observations thus revealed that the particularities of the topography of the deep cortex of a given node are influenced by those of the

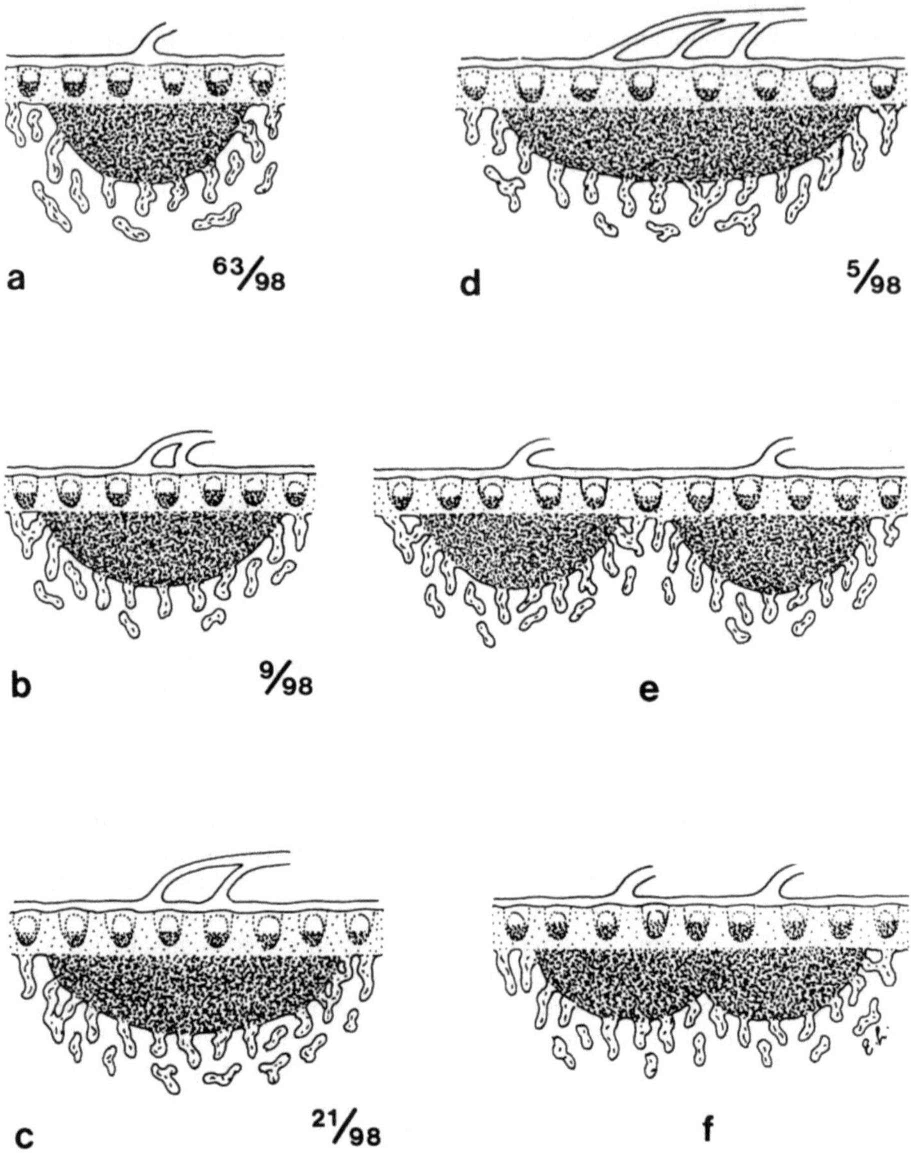

Fig. 5a–f. Relationship between the appearance of a deep cortex unit and the pattern of the opening(s) of the related afferent lymphatic vessel. Semispherical units are associated with one (**a**) or two very close openings (**b**) of the same vessel. Semiovoid units are associated with two (**c**) or a few distant openings (**d**) of a single vessel. In (**e**), two neighboring but still isolated units are associated with the close opening of two lymphatics while (**f**) shows the fusion, into a complex, of two neighboring units but associated with lymphatic openings closer than in (**e**). The ratios give the frequency of the patterns **a–d**, in a total of 98 analyzed units

opening(s) of its afferent lymphatics. While an afferent lymphatic (or a prenodal branch) can abut on a subcapsular sinus by way of more than one opening, we will mention only one opening from now on, for the sake of simplicity.

Another general relationship concerns the diameter of an afferent lymphatic and the width of the related unit. As stated above, the wider units are present in the large cervical and mesenteric nodes which receive the larger lymphatics. The importance of the antigenic presence in the tissues drained by these nodes can explain the larger size and the more frequent terminal branching of their afferent lymphatics at a node's capsule; the consequences are wider units, a higher proportion of semiovoid units, and a higher frequency of complexes in these nodes. Indeed, antigenic invasion enhances the pressure of the interstitial fluid at the site of injury and increases the flow of lymph to a draining node (YOFFEY and COURTICE 1970). In the case of sites of early and persistent invasion, the greater lymph flow will cause the afferent lymphatics to enlarge and/or divide, thus provoking the formation of wider semiovoid units and/or the enlargement and fusion of units into complexes. It will be seen later that, accordingly, the formation of complexes can be observed soon after birth. A study of nodes of bovines of various ages indicated that complexes can also form later (AIJIMA et al. 1986).

2.3 Morphology of the Deep Cortex Unit

Each unit has been shown to comprise a center and a periphery with distinct features (BÉLISLE and SAINTE-MARIE 1981c). The unit center is contiguous to peripheral cortex. The unit periphery covers the semispherical portion of the margin of the unit center; it is also contiguous to peripheral cortex but mostly to medulla (Fig. 1). In tissue sections stained with standard methods, the outline between the center and the periphery of a unit, as well as that between the unit periphery and the medulla, is more or less clearly demarcated. These outlines are clearer where there is a marked difference in the density and the nature of the cell population of one of these constituents compared with that of the nearby constituents. Since the immunological conditions prevailing in a given compartment influence the density and the nature of the cell population of its constituents, variations in these conditions account for the degree of clarity of the outlines of its unit.

2.3.1 Reticular Fiber Framework

Silver impregnation improves the demarcation of the unit center and periphery. Indeed, the unit center contains few fibers so that most of its lymphoid nuclei are blackened. By contrast, the unit periphery has a dense framework of fibers so that very few of its lymphoid nuclei are darkened. Hence, the tissue background of the periphery appears lighter than the center of a unit. As a result, the boundary between the two elements of a unit is rather sharp. It corresponds to an almost abrupt increase in the concentration of fibers in the unit periphery, many of which are coarse and run in a grossly parallel manner. As for the boundary between the unit periphery and the medulla, it is also generally clear, partly due to the presence of the pale medullary sinuses. But the boundary between the unit center and the peripheral cortex, while more neatly demarcated than with standard staining methods, is often still poorly delineated. Commonly, this boundary runs slightly below the folliculonodules (Fig. 1), corresponding to the line of disappearance of the characteristic network of coarse fibers crossing the depth of the extrafollicular zone (SAINTE-MARIE and SIN 1970). At times, the same boundary shows a wavy appearance, as it rises between folliculonodules.

2.3.2 Network of High Endothelial Venules

The peculiar vessels termed high endothelial venules or postcapillary venules have an endothelium of hypertrophied cells crossed by lymphocytes. High endothelial venules were once thought to occur only in the deep cortex. However, studies confirmed their presence in the extrafollicular zone (SAINTE-MARIE and SIN 1970; KOJIMA et al. 1971; HERMAN et al. 1972). High endothelial venules were also said to be randomly scattered in the deep cortex (ANDERSON and ANDERSON 1975). It was demonstrated that instead they are almost restricted to the unit periphery, where they continue the high endothelial venules of the extrafollicular zone associated with the unit (BÉLISLE and SAINTE-MARIE 1981c). First, high endothelial venules from the extrafollicular zone above the unit center curve toward the unit periphery while running along the outer margin of the unit center (Fig. 1). Due to this fact, high endothelial venules appear distributed almost throughout the unit center in transverse sections grazing the peripheral cortex. Second, high endothelial venules from the extrafollicular zone above the unit periphery enter the latter directly. Third, some high endothelial venules from the extrafollicular zone neighboring the peripheral cortex above the unit also join the unit periphery. As they penetrate deeper into the unit periphery, these vessels form larger collecting venules. The latter give off lateral branches which extend into contiguous medullary cords. At this point, a high endothelial venule transforms into a regular venule. Note that, at times, a high endothelial venule of the extrafollicular zone above a unit center runs instead across the unit center to reach a deep part of the unit periphery. This seems to be the result of an accident occurring during the postnatal formation of the units as explained in Sect. 4.3.

2.3.3 Lymphatic Sinuses

The unit periphery contains characteristic sinuses whose number varies from zero to ten in single sections of a unit, depending on its size (BÉLISLE and SAINTE-MARIE 1981c). These "unit sinuses" originate locally as culs-de-sac, not being connected with the subcapsular sinus (Fig. 1). A unit sinus differs from the continuing medullary sinus in that it is commonly narrower and loaded with lymphocytes. Segments of medullary sinuses immediately extending unit sinuses can contain a relatively large number of lymphocytes, the concentration diminishing gradually as these sinuses reach deeper in the medulla. The average width of the unit sinuses and the density of their lymphocyte content tend to vary with the size of a unit. Wide and heavily loaded sinuses are encountered most often in the large units. In the small units, the sinuses are narrow and contain few lymphocytes, which are hardly detectable.

On sections stained with standard methods, it is generally difficult to distinguish the unit sinuses, for their dense cell content resembles that of the unit. But on silver-impregnated sections, the more darkened sinuses contrast with the paler unit periphery. The darker aspect of the unit sinuses results from the blackening of most nuclei of the contained lymphocytes, due to a scarcity of intrasinusal fibers. Hence, the greater the lymphocyte content of a unit sinus, the more obvious the sinus.

2.3.4 Cell Population

The unit is populated by lymphocytes with a small minority of proliferative precursor forms; lymphocyte subsets will be considered later. The unit also contains some reticular, dendritic, or macrophagic cells. In the unit center, the lymphocyte population is variably dense and presents a uniform to marble-like pattern of distribution. The unit periphery commonly has a lower concentration of lymphocytes and is thus often paler than the unit center.

Neonatal thymectomy revealed that the lymphocytes of the deep cortex are T cells, for it is subsequently almost completely devoid of lymphocytes (WAKSMAN et al. 1962; PARROTT et al. 1966). However, a later study showed that only the center of a unit is devoid of lymphocytes under the athymic state, which demonstrates that, unlike the unit center, the unit periphery is not exclusively thymus dependent (SAINTE-MARIE and PENG 1983). This is in line with the fact that the unit periphery has a function distinct from that of the unit center, serving as a route for migration of incoming circulating lymphocytes of B and T types, which will be discussed below. The unit periphery is hence not devoid of lymphocytes under the athymic state since B cells continue to migrate there. While the lymphocytes present in the periphery of units of nodes of nude animals are presumably B cells, some of them might be T cells, for a small fraction of the lymphocytes in nude animals bear surface markers considered to be specific for T cells (FOSSUM 1983).

In the unit periphery, each high endothelial venule is cuffed by one to three vaguely concentric "perivascular channels" or spaces containing lymphocytes (SAINTE-MARIE 1966). Where a high endothelial venule occasionally runs across a unit center in a node of an athymic animal, one accordingly observes a dense cuff of lymphocytes immediately around this venule whereas the surrounding tissue is devoid of lymphocytes (SAINTE-MARIE et al. 1984c). This observation reveals that the space occupied by the perivascular channels of such a venule constitutes a milieu similar to that of the unit periphery although it is located in a unit center, and that the cell population in these latter channels is similar to that in the unit periphery. This may be of interest for studies analyzing types or subsets of lymphocytes in the deep cortex. Hence, BARCLAY (1981) observed the presence of rare Ig^+ cells in probable unit centers but did not determine their precise location.

3 The Deep Cortex in Various Mammal Species

It was wondered whether the deep cortex, in nodes of other species, is similar to that of the rat. Therefore, a total of 181 nodes from mice, guinea pigs, hamsters, rabbits, dogs, sheep, and humans were examined (BÉLISLE and SAINTE-MARIE 1981e). The examination of sections from these serially cut nodes revealed the presence of deep cortex units in all species. Deep cortex complexes occur as well, and are also more frequent in the large cervical and mesenteric nodes. Moreover, the morphological features of the units and complexes resemble those of the rat.

The largest units are observed in the rabbit, reaching almost 3 mm in thickness. In the dog, the units are often not much wider than the individual overlying folliculonodules, which, however, are commonly larger than in the other species. In the other large species studied, the units rarely exceed 1 mm in thickness, as is the case in the rat. On the whole, the absolute size of the units is thus rather comparable in these different species, not varying in a manner directly proportional to the size of the animals or of their nodes. In comparison to the size of the nodes, therefore, the units of the larger species studied are relatively small and may not be noticed at first glance. The units correspondingly occupy a much lesser volume of the nodes in the larger than in the smaller species, most of the volume of a node comprising medullary sinuses.

4 Function of the Deep Cortex

Distinct morphological features characterize the periphery and the center of the deep cortex unit. Clearly, such morphological division of the unit into two constituents should reflect distinct functions, which is the case.

4.1 The Periphery of the Deep Cortex Unit

Except for the presence of unit sinuses, the unit periphery has the same constitution as the extrafollicular zone, and represents an extension of this zone beneath the unit center (SAINTE-MARIE and PENG 1979). Accordingly, the extrafollicular zone and the unit periphery are both routes for the migration of circulating lymphocytes having entered a node via the blood at the high endothelial venules (Gowans and Knight 1964) or via the afferent lymph at the subcapsular sinus (Sainte-Marie et al. 1975). These routes allow an incoming cell to reach, as directly as possible, the proper structure of the node where the nodal processes of the immune response in which it is to participate will take place. Hence, having left the subcapsular sinus or a high endothelial venule of the peripheral cortex above the unit center, a lymphocyte involved in a cellular immune response migrates directly to the unit center, where such a response develops as is described below, whereas a lymphocyte involved in humoral immune response reaches a medullary cord contiguous to the unit by migrating to its periphery (Fig. 1). A cell involved in a humoral immune response, but having left the subcapsular sinus or a high endothelial venule beyond the unit, migrates directly to an underlying medullary cord. These patterns of migration of incoming lymphocytes imply topographically selective activity of the inner wall of the subcapsular sinus and of the high endothelial venules of the peripheral cortex in the recruitment of circulating lymphocytes, at least in the case of those involved in cellular immune responses and having to reach a unit center. This was supported by findings in nodes of nude animals (Sainte-Marie and Peng 1983). Partly due to the presence of dense fiber networks, it would indeed be hardly possible for circulating lymphocytes concerned with cellular immune responses to reach a unit center if they were to enter the extrafollicular zone at a distance beyond a unit instead of above a unit center. Also, these patterns of migration prevent cells which are not involved in the activities of the folliculonodules or the unit centers from migrating through these structures; this contributes to the maintenance of the integrity of their milieu. The concentration of incoming cells into restricted routes of migration might further favor the encounter and interaction of some of these cells with appropriate elements present there.

The common role of the unit periphery and the extrafollicular zone was shown by experiments in which labeled thymic lymphocytes were injected locally or transfused (Sainte-Marie and Peng 1975, 1976). A few hours after transfer, labeled lymphocytes were present in the extrafollicular zone and the unit peripheries. After 24 h, labeled cells were scarcely observed there, but were concentrated in unit centers. The common role of the unit peripheries and the extrafollicular zone is also supported by diverse observations. First, unlike the unit centers but like the extrafollicular zone, the unit peripheries are not devoid of lymphocytes under the athymic state, a condition which further reveals that B cells use the unit peripheries to reach those medullary cords located beneath units. Second, in germ-free animals, the unit peripheries are populated by lymphocytes similarly to the extrafollicular zone above the units but unlike that present beyond the units. Moreover, only the segments of medullary cords contiguous to units are usually developed. All of this indicates that cells reach the developed cords via the unit peripheries. Third, findings in postnatal nodes similarly indicate that the precursors of the eventual plasmacytes of the medullary cords contiguous to units enter these cords from the unit peripheries. Indeed, at 1 week after birth, a concentration of blasts occurs in the peripheries of the forming units whereas blasts are scarce elsewhere in a same node (BÉLISLE and SAINTE-MARIE 1981 d). At 2 weeks, blast concentrations in the unit peripheries are matched by similar concentrations in the contiguous segments of medullary cords whereas the cords distant from the units have few blasts. At 3 weeks, there are few blasts in the unit peripheries, but the adjacent cords are populated by many plasmacytes, unlike the distant cords. Lastly, that cortical B cells follow the unit peripheries to reach the medullary cords below, where they become plasmacytes, is supported by observations made during studies using immunofluorescence (VAN ROOJEN 1987).

Besides supporting numerous vessels, the dense network of coarse parallel fibers of the unit periphery, as of the extrafollicular zone, contributes to the guidance of incoming cells toward the unit center or medullary cords (SAINTE-MARIE and PENG 1980).

The sinuses of the unit periphery represent an exit by which lymphocytes can leave the unit. The loading of these sinuses with lymphocytes was initially proposed to reflect an increase in cell traffic following antigenic challenge (SÖDERSTROM and STERNSTRÖM 1969) or a traffic jam caused by lymphocyte adherence there (KELLY et al. 1972). However, the simple fact that the unit sinuses originate locally and do not receive lymph from the subcapsular sinus can account for their filling with lymphocytes (BÉLISLE and SAINTE-MARIE 1981 c). Indeed, the unit sinuses drain a limited volume of interstitial fluid and, therefore, more lymphocytes than fluid may enter them, resulting in a high cell concentration in these sinuses. Moreover, the unit sinuses are continued by segments of medullary sinuses in which the lymph flows indirectly, and less actively, than in medullary sinuses connected directly with the subcapsular sinus. Hence, lymphocytes of the unit sinuses are somewhat passively drawn by the slow flow occurring in the continuing segments of medullary sinuses. Since the importance of this flow increases, as expected, with proximity to the hilus, the concentration of lymphocytes in the medullary sinuses concerned decreases as they are drawn away from a unit periphery.

4.2 The Center of the Deep Cortex Unit

SCOTHORNE and MCGREGOR (1955) investigated the effects of a homograft on the structures of draining nodes, and OORT and TURK (1965) studied the effects caused by oxazolone painting, which induces delayed hypersensitivity. It was found that both stimuli rapidly enlarge the deep cortex but have almost no effect on the folliculonodules and medullary cords, leading to the conclusion that such treatments stimulate almost exclusively the deep cortex, where, therefore, the resulting immune activity occurs. That the stimulated deep cortical elements are indeed units is particularly obvious in the work of SCOTHORNE and MCGREGOR (1955), who used rabbits. As stated above, units can become very large in this species and, thus, very obvious, as is evident in SCOTHORNE and MCGREGOR's figures. Both teams of workers further observed that the increase in the lymphocytic population of the deep cortex is accompanied by an increase in its content of blasts. Following labeling with ^{3}H-thymidine, OORT and TURK (1965) found that these blasts transform into lymphocytes and related them to cellular immunity. Later, HALL et al. (1980) demonstrated that oxazolone painting provokes cellular and humoral changes in the efferent lymph of the draining nodes similar to those occurring after challenge with conventional antigens. This does not support the view that oxazolone almost exclusively stimulates the components of cell-mediated immunity. The likely explanation for this discrepancy is that OORT and TURK (1965) did not carry out a sufficiently detailed analysis of the nodal structures concerned with humoral immunity, so that they could not detect an influence of oxazolone on them.

The role of the unit center, as the site of the nodal processes of cellular immune responses, was evidenced by the finding that it is the sole nodal constituent which is almost totally devoid of lymphocytes under the athymic state. In addition, cell transfer experiments demonstrated that T cells stay for a relatively long time in the unit centers (SAINTE-MARIE and PENG 1975, 1976), this long residency being in concordance with the absence of high endothelial venules and sinuses there. Such a stay allows cell proliferation, an essential process in an immune response. Newborn lymphocytes can leave the unit by way of the unit sinuses. The importance of the lymphocyte content of these sinuses thus could usually reflect the intensity of the immune activity of a given unit center, since heavily loaded unit sinuses are most often encountered in the greatly challenged large cervical and mesenteric nodes.

As stated above, lymphocytes can stay for a relatively long time in unit centers. It is probable that many of these cells are not actually involved in ongoing immune responses. Lymphocytes indeed accumulate in unit centers of nodes of young germ-free animals (BÉLISLE and SAINTE-MARIE 1982), in spite of a virtual absence of immune responses in such animals. It thus appears that unit centers are also places of sojourn of circulating T-cells. We suggested earlier that such sojourn might allow lymphocytes, modified by their passage in a drained tissue, to somewhat recover their original state. This is in line with the finding that circulating lymphocytes are modified by their passage in nodes (TRAVELLA and MORRIS 1980).

Studies with monoclonal antibodies confirmed that the deep cortex, i.e., probably the unit center since the existence of the unit periphery was then unknown, contains practically only T cells (POPPEMA et al. 1981). The vast majority of these T cells stain with antibodies reacting with all mature peripheral T cells, while none stain with T-6 antibody reacting with most immature thymocytes but not with mature peripheral T cells (POPPEMA et al. 1981). Only a minority of the lymphocytes of the unit center are suppressor/cytotoxic cells (POPPEMA et al. 1981; VAN DEN OORD et al. 1985); the vast majority belong to the inducer/helper subset, as is the case for circulating T cells (REINHERZ et al. 1979). The abundance of T helper cells in the unit center raises the question as to whether or not the unit center plays a role other than that of being the site of nodal processes of cellular immune responses. It was proposed by VAN DEN

OORD et al. (1985) that transformed B cells of a folliculonodule enter the underlying unit, where they are stimulated by T helper cells before migrating into medullary cords and becoming plasmacytes. No evidence was presented to support this proposal, which is most questionable, since a large fraction of the folliculonodules and of the plasmacytic medullary cords are not connected by a unit. Moreover, this proposal derived from a morphological concept, suggested by the same authors, which is untenable, as will be seen in Sect. 5.2.

4.3 Postnatal Formation of the Deep Cortex Units

We will briefly consider observations made in a study of the postnatal formation of the units, for some of them are of functional relevance (BÉLISLE and SAINTE-MARIE 1981 d). The study was performed on serial sections of 60 rat nodes fixed "in situ" and silver impregnated or stained with the May-Grünewald-Giemsa technique. One minute after birth, the nodal parenchyma can be distinguished into a medulla and a cortex. The cortex then consists of a regular framework of reticular fibers containing only a few small lymphocytes. Twenty-four hours later, the cortex may show tiny rounded areas, each related to an afferent lymphatic and populated by small lymphocytes and relatively numerous blasts. At 1 week, a peripheral and a deep cortex are discernible. The deep cortex consists of the above lymphocytic areas, which enlarge and acquire the features of units. Hence, the local fibers and venules are compressed at the periphery of these areas, which become the unit centers. It appears that, at times, a venule escapes this process and remains located in a unit center. Structures apparently corresponding to units were also observed by EIKELENBOOM et al. (1978, 1979), who, using specific markers, further showed that only T cells occur in nodes for a few days after birth.

In the rat, units can arise soon after birth, when the nodes are challenged by extraneous antigens. That units arise as a result of antigenic stimulation is indicated by the fact that their earliest forms have a high content of blasts. It is also indicated by the differences in the timing of formation of units in diverse nodes of an animal, as this probably reflects site-related variations in the timing of the occurrence of antigenic challenges. A more rapid formation was observed in cervical and mesenteric nodes, which can be expected to be the nodes first stimulated. The fact that units can form 1–2 weeks earlier than folliculonodules and plasmacytic medullary cords tends to corroborate the function of the unit as the site of occurrence of the nodal processes of cellular immune responses. It is most probable that extraneous antigens for humoral immune responses occur after birth simultaneously with antigens causing cellular immune responses. But it is likely that the former antigens are processed by antibodies of maternal origin, allowing almost only antigens causing cellular immunity to stimulate nodes and thus the initial formation of the units.

4.4 Differential Labeling of the Deep Cortex Units with ^{3}H-Uridine

Following transfusion of rat lymphocytes, incubated in vitro with ^{3}H-uridine, the more heavily labeled cells were observed to concentrate in components of nodes referred to as the mid and deep cortex by HOWARD et al. (1972). Because these components appeared to us to correspond to the actual deep cortex, the question arose as to whether ^{3}H-uridine could permit a physiological outlining of the units.

Differential labeling of the units was observed on the radioautographs of nodes from rats given ^{3}H-uridine intravenously and sacrificed 24 h thereafter (SAINTE-MARIE et al. 1981). This differential labeling was characterized by a markedly greater intensity of the radioautographic reaction of the units as compared with that of the nearby structures (Figs. 6, 8). The labeling intensity of the units, however, is not constant among the nodes of an animal, and it can also differ among units of a node. On day 3, such differential labeling of the units is no longer present in most nodes, but it persists in popliteal nodes stimulated with DNCB previous to labeling. In fact, the labeling intensity of the DNCB-stimulated units is initially about twice as great as that of the units of the control nodes. It should be noted that some nonexperimentally stimulated units, in nodes of diverse sites, can be as intensely labeled as DNCB-stimulated units.

This differential labeling of the units may be interpreted as meaning that their lymphocytes are of a different origin than those of the peripheral cortex. This would be in line with the conclusion of previous investigators that rat lymphocytes heavily labeled in vitro with ^{3}H-uridine are T-cells since, when transfused, they were observed to accumulate in the so-called thymic-dependent area of nodes (HOWARD et al. 1972; SPRENT 1973; HOLLINGSWORTH and CARR 1973; SCOTT and JOSEPHS 1975). The lightly labeled lymphocytes observed in the extrafollicular zone were thus concluded to be B cells (HOWARD et al. 1972). However, an alternative explanation was also proposed, namely that the heavier labeling of some rat lymphocytes is due to the intensity of their activity rather than to their origin (BOTTOMLY et al. 1975; DENNISON and CLANCY 1979). This agrees with the finding that the lymphocytes of the DNCB-stimulated units are much more intensely labeled than those of the control units, and with a corresponding variation in labeling intensity among the units of poorly or highly naturally stimulated nodes of the same animal (SAINTE-MARIE et al. 1981). Hence, the intensity of the labeling of units with ^{3}H-uridine might indicate the intensity of their stimulation or their ongoing immune activity.

The outer margin of the heavily labeled lymphocyte population of a unit commonly runs slightly beneath the inner limit of the subjacent folliculonodules; alternatively it undulates between these structures. It is of particular interest that the extrafollicular zone above some units mostly contains heavily labeled lymphocytes similar to those of the units, but unlike those of the extrafollicular zone present beyond the same units (Figs. 6, 8). To confirm that such areas present above units and containing heavily labeled lymphocytes

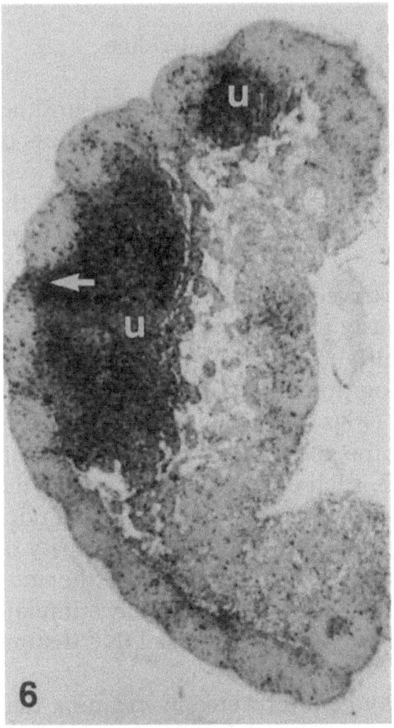

6

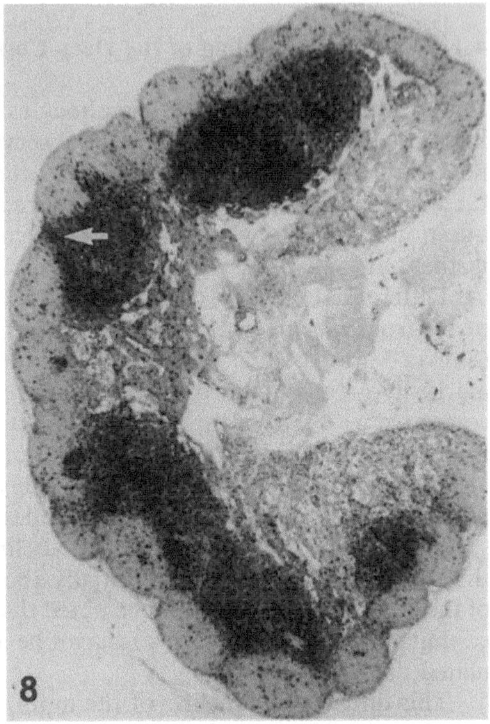
8

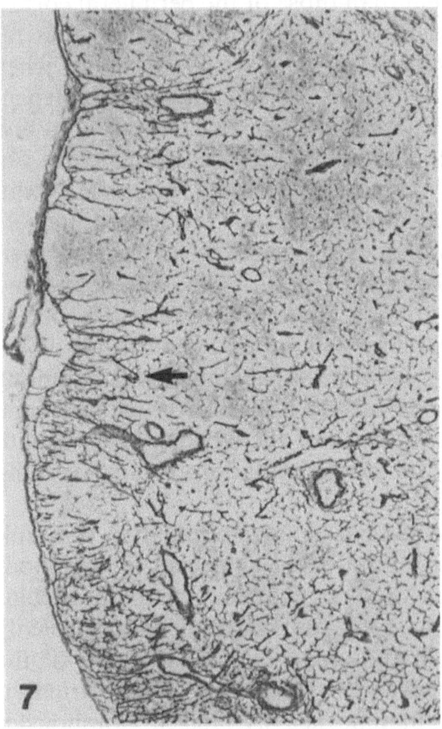
7

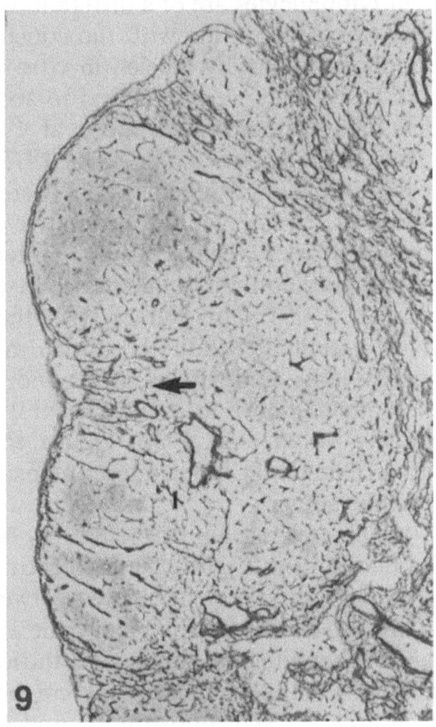
9

were truly areas of extrafollicular zone, the consecutive sections were silver impregnated. The features of the fiber network of these areas were characteristically those of areas of extrafollicular zone (Figs. 7, 9). The concentration of heavily labeled lymphocytes in these same areas can be explained by the fact that the extrafollicular zone above a unit is the site of arrival of incoming T cells, from the subcapsular sinus or local high endothelial venules, that have to reach the underlying units. Hence, the presence of greater numbers of heavily labeled lymphocytes in these areas of extrafollicular zone should reflect an increased arrival of stimulated T cells which eventually migrate to a unit center. Antigenic stimulation indeed provokes a greater influx of cells into a node (KELLY 1970; CAHILL et al. 1976). Given that cells destined to migrate into a unit first enter the extrafollicular zone above, the greater concentration of heavily labeled lymphocytes that occurs there after appropriate stimulation is expected. This suggests that the units concerned were probably naturally stimulated at the time of the labeling. HALL (1979) demonstrated a marked increase in the lymphocytic content in the drained lymph from an area of skin painted with oxazolone. The fact that cells of the afferent lymph enter the extrafollicular zone by migrating across the inner wall of the subcapsular sinus explains how heavily labeled, or stimulated, lymphocytes can be present even beneath this sinus wall.

The above considerations should be borne in mind in studies analyzing the types and subsets of lymphocytes in nodal structures. The fact that the same subsets may be encountered in the extrafollicular zone overlying some unit centers as in the unit centers themselves could be misleading in the absence of proper morphological consideration, as it could incorrectly suggest that the area of extrafollicular zone in question is an element of the deep cortex. We will see in Sect. 5.2 that such a line of thinking appears to account for an erroneous proposal on the morphology of the deep cortex based on immunohistochemical observations.

◀ **Fig. 6.** Radioautograph of a cervical lymph node from a 10-week-old normal rat injected intravenously with ^{3}H-uridine. The lymphocytes of the two deep cortex units (*u*) are strongly reactive. The *arrow* points to an area of extrafollicular zone present above a unit, which has a dense content of lymphocytes as heavily labeled as those in the unit. The extrafollicular zone beyond the units does not show this penomenon. ×23

Fig. 7. Section consecutive to that in Fig. 6, but silver impregnated. The enlargement of the area pointed in Fig. 6 shows the presence there of a reticular fiber meshwork characteristic of the extrafollicular zone. ×50

Figs. 8, 9. Cervical lymph node from a 10-week-old normal rat. The figures show the same phenomena observed in Figs. 6 and 7, except that the node has more deep cortex units. Fig. 8, ×23; Fig. 9, ×50

5 Variations of the Deep Cortex Units with Stimulation

Morphological variations of the structure of a draining node compartment result from stimulation by an antigen or the emergence of a local pathological condition.

5.1 Antigenic Stimulation

The variations caused by an antigen of a given type are bascially the same under all conditions, i.e., regardless of whether the antigen is of pathological origin. The extent of these variations differs in relation to the intensity of the challenge; their nature depends on whether or not a draining node functions normally.

5.1.1 Normal Lymph Nodes

Antigenic stimulation of a normally functioning node causes the diverse variations in the degree of development or activity of nodal structures usually observed in nodes of different anatomical sites. In the case of the deep cortex, these variations relate to the size of the units and of their lymphocytic population, and to the percentage of proliferative cells among this population (SCOTHORNE and MCGREGOR 1955; OORT and TURK 1965). Variations in the percentages of T-cell subsets are likely but remain to be shown. This could constitute a great task, considering the difficulties involved in obtaining such valid quantitative data and the pitfalls of the required techniques (HAAIJMAN et al. 1984). The interpretation of such data would be complicated, e.g., because a given unit can be the site of more than one cellular immune response at a time, with the responses being of different intensity and/or at different stages of development.

To further appreciate aspects of the variations in the deep cortex induced by antigenic stimulation, BÉLISLE et al. (1982) examined 60 nodes of diverse sites in germ-free rats. Their nodes were smaller than those of standard animals, and the units measured 0.2–0.9 mm in thickness as compared with 0.7–1.5 mm in standard animals. Moreover, the unit centers were paler than usual, having a less dense lymphocytic population composed almost only of small lymphocytes. These facts agree with the finding that stimulation increases the size of units and their blastic content (SCOTHORNE and MCGREGOR 1955). In addition, lymphocyte distribution is most generally homogeneous in the unit centers of germ-free rats, while it is usually marble-like in unit centers of standard rats (BÉLISLE et al. 1982). A marble-like pattern might thus reflect a state of stimulation and/or of ongoing cellular immune responses. An additional difference is that the unit peripheries of germ-free rats contain few lymphocytes, reflecting a lesser migration of incoming circulating lymphocytes there. Other differences compared with nodes of standard animals are: less development of the network of high endothelial venules in the unit peripheries, less hypertrophy of the endothelial cells of these venules, and a lesser number of lymphocytes associated with their endothelium. These latter differences are due to a weak recruitment of circulating lymphocytes via the blood, in line with the fact that stimulation increases lymphocyte entry into a node (KELLY 1970). However, it is not known whether these differences relate to a lack of stimulation for cellular immune responses only. Interestingly, the few lymphocytes present in the unit peripheries are concentrated in the perivascular channels of the high endothelial venules while only the medullary cords contiguous to units are developed. Both facts fit with the conclusion that these channels serve for the migration of incoming circulating lymphocytes toward medullary cords (SAINTE-MARIE and PENG 1980). Lastly, the unit sinuses are fewer and smaller in germ-free rats than usual, indicating that their degree of development in a given unit reflects the intensity of ongoing immune activity in that unit. Hence, besides the variations reported by earlier investigators, antigenic stimulation causes additional variations of the deep cortex that may not be obvious when comparing with the standard situation, in which the units have already undergone a variable degree of natural stimulation. Variations are better evidenced by comparison with the situation in the nodes of germ-free animals.

5.1.2 Deficient Lymph Nodes

A state of deficiency of the immune or lymphoid system, involving certain antigens, may emerge in a standard individual, for instance with aging (HANNA et al. 1967). Immunodeficiency is taken here in its broad sense, being due to a variety of possible weaknesses or failures of the immune system (HAYWARD 1977). Under such a state, challenge of a node by an antigen for which the organism is immunodeficient causes the emergence of "unusual features," which we have just started to recognize, instead of regular variations (SAINTE-MARIE and PENG 1983). The nature of these unusual features depends on the mechanism(s) responsible for the immunodeficiency, and on the type of antigen. Their degree of development depends on the importance of the deficiency and on the intensity of the challenge. This was shown by comparing such unusual features in diverse nodes of animals affected by variants of the athymic state (SAINTE-MARIE et al. 1984a–c). Incidentally, our study of athymic animals revealed that a state of immunodeficiency does not per se induce the formation of most of these unusual features, many types arising only upon overstimulation of a node by an antigen. Indeed, they can be greatly developed in the much challenged nodes but be absent in the nodes draining weakly challenged sites of the same animal.

It is the rather recent study of the athymic condition that has revealed the existence and the significance of the unusual nodal features accompanying a state of immunodeficiency. The most studied of such features are thus those due to a lack of T cells. In the absence of T cells and with respect to the deep cortex, solely the unit centers are devoid of lymphocytes, whereas, with a combined lack of B cells, the unit peripheries are quite devoid of lymphocytes as well (SAINTE-MARIE and PENG 1985). It has further been demonstrated that the unusual features occurring in the units of much challenged nodes of an athymic animal do not relate solely to their usual population of T cells involved in cellular immunity. For instance, the concomitant failing of T-dependent humoral immune responses provokes a compensatory increase in nodal B-cells (SAINTE-MARIE and PENG 1983). This is manifested by an unusually pronounced hypertrophy of follicles and often by the formation of "lymphocyte clusters" which are actually follicles forming elsewhere than in the peripheral cortex, as is usual. [Note that athymic animals lack nodules (germinal centers) and thus have only follicles instead of folliculonodules.] Such a lymphocyte cluster forms in association with a high endothelial venule, at a point where a cuffing perivascular channel is distended by a B-cell accumulation. Their location is species influenced. In the athymic mouse they form in medullary cords whose regular venules transform into high endothelial venules (SAINTE-MARIE and PENG 1983). In the athymic rat they form in the unit peripheries but also in unit centers unusually crossed by a high endothelial venule (SAINTE-MARIE et al. 1984c). There, a lymphocyte cluster contrasts with the surrounding lymphocyte-devoid center. Hence, a state of immunodeficiency due to a lack of T cells can increase the occupation of the T-dependent unit centers by spaces containing B cells. These findings reveal that the organism reacts under certain conditions in a manner detectable only by a detailed analysis of the lymphoid organs or by an in vivo investigation. Incidentally, while the hypertrophy of a nodal structure or cell population was hitherto thought to reflect the occurrence or greater intensity of an ongoing immune response, these findings further reveal that under certain conditions such hypertrophy instead reflects a state of immunodeficiency or the failure of a solicited immune response.

Additional unusual features due to the athymic state or to the stimulation of a node by antigens for which the organism is immunodeficient can form in the deep cortex but their description is not the subject of this chapter. It should nevertheless be pointed out that the development of such unusual features can eventually attain such proportions that they greatly distort the architecture of a compartment or of a node, rendering it almost unrecognizable. In some cases more or less complete atrophy of an affected node compartment may result, which then worsens the immunodeficient state of an individual (SAINTE-MARIE and PENG 1990). In contrast, an unusual feature can instead occur which represents an attempt to compensate for the partial atrophy or deficiency of a compartment, including that of its unit – hence the formation of a "compartment replica" which constitutes a more or less exact copy of an affected compartment above the outer wall of the subcapsular sinus (SAINTE-MARIE and PENG 1987a). The unusual features that weaken or strengthen the immune system can be observed simultaneously in the same animal, but in nodes of different sites.

5.2 Pathological Conditions

Antigens of a pathological origin induce variations in a draining node which are similar to those caused by common antigens, as long as a node functions normally. If, however, the immune system is locally overcome by a prevailing pathological condition, or if a draining node is invaded by elements of such a condition, the nodal morphology can be disturbed. It is not within the scope of the present paper to consider the abnormal morphological changes which characterize pathological conditions. However, it is appropriate to point out that some of the nodal changes observed under a pathological condition might not be specific features of this condition but instead be unusual features reflecting an accompanying state of immunodeficiency. Indeed, the emergence of some pathological conditions can result from, or be accompanied by, that of a certain state of immunodeficiency (HAYWARD 1977). With the progress in our knowledge of the unusual nodal features reflecting immunodeficiency, attempts should be made to distinguish such features from the abnormal changes specific to a given pathological condition in order to place the observations into better perspective.

Although the present paper does not deal with pathological conditions, the following discussion considers three reports of changes of the deep cortex claimed to occur in "reactive" human nodes under a variety of such conditions. This is relevant, for these reports led to the proposal of morphological and functional concepts regarding the deep cortex which are unjustified and misleading. Incidentally, the term "reactive" is used in these reports to refer to nodes whose morphology has been modified by pathological conditions. This seems inappropriate, for the node is in essence a reactive organ, modifying aspects of its morphology in reaction to even common antigenic stimuli.

REE and FANGER (1975) reported that a process of "nodular alteration" of the deep cortex occurs in reactive human nodes under a variety of pathological conditions. They explained that a nodular alteration of ill-defined deep cortex consists in its "expansion," which gives rise to well-defined and rather large "T nodules." Now, the T nodules shown in their Figs. 2 and 7 are, in fact, typical units. The problem is that their view implies that such units are not normally present in nodes, which is not the case. Actually, the latter authors made no comparison with the usual situation, so that no transformation of a presumed ill-defined deep cortex into clear nodular structures was demonstrated.

More recently, VAN DEN OORD et al. (1986) reported having identified a new type of structure, the "composite nodule," in reactive nodes from humans affected by various pathological conditions. A composite nodule was said to comprise a "small T nodule" and a single folliculo-nodule. They suggested that a composite nodule represents the "morphological and functional unit of the cortex" of the reactive nodes. They explained that the small T nodules arise from the process of nodular alteration of the deep cortex described by REE and FANGER (1975). But REE and FANGER (1975) had instead stated that nodular alteration gives rise to large T nodules. In fact, the small T nodules reported by VAN DEN OORD et al. (1986) correspond to the smallest units which occasionally occur even in normal nodes, including those of humans (BÉLISLE and SAINTE-MARIE 1981 e). Accordingly, VAN DEN OORD et al. (1986) observed small T nodules in only a minority (43%) of the nodes studied. Moreover, they did not estimate their relative importance with respect to larger forms of such structures and they did not consider the influence of the cutting incidence on the apparent size of a structure. Even more surprising is their statement that the composite nodules are most frequent in nodes manifesting "T-zone hyperplasia." Now, the structure illustrating this condition in their Fig. 4 is a typical deep cortex unit overlaid by several folliculo-nodules as is usual, but which they reported having observed only in nodes with T-zone hyperplasia. They provided no justification for this diagnosis and statement, not having studied the usual situation. The structure shown in their Fig. 4, not fitting the definition of a composite nodule, was interpreted as resulting from the fusion of small T nodules. Again, however, the authors provided no evidence for such a fusion, nor for an actual difference between the observed structure and a usual deep cortex unit. In fact, the regular semispherical outline and the concentration of high endothelial venules in the periphery of this structure confirm that it is indeed a usual deep cortex unit. Since such a unit and the overlying folliculo-nodules were considered by them as composite nodules and were said to account for a large fraction of the composite nodules, truly small T nodules (or smallest units) represented only a minor fraction of the deep cortex structures, as is usual. Hence, it was not demonstrated that association of a small deep cortex unit with a folliculo-nodule is the rule in reactive human nodes, and it is not in usual nodes. Consequently, the derived concept that such an association forms the "functional unit of the cortex" is not valid.

Observations made in immunohistochemically stained sections of the same reactive nodes further led VAN DEN OORD et al. (1985) to claim the existence of primary, secondary, and tertiary T nodules. They proposed that a T nodule undergoes maturation stages, each related to a phase in the development of a cellular immune response, but they presented no data on their relative frequency. Primary T nodules were said to occur often in the peripheral cortex. The related Fig. 1 b shows an area lateral to a folliculo-nodule and populated mainly by $OKT4^+$ and Leu-3 a^+ helper/inducer cells. But this area has no nodular shape, and it appears as an area of extrafollicular zone neighboring a folliculonodule, which is usual. Their Figs. 1 a, 1 c, and 1 d are intended to illustrate a primary T nodule stained for S-100 β^+ cells, for reticulin, or with H&E. The structures in these figures are indeed nodular-like but do not correspond to that in Fig. 1 b. They can be recognized as cross-cut folliculo-nodules, being typically round and outlined by high endothelial venules (SAINTE-MARIE and SIN 1970). The secondary T nodules are vaguely described and said to occur in the outer or deeper part of a node. The related Fig. 2 b shows an area present between the bottom portion of two folliculo-nodules and populated by the same lymphocyte subsets as the primary T nodules. What is shown in this Fig. 2 b appears to be part of a unit slightly extending between two folliculo-nodules, as often occurs. Figures 2 a, 2 c, and 2 d are meant to illustrate differently stained secondary T nodules but, again, the shown structures do not correspond to that in Fig. 2b. The tertiary T nodules are described as large aggregates of S-100β$^+$ dendritic cells with relatively few lymphocytes of unmentioned subsets. S-100β$^+$ cells were observed in secondary T nodules as well, and the difference between secondary and tertiary T nodules is not explained. Therefore, we must conclude that they gave no evidence for the existence of three types of T nodule. These authors furthermore did not mention three types of T nodule in their above-discussed histological study of the deep cortex of the same nodes (VAN DEN OORD et al. 1986). Moreover, the standard deep cortex units, filled with lymphocytes and described in the same histological study, are surprisingly not mentioned in their present study using immunohistochemical stains.

One observation which led VAN DEN OORD et al. (1985) to make their proposal was apparently the occasional presence of large numbers of T cells in areas of extrafollicular zone (so-called primary T nodules) above a deep cortex unit. But this can be accounted for in the same manner as the occasional presence there of a high percentage of lymphocytes as heavily labeled with ^{3}H-uridine as those of the underlying unit. As discussed above, this situation probably reflects an increased arrival of T cells in the overlying extrafollicular zone. This also explains the reported almost constant association of a primary and a so-called secondary T nodule, an area of extrafollicular zone (primary T nodule) being the site of such an increased arrival of T cells above a deep cortex unit (so-called secondary T nodule). In their Fig. 2b, moreover, the cell population of an apparent unit extends about halfway between two folliculo-nodules. This fits the fact, also observed with ^{3}H-uridine labeling, that the outer margin of the heavily labeled lymphocytic population of a unit may undulate between folliculo-nodules. Another observation that contributed to VAN DEN OORD et al.'s proposal is that of units (tertiary nodules) having mostly dendritic cells. As discussed above, this is common under the athymic state. The presence of such units in the studied nodes could simply reflect a certain state of immunodeficiency accompanying some pathological conditions. Hence, consideration of the normal histology of the node and of the possible variations of its structures following stimulation or accompanying a state of immunodeficiency is necessary for the interpretation of immunohistochemical observations.

6 Conclusion

The deep cortex consists of semispherical "units" which are contiguous to the peripheral cortex. There exists one unit per node compartment, the unit being centered on the opening of the afferent lymphatic vessel (or one of its prenodal branches) related to each compartment. A unit has a periphery and a center. The "unit center" is the site of nodal processes of cellular immune responses; the "unit periphery" shares, with the extrafollicular zone of the peripheral cortex, the function of being a migration route for incoming circulating B and

T cells. Antigenic stimulation of units of normally functioning nodes increases the size of the units as well as that of their lymphocytic and blastic content. It also induces greater development and activity of the network of high endothelial venules of the unit peripheries, contributing to increased recruitment of circulating lymphocytes. The stimulation of units by an antigen for which the organism is immunodeficient causes the formation of "unusual features" which can attain a very pronounced degree of development. Some of these unusual features reflect the nature of the deficiency, such as a lack of lymphocytes in the unit centers under the athymic state. Other unusual features reflect detrimental secondary effects which can result in the atrophy of the challenged units and even of whole node compartments. Still others reflect a compensatory or beneficial reaction of the organism, such as the formation of "lymphocyte clusters" (or follicles) in the units and a partial duplication of deficient units by way of the de novo formation of "compartment replicas." Both the detrimental and the beneficial unusual features can be observed in the same animal but in nodes of different sites. Lastly, it is suggested that some of the modifications of nodal components, including the deep cortex, which are observed in draining nodes under prevailing local pathological conditions might reflect an accompanying state of immunodeficiency instead of being abnormal modifications specific to a given pathological condition.

Acknowledgement. This work was funded by La Direction Générale de l'Enseignement Supérieur du Québec and by the Medical Research Council of Canada.

References

Aijima H, Horie K, Nagata H, Hoshi H (1986) Cortical structure of bovine lymph nodes. Acta Anat Nippon 61:173–185

Anderson AD, Anderson ND (1975) Studies on the structure and permeability of the microvasculature in normal rat lymph nodes. Am J Pathol 80:387–418

Barclay AN (1981) The localization of populations of lymphocytes defined by monoclonal antibodies in rat lymphoid tissues. Immunology 42:594–600

Bélisle C, Sainte-Marie G (1981 a) Tridimensional study of the deep cortex of the rat lymph node. I. Topography of the deep cortex. Anat Rec 199:45–59

Bélisle C, Sainte-Marie G (1981 b) Tridimensional study of the deep cortex of the rat lymph node. II. Relation of deep cortex units to afferent lymphatic vessels. Anat Rec 199:61–72

Bélisle C, Sainte-Marie G (1981 c) Tridimensional study of the deep cortex of the rat lymph node. III. Morphology of the deep cortex units. Anat Rec 199:213–226

Bélisle C, Sainte-Marie G (1981 d) Tridimensional study of the deep cortex of the rat lymph node. V. Postnatal development of the deep cortex units. Anat Rec 200:207–220

Bélisle C, Sainte-Marie G (1981 e) Topography of the deep cortex of the lymph nodes of various mammalian species. Anat Rec 201:553–561

Bélisle C, Sainte-Marie G, Peng FS (1982) Tridimensional study of the deep cortex of the rat lymph node. VI. The deep cortex units of the germ-free rat. Am J Pathol 107:70–78

Bottomly HK, Perkins WD, Schwarz MR (1975) ^{3}H-uridine incorporation by small lymphocytes of tolerant rats: relationship to T and B lymphocytes. J Immunol 115:648–652

Cahill RNP, Frost N, Trnka Z (1976) The effects of antigen on the migration of recirculating lymphocytes through single lymph nodes. J Exp Med 143:870–888

Cottier H, Turk J, Sobin L (1973) A proposal for a standardized system of reporting human lymph node morphology in relation to immunological function. J Clin Pathol 26:317–331
Dennison DK, Clancy J (1979) ^{3}H-5-uridine incorporation by small lymphocytes from transplantation-tolerant and tolerance-reversed rats. J Immunol 122:1376–1382
Denz FA (1947) Age changes in lymph nodes. J Pathol Bact 59:564–591
Drinker CK, Wislocki GB, Field ME (1933) The structure of the sinuses in the lymph nodes. Anat Rec 56:261–273
Ehrich W (1929) Studies of the lymphatic tissue. I. The anatomy of the secondary nodules and some remarks on the lymphocytic and lymphoid tissue. Am J Anat 43:347–371
Ehrich WE (1946) The role of the lymphocyte in the circulation of the lymph. Ann NY Acad Sci 46:823–857
Eikelenboom P, Nassy JJJ, Post J, Versteeg JCMB, Langevoort HL (1978) The histogenesis of lymph nodes in rat and rabbit. Anat Rec 190:201–216
Eikelenboom P, Levenbach MGE, van den Brink HR, Streefkerk JG (1979) Development of T and B cell areas in peripheral lymphoid organs of rats. Anat Rec 194:523–537
Fossum S (1983) The density and distribution of W3/13, OX19, W3/25 and OX8 positive cells in nude rat (rnu) lymph nodes. Transplant Proc 15:1638–1639
Goldschneider I, McGregor DD (1968) Migration of lymphocytes and thymocytes in the rat. I. The route of migration from blood to spleen and lymph nodes. J Exp Med 127:155–157
Goldschneider I, McGregor DD (1973) Anatomical distribution of T and B lymphocytes in the rat. J Exp Med 138:1443–1465
Gowans JL, Knight EJ (1964) The route of recirculation of lymphocytes in the rat. Proc R Soc Lond [Biol] 159:257–282
Greaves MF, Owen JJT, Raff MC (1974) T and B lymphocytes: origins, properties and roles in immune responses. Excerpta Medica, Amsterdam. American Elsevier, New York
Gutman GA, Weismann IL (1972) Lymphoid tissue architecture. Experimental analysis of the origin and distribution of T-cells and B-cells. Immunology 23:465–479
Haaijman JJ, Deen C, Kröse CJM, Zijlstra JJ, Coolen J, Radl J (1984) Monoclonal antibodies in immunocytology: a jungle full of pitfalls. Immunol Today 5:56–58
Hall JG (1979) Effect of skin painting with oxazolone on the local extravasation of mononuclear cells in sheep. In: Blood cells and vessel walls: functional interactions. Ciba Found Symp 71:197–209
Hall JG, Hopkins J, Reynolds J (1980) Studies on efferent lymph cells from nodes stimulated with oxazolone. Immunology 39:141–149
Hanna MG, Nettesheim LO, Makinodan T (1967) Reduced immune potentiality of aged mice: significance of morphologic changes in lymphatic tissue. Proc Soc Exp Biol Med 125:882–886
Hayward AR (1977) Immunodeficiency. Edward Arnold, London
Heath T, Brandon R (1983) Lymphatic and blood vessels of the popliteal node in sheep. Anat Rec 207:461–472
Herman PG, Benninghoff DL, Mellins HZ (1968) Radiation effect on the barrier function of the lymph node. An experimental study. Radiology 91:698–702
Herman PG, Yamamoto I, Mellins HZ (1972) Blood microcirculation in the lymph node during primary immune response. J Exp Med 136:692–714
Hobbs BB, Davidson JW (1976) The microcirculation of the mammalian lymph node. Lymphology 9:155–157
Hollingsworth JW, Carr J (1973) ^{3}H-Uridine incorporation as a T lymphocyte indicator in the rat. Cell Immunol 8:270–279
Howard JC, Hunt SV, Gowans JL (1972) Identification of marrow-derived and thymus-derived small lymphocytes in the lymphoid tissues of normal rats. J Exp Med 135:200–219
Kearney JF (1974) T and B lymphocytes. J Oral Pathol 3:151–166
Kelly RH (1970) Localization of afferent lymph cells within the draining node during a primary immune response. Nature 227:510–513
Kelly RH (1975) Functional anatomy of lymph nodes. I: The paracortical cords. Int Arch Allergy Appl Immunol 48:836–849
Kelly RH, Wolstencroft RA, Dumonde DC, Balfour BM (1972) Role of lymphocyte activation products (LAP) in cell mediated immunity. II. Effects of lymphocyte activation products on the

lymph node architecture and evidence for peripheral release of LAP following antigenic stimulation. Clin Exp Immunol 10:49–65
Kett K, Illényi L, Lukacs L, Nyarady J (1978) Passage through the lymph node. Studies with watered and oiled contrast medium given into an afferent lymphatic. Lymphology 11:75–80
Kojima M, Takahashi K, Sue A, Imai Y (1971) Study on the function and structure of blood vessels of the secondary nodule in lymph node. Acta Pathol Jpn 21:369–386
Meyer EM, Schlake W, Grundmann E (1979) Comparative histology, histochemical, and histomorphometric studies of T and B cell areas in peripheral lymphoid organs of normal young adult BALB/c mice. Pathol Res Pract 164:141–156
Nordman M (1928) Studien an Lymphknoten bei akuten und chronischen Allgemeininfektionen. Virchows Arch [A] 267:158–203
Nossal GJV, Ada GL (eds) (1971) Antigens, lymphoid cells and the immune response. Academic, New York
Oort J, Turk JL (1965) A histological and autoradiographic study of lymph nodes during the development of contact sensitivity in the guinea-pig. Br J Exp Pathol 46:147–154
Osoba D, Miller JFAP (1964) The lymphoid tissues and immune responses of neonatally thymectomized mice bearing thymus tissue in millipore diffusion chambers. J Exp Med 119:177–194
Parrott DMV, de Sousa MAB, East JE (1966) Thymus-dependent areas in the lymphoid organs of neonatally thymectomized mice. J Exp Med 123:191–204
Poppema S, Bhan AK, Reinherz EL, McCluskey RT, Schlossman SF (1981) Distribution of T cell subsets in human lymph nodes. J Exp Med 153:30–41
Ree H, Fanger H (1975) Paracortical alteration in lympadenophatic and tumor draining lymph nodes: histologic study. Hum Pathol 6:363–372
Reinherz EL, Kung PC, Goldstein G, Schlossman SF (1979) Further characterization of the human inducer T cell subset defined by a monoclonal antibody. J Immunol 123:2894–2896
Ringertz N, Adamson CA (1950) The lymph node response to various antigens. An experimental morphological study. Acta Pathol Microbiol Scand [Suppl] 86:1–69
Sainte-Marie G (1966) The postcapillary venules in the mediastinal lymph node of ten-week-old rats. Rev Can Biol 25:263–284
Sainte-Marie G, Peng FS (1975) Migration into pseudo-follicles of draining lymph nodes of medullary small thymocytes injected in the mediastinal cavity. Rev Can Biol 34:205–212
Sainte-Marie G, Peng FS (1976) Migration into pseudo-follicles of lymph nodes of transfused medullary small thymocytes. J Ret Reticuloendothelial Soc 20:51–54
Sainte-Marie G, Peng FS (1979) Morphology of the extrafollicular zone and pseud-follicles of the rat lymph node, and their role in lymphocyte traffic. In: Müller Ruchholz W, Müller-Hermeling HK (eds) Function and structure of the immune system. Plenum, New York, p 59
Sainte-Marie G, Peng FS (1980) Thymic cell migration in the subnodular spaces of draining lymph nodes of rats. Cell Immunol 52:211–217
Sainte-Marie G, Peng FS (1981) Histological observations on the deep cortex of the lymph nodes of the germ-free mouse. Ann Inst Pasteur Immunol D132:55–63
Sainte-Marie G, Peng FS (1983) Structural and cell population changes in the lymph nodes of the athymic nude mouse. Lab Invest 49:420–429
Sainte-Marie G, Peng FS (1985) The lymph nodes of the N:NIH(S)-nu/nu mouse. Lab Invest 52:631–637
Sainte-Marie G, Peng FS (1986) Diffusion of a lymph carried antigen in the fiber network of the lymph node of rat. Cell Tissue Res 245:481–486
Sainte-Marie G, Peng FS (1987 a) The formation of "compartment replicas" in the lymph nodes of athymic animals. Cell Tissue Res 248:323–333
Sainte-Marie G, Peng FS (1987 b) Morphological anomalies associated with immunodeficiencies in the lymph nodes of aging mice. Lab Invest 56:598–610
Sainte-Marie G, Peng FS (1990) Mast cells and fibrosis in compartments of lymph nodes of normal, gnotobiotic, and athymic rats. Cell Tissue Res (in press)
Sainte-Marie G, Sin YM (1970) The lymph node: structures and their possible function during the immune response. In: Gordon AS (ed) Regulation of haematopoiesis, vol 2. Appleton-Century-Crofts, New York, pp 1339–1383

Sainte-Marie G, Peng FS, Denis G (1975) A study of the mode of lymphocyte recirculation in the dog. Ann Inst Pasteur Immunol 126C:481–500

Sainte-Marie G, Peng FS, Bélisle C (1981) Tridimensional study of the deep cortex of the rat lymph node. IV. Differential labelling of the deep cortex units with ^{3}H-uridine. Anat Rec 199:227–237

Sainte-Marie G, Peng FS, Bélisle C (1982) Overall architecture and pattern of lymph flow in the rat lymph node. Am J Anat 164:275–309

Saint-Marie G, Pelletier M, Peng FS (1984a) Modifications of the structures of the rat lymph nodes by neonatal thymectomy. Thymus 6:309–323

Sainte-Marie G, Peng FS, Pelletier M (1984b) Development of the lymph nodes in the very young, and their evolution in the mature, nude rat. Dev Comp Immunol 8:695–710

Sainte-Marie G, Peng FS, Pritchard D (1984c) Tridimensional study of the deep cortex of the rat lymph node. VIII. The deep cortex units of athymic nude rats. Anat Rec 209:95–104

Scothorne RJ, McGregor IA (1955) Cellular changes in lymph nodes and spleen following skin homografting in the rabbit. J Anat 89:283–292

Scott DW, Josephs SH (1975) Uridine labelling of human lymphocytes: differential uptake by T and B cells. Cell Immunol 20:64–68

Sin YM (1972) Histological and topographical studies of germinal centers of rabbit lymph nodes. J Anat 112:151–163

Söderström N, Sternström A (1969) Outflow paths of cells from the lymph node parenchyma to the efferent lymphatics. Scand J Haematol 6:186–196

Sprent J (1973) Circulating T and B lymphocytes of the mouse. I. Migratory properties. Cell Immunol 7:10–39

Travella W, Morris B (1980) Reassortment of cell populations within the lymphoid apparatus of the sheep. In: Blood cells and vessel walls: functional interactions. Ciba Found Symp 71:127–139

van den Oord JJ, Wolf-Peters de C, Desmet VJ, Takahashi K, Ohtsuki Y, Akagi T (1985) Nodular alteration of the paracortical aera. An in situ immunohistochemical analysis of primary, secondary and tertiary T-nodules. Am J Pathol 120:55–66

van den Oord JJ, Wolf-Peters de C, Desmet VJ (1986) The composite nodule. A structural and functional unit of the reactive lymph node. Am J Pathol 122:83–91

van Roojen N (1987) The "in situ" immune response in lymph nodes: a review. Anat Rec 218:359–364

Waksman BH, Arnason BG, Jankovic BD (1962) Role of the thymus in immune reactions in rats. III. Changes in the lymphoid organs of thymectomized rats. J Exp Med 116:187–206

Weissman IL (1967) Thymus cell migration. J Exp Med 126:291–304

Weissman IL, Warnke R, Butcher EC, Rouse R, Levy R (1978) The lymphoid system – its normal architecture and the potential for understanding the system through the study of lymphoproliferative diseases. Hum Pathol 9:25–46

Yoffey JM, Courtice FC (eds) (1970) Lymphatics, lymph and the lymphomyeloid complex. Academic, New York, pp 517–619

Differences Between Lymph Node Structure and Function in Normal and Athymic Rats

S. Fossum

1 Introduction

1.1 The Nude Rat (rnu)

The congenitally athymic, nude mouse strain could hardly have arrived at a more opportune time than in the mid 1960s (Flanagan 1966; Pantelouris 1968). Only a few years earlier neonatally thymectomized mice had been shown to develop immunodeficiency (Miller 1961), the dual nature of the immune system was indicated by studies of chicken lacking either a bursa of Fabricius or both a bursa and thymus (Warner et al. 1962), and lymphocytes had been proven to be the immunocompetent cells of the body (Gowans and McGregor 1965). The selective absence of T cells rendered the nude mouse an invaluable animal model for tumor research and many areas of immunological research. For almost a decade it ruled the ground alone before the nude rat entered the stage. Hairless rats had incidentally been bred at the Rowett Research Institute since 1953, but were apparently not realized to be athymic and were subsequently lost, until they reemerged in the same breeding colony in 1975. This time they were found to be congenitally athymic, and were assigned the symbol rnu (Festing et al. 1978). At about the same time, another nude rat strain, designated nznu, was discovered in New Zealand (reviewed in Festing 1981). Although they arrived late, the role of these athymic rats has not been restricted to duplicating research on the nude mouse. Due to their larger size rats are often better suited than mice for in vivo physiological studies of lymphocytes and other leukocytes. It is also possible that a pleiotropic gene such as rnu will have other functional consequences immunologically than the absence of a thymus.

In this article I shall describe the nude rat lymph nodes with the primary aim of elucidating the role of the thymus and thymus-processed cells in creating and maintaining the lymph node morphology and function. Secondly, I shall briefly discuss the T-like cells present in the lymphoid tissues of nude animals. The presence of these cells means that the nude animals are not as absolutely T deficient as originally thought. On the other hand, their existence provides us with opportunities for studying the requirements for the development of a mature T-cell population possessing a wide repertoire of MHC-restricted antigen receptors. Finally, I shall consider some of the nonlymphoid cells present in nude rat lymph nodes, in particular NK cells and dendritic leukocytes. The immune functions of NK cells stand out more clearly in the absence of T-cell immunity, while dendritic cells are interesting partly because they are so strikingly numerous. Unless otherwise stated, comparisons are made between rnu/rnu rats and their euthymic littermates (+/rnu or +/+). For brevity the organs and tissues from these rats will be referred to simply as nude and euthymic, respectively.

1.2 How Athymic Is the Nude Rat?

The rnu nude rats are not completely hairless; in particular adult males usually have some fur, whereas the nznu nude rats and the nude mice are almost completely nude. The nznu nude rats and the nude mice also seem to be more susceptible to infections than the rnu nude rats (Festing 1981). However, rnu nude rats are equally as athymic as nznu nude rats and nude mice: the mutations in the two rat strains are in the same gene (Festing 1981) and the rnu nude rat has only got a small thymic rudiment, similar to the one described in the nude mouse (Fossum et al. 1980). The nude mouse thymic rudiment consists of small cysts lined with ciliated cells, mucous cells, undifferentiated cells, and glandular cells. Most authors have failed to detect lymphocytes associated with these rudiments (see review in Kindred 1979), but Ikehara et al. (1987) have recently described the presence of clusters of Thy-1$^+$ lymphocytes enmeshed with epithelial cells surrounding fluid-filled cystic spaces in the rudiments. Cystic, gland-like structures with ciliated cells are also found in the thymic rudiments of the rnu nude rat, but without any sign of infiltration by lymphoid cells (Fossum et al. 1980). [It should be added that the studies from Fossum et al. (1980) were only performed on rats up to 3–4 months of age.] Serial sections through the neck region and mediastinum of newborn nude rats did not reveal any sign of ectopic thymic tissue (unpublished).

As regards thymic hormones, some measurements have been made in the nude mouse, whereas published results are scant in the rat. In the nude mouse, circulating thymulin is absent, but the serum levels of thymosin α_1 are only diminished. Although there is some evidence that this hormone has additional, extrathymic sources (see review in SAFIEH and KENDALL 1988), the possibility that the rudiments produce some thymic hormones cannot as yet be ruled out. Whether the nude T-like cells (see Sect. 3.1), which increase in number with age, have developed under the influence of the thymic rudiments or by an extrathymic pathway, they are usually extremely few, and therefore most likely functionally insignificant, in most young animals. Consequently, to minimize complications in interpretations of results the following descriptions are largely from work on young rats, i.e., from 6 to 12 weeks old. However, one should be aware that occasional young rats do contain larger than normal amounts of T-like cells (Fig. 1).

2 The Morphology of Nude Rat Lymph Nodes

2.1 Macroscopic Appearance and Cellularity

The relative weights of nude lymph nodes compared with euthymic nodes show great variation among different regional groups. Whereas the nude mesenteric, celiac, inguinal, and popliteal nodes usually are small, often less than half the weight of the corresponding euthymic nodes, the nude cervical lymph nodes, both the deep and the superficial, are often as large as or even larger than the euthymic nodes, and the brachial and axillary nodes may sometimes be grossly hypertrophic (FOSSUM et al. 1980). Quantitative measurements on the various regions in lymph node sections were not made, but the paracortical nodules seemed to be particularly enlarged in the hypertrophic nodes (unpublished). These studies were performed on nude rats kept under normal animal house conditions, so persistent antigenic stimulation may be the cause of this hypertrophy, but it is unclear why this should preferentially affect only some nodes.

Fig. 1a–h. Frozen serial sections of an axillary lymph node from a 3-month-old nude rat. The sections were stained with a panel of monoclonal antibodies labeling the following cell types: **a** B cells and plasma cells (χ light chains – MRC OX12); **b** B cells and subset of T cells (CD45R – MRC OX22); **c** all T cells, plasma cells, and possibly some macrophages (leucosialin – W3/13); **d** all T cells and some B cells (CD5 – MRC OX19); **e** $T_{c/s}$ cells and NK cells (CD8 – MRC OX8); **f** T_h cells and macrophages (CD4 – W3/25); **g** B cells, dendritic leukocytes, and activated macrophages (MHC class II – MRC OX6); **h** pericytes or basement membrane material and some dendritic leukocytes (Thy-1 – MRC OX7). (The surface antigens and monoclonal antibodies are indicated in parentheses; for further information on antibody specificity, see MASON et al. 1983 and PUGH et al. 1983.) The regions are indicated in **a**: *F*, follicle; *P*, paracortical nodule; *M*, medulla. For a 3-month-old nude rat, this node contains unusually many $CD5^+$ T-like cells **d**. A small germinal center can be discerned in **b**. Note the almost confluent staining of the paracortical IDCs in **g**

▶

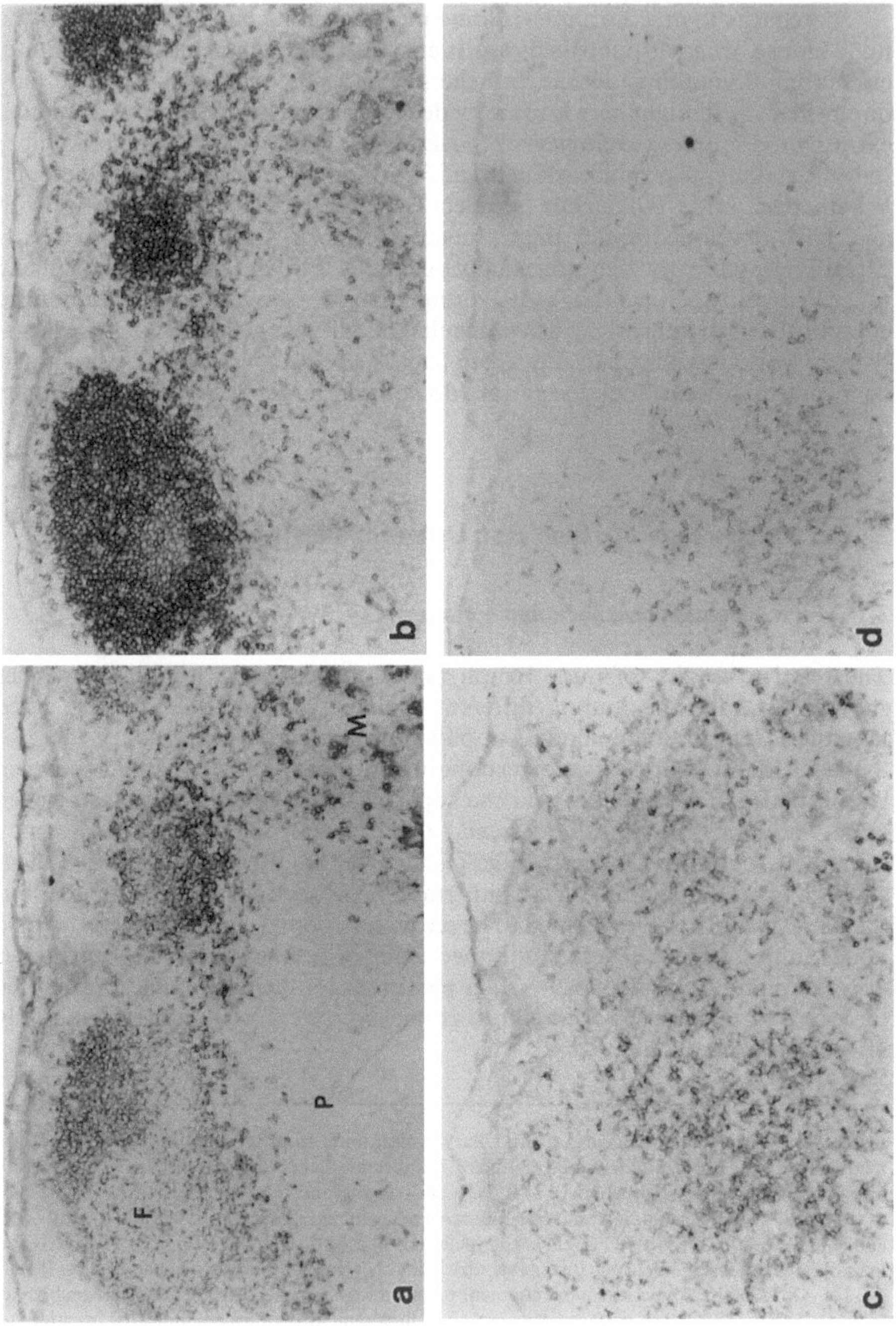
a
b
c
d
F
P
M

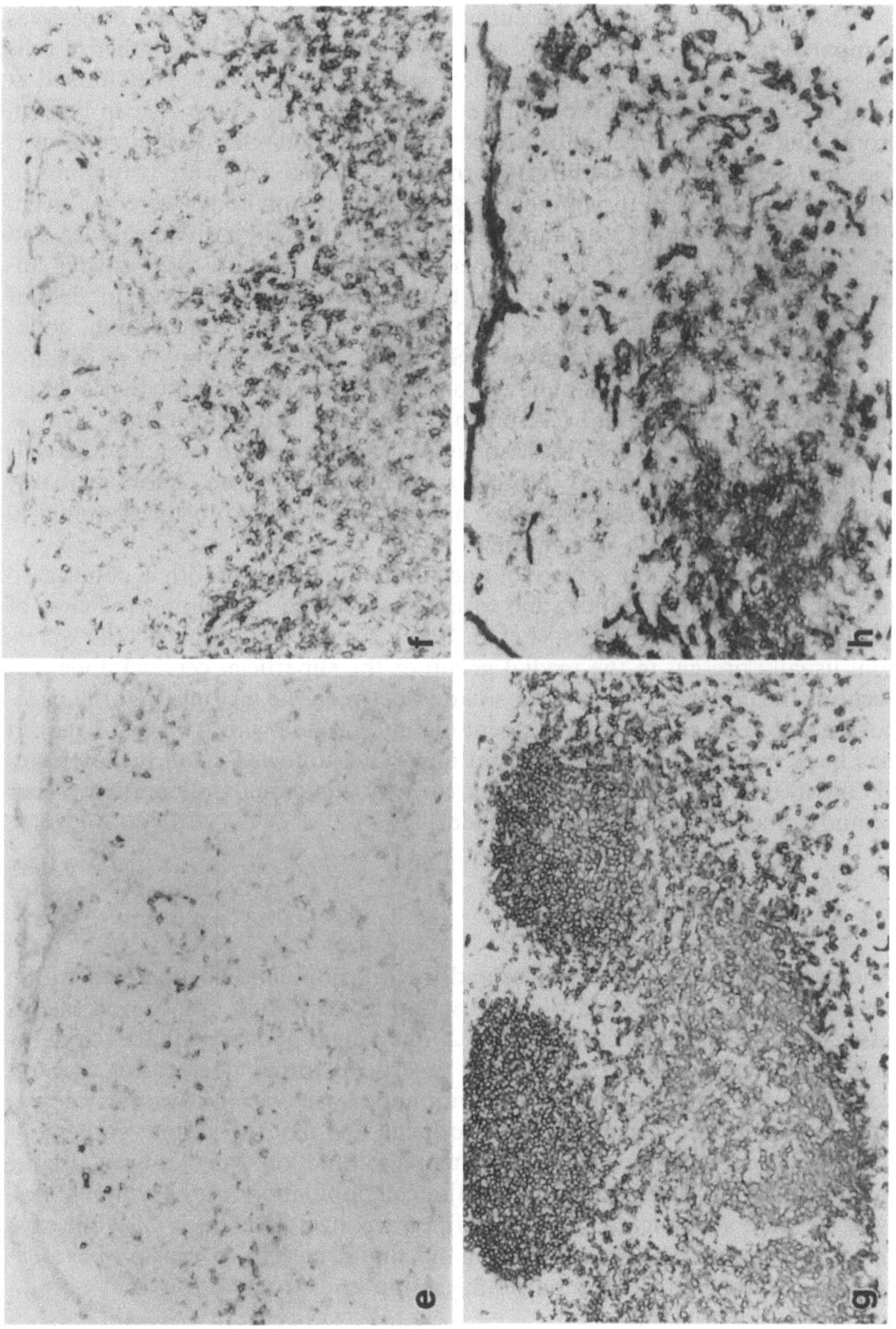

The cellularity of nude and euthymic LEW (RT1[l]) rat lymph nodes was compared by Klausen and Hougen (1987), as scored by the number of cells teased out of the tissue into suspension per mg lymph nodes. They looked at both specified pathogen-free (SPF) and germ-free (GF) rats. As can be seen from Table 1, the number of cells recovered from nude SPF lymph nodes was less than half that recovered from normal SPF nodes. There are two points to be made: Firstly, even though the weights of the lymph nodes were not given, these nude lymph nodes were most likely smaller than the euthymic nodes, and the differences in absolute cell numbers recovered therefore even greater. Indeed, Brooks et al. (1980) reported a more than sixfold difference in yield of mononuclear cells from nude as compared with euthymic lymph nodes (15×10^6 and 98×10^6, respectively). Secondly, the lower number of cells recovered per mg tissue from nude lymph nodes must mean that either a larger proportion of the weights were taken up by extracellular elements, such as fibers or lymph, or the cells in these nodes were on average larger; or the cells were not so easily extracted into cell suspension. All three factors probably contribute to the differences found, as will be evident from the histological description of the nude lymph nodes.

Macroscopically, the surface of nude lymph nodes is smooth in contrast to the cobblestone appearance, due to the many large protruding follicles, of euthymic lymph nodes (Fossum et al. 1980). A curious finding is a dark crescent usually present in the medial group of the superficial cervical nodes. In sections the crescent is seen to be situated between the medulla and the paracortex and to be caused by a pigment mainly situated within macrophages. It has been suggested that the pigment may have followed small hemorrhages (Fossum et al. 1980), but if so, it is unclear why this should preferentially occur in nude rats and in this group of nodes.

2.2 General Architecture

The organization of lymph nodes and the cell populations contained within them was recently reviewed by Fossum and Ford (1985). The compartments of the nodes are summarized in Table 2. The salient points are that each of the "classical" regions of a lymph node – superficial cortex, deep cortex or paracortex, and medullla – has an intralymphatic space, an intravascular space, and an interstitium, separated by endothelia, and that the various subregions are specialized with respect to cell content and function. Furthermore, despite an extremely rapid exchange of the major cell populations of the lymph nodes, they preserve an intricate, but well-defined architecture. This implies the existence of effective mechanisms guiding the migrating cells to their proper location and strict control of input/immigration and proliferation, and output/emigration and death.

T cells not only constitute the major part of the recirculating lymphocyte pool, but are also the main regulatory cells of the immune system. Lymphoid tissues in animals completely lacking thymus-processed cells would therefore

Table 1. Cellularity of nude and euthymic rat lymph nodes (cells × 10^6/mg tissue) (KLAUSEN and HOUGEN 1987)

Group	Mesenteric lymph nodes	Inguinal lymph nodes
A rnu/rnu GF	0.16±0.05	0.04±0.01
B rnu/rnu SPF	0.18±0.08	0.08±0.03
C rnu/+GF	0.26±0.02	0.13±0.04
D rnu/+SPF	0.41±0.05	0.17±0.06
Statistics (Mann-Whitney test)	C vs D: $P<0.05$ A+B vs C+D: $P<0.01$	A+B vs C+D: $P<0.05$

Table 2. Lymph node compartments with predominant cell types (cell types in parentheses; areas showing clear differences between lymph nodes of nude and euthymic rats italicized)

	Lymphatic spaces	Blood vessels	Interstitium or extravascular space
Superficial cortex	Marginal and cortical sinuses (VCs)	Not known to be specialized	Follicles (B cells, FDCs) *Germinal centers* (B blasts, FDCs, TBMØ) Interfollicular areas (VCs/DCs, T cells, MØ)
Deep cortes or paracortex	Deep cortical sinuses (emigrating lymphocytes)	*High endothelial venules* (immigrating lymphocytes)	*Paracortical nodules – traffic areas for T and B cells* (T cells, IDCs, MØ)
Medulla	Medullary sinuses (sinus MØ)	Not known to be specialized	Medullary cords (plasma cells)

VCs, veiled cells; DCs, dendritic cells; FDCs, follicular dendritic cells; MØ, macrophages; TBMØ, tingible body macrophages

perhaps be expected to be grossly anomalous. However, in most aspects nude lymph nodes are surprisingly normal. Firstly, the regional organization as delineated in Table 2 is identical in nude and euthymic lymph nodes. Secondly, all the subregions contain the same sets of cells as in the euthymic lymph nodes, with the one evident exception, the paracortex, which invariably shows extreme depletion of lymphocytes (BROOKS et al. 1980; FOSSUM et al. 1980).

The unmistakable presence of a paracortex, although T-cell depleted, illustrates that the designation "T-dependent or thymus-dependent area" is a misnomer (FOSSUM 1989). The designation was originally used in the sense that the paracortex contains thymus-matured cells and is depleted of cells by neonatal thymectomy, but it carries the connotation that the emergence of this area depends on the presence of a thymus or T cells, which is not true. As will be shown below, the nude paracortex can attract and retain injected donor T cells from euthymic littermates, and is in this respect functionally mature. The paracortical localization of T cells is therefore secondary to the creation of the microenvironment. The predominant cell types in the nude paracortex are the interdigitating cells and the reticular fibroblasts (see Sect. 2.2.2), and one of these cell types, or an interaction between them, is probably responsible for creating the typical paracortical microenvironment. The same argument goes for the T-dependent areas in other lymphoid tissues (Fossum 1989).

The basic design and the depletion of lymphocytes within the paracortex are, however, the only constant features of the nude lymph nodes; in other respects there are large variations in histological appearance of the nodes even within the same individual. Some of the lymph nodes have only a thin rim of cortical tissue with tiny primary follicles, no germinal centers, and little discernible paracortex. These lymph nodes are dominated by wide, anastomosing medullary sinuses and slender medullary cords. Other lymph nodes contain a normal proportion of cortical tissue, with prominent, pale paracortical nodules. Some of these contain secondary follicles with definite germinal centers, or wide medullary cords engorged with numerous plasma cells, or both (Fossum et al. 1980).

2.2.1 The Superficial Cortex, Follicles, and Germinal Centers

The marginal sinus of nude lymph nodes contains abundant veiled cells, but usually smaller concentrations of small lymphocytes than normal nodes. As in the normal lymph nodes, the veiled cells adhere to and penetrate the inner lymphendothelium, the penetrating cells usually being seen with irregular bulbous masses of trailing cytoplasm covering the sinus side of the lymphendothelium (Fossum 1980). The majority of these cells represent dendritic leukocytes (DLs) en route from the afferent lymphatics to the paracortex (see Sect. 4.2), but some of the cells may participate in the "alternative antigen pathway" (Tew et al. 1984, 1989).

Primary follicles appear to be just as numerous and to have the same appearance as in normal lymph nodes, apart from some difference in size. In addition to numerous small lymphocytes, they also contain follicular dendritic cells (FDCs) (Mjaaland and Fossum 1987). The morphology of the nude FDCs is similar to that of euthymic FDCs, with the exception that the conspicuous electron-dense deposits covering the long convoluted extensions of euthymic FDCs are less prominent in the nude follicles. Antigen injected into the footpads of passively immunized nude recipients localized normally in the follicles onto the FDC processes. However, without passive administration of antibody there was no detectable follicular localization of antigen, even after repeated administration of antigen (Mjaaland and Fossum 1987), whereas distinct follicular localization was obtained in euthymic littermate controls. This demonstrates that nude FDCs can capture and retain complexes, but that antigenic stimulation fails to elicit sufficient antibody of the isotype necessary for follicular localization.

In contrast, secondary follicles containing germinal centers are much less frequently observed than in normal lymph nodes. When present, they are usually found in cervical lymph nodes, only occasionally in other nodes (BROOKS et al. 1980; FOSSUM et al. 1980). The germinal centers are on average much smaller than normal, frequently lacking both tingible body macrophages and a distinct boundary (FOSSUM et al. 1980) (Fig. 1). However, larger germinal centers with tingible body macrophages and a typical boundary layer are also seen. These germinal centers are indistinguishable from germinal centers in lymph nodes of normal rats in terms of structure and cell content (BROOKS et al. 1980; FOSSUM et al. 1980).

The importance of the presence of germinal centers in nude rats is that these structures have been proposed to be absolutely T dependent. Thus, DE SOUSA et al. (1969) reported that nude mice contained no germinal centers. Later, VAESSEN et al. (1986) failed to find germinal centers in the nude rat, even in cervical lymph nodes. Their material included 40 nude rats, spanning from 2 to 17 months of age. Some germinal centers observed in the nude rats investigated by BROOKS et al. (1980) and FOSSUM et al. (1980) could possibly have been elicited with the help of the T-like cells that increasingly appear with age in the nude rat (see Sect. 3.1), although in both instances the animals investigated were young (<12 weeks), i.e., at an age when T-like cells are still rare in most animals. The observed germinal centers were all spontaneous, i.e., not the result of deliberate immunization. On the contrary, injection of sheep erythrocytes and the thymus-independent antigen levan failed to provoke germinal center formation in the draining (popliteal) lymph node (and in the spleen after intravenous injection) of nude rats (FOSSUM and FORD, unpublished results). The conclusion is that T cells normally contribute to the events that elicit germinal center formation, but that the T-cell requirement under some circumstances may be bypassed.

2.2.2 The Paracortex

The paracortex of nude rat lymph nodes can be discerned even in thick lymph node slices under the dissecting microscope and stands out clearly under low power in sections because of its exeeptionally light appearance. It usually takes the form of contiguous nodules. The majority of the cells are nonlymphoid, of which there are three different main types. The first and most prominent are the interdigitating cells (IDCs). These are large cells with light, irregular nuclei, a dark cytocenter containing most of the organelles, and a strikingly pale peripheral cytoplasm with numerous bulbous elongations and protrusions interlocked with protrusions from similar neighboring cells (VELDMAN 1970). IDCs belong to the family of dendritic leukocytes thought to function primarily as antigen-presenting cells (reviewed in STEINMAN 1981 and AUSTYN 1987; see also Sect. 4.2). They are constitutively MHC class II$^+$. In immunohistochemical sections stained with antibodies to MHC class II, the paracortex is seen as areas with almost confluent staining (Fig. 1) (see below). The importance of the presence of normal-looking IDCs in the nude rat is that it refutes the proposal (VEERMAN 1974) that IDCs represent macrophages that attain their peculiar phenotype due to T-cell influences (reviewed in FOSSUM 1989).

The second nonlymphoid cell type is the reticular fibroblast, a dark stellate cell associated with fibrillar collagen. These cells usually completely surround the collagen bundles and send out slender extensions connecting with other similar cells, thus forming a cellular reticulum. They are indistinguishable from the reticular fibroblasts found in normal nodes, but their network is more readily apparent, because they are usually less separated from each other due to the lower cellularity of the nude paracortex. The third nonlymphoid cell type, referred to as a "laden macrophage," resembles the tingible body macrophages, which are only infrequently found in the paracortex of normal lymph nodes. In contrast to tingible macrophages of germinal centers, most of the laden macrophage phagolysosomes contain not nuclear remnants but lipid material. If the laden macrophages indeed correspond to germinal center tingible body macrophages, it is unclear why they contain so much more lipid. A possibility is that their diet may be different: whereas germinal center tingible body macrophages ingest lymphoblasts (reviewed in Fossum and Ford 1985), the laden macrophages may phagocytose mainly IDCs, which have a very rapid turnover (see Sect. 4.2) and which, due to their large surface and abundant organelles, are rich in membrane lipids. Finally, some lymphoid cells – both lymphoblasts and small lymphocytes – are found in the nude rat paracortex. In young nude rats most small lymphocytes are B cells, probably en route from the high endothelial venules to the follicles, but T-like cells increasingly accumulate in older animals (see Sect. 3.1).

2.2.3 *High Endothelial Venules*

Blood-borne cells entering the lymph nodes suffer two possible fates: the majority are led through the lymph node confined to the vessel lumen, and a minority, almost exclusively lymphocytes, are directed into the lymph node interstitium. These recirculating lymphocytes leave the bloodstream via specialized postcapillary venules (Gowans and Knight 1964). Thus the endothelium of these venules can be regarded as a natural cell-sorting apparatus, equipped with special adhesion molecules, operating on complementary ligands on the lymphocyte surface (reviewed in Yednock and Rosen 1989). The endothelial cells of these postcapillary venules are normally conspicuously plump (Marchesi and Gowans 1964), hence the designation high endothelial venules (HEVs). It has been debated whether the plumpness of the endothelium is a prerequisite for the adherence and passage of lymphocytes or whether it is secondary to a high rate of migration across the endothelium (reviewed in Ford et al. 1984).

In nude rat lymph nodes, the endothelial cells of the HEVs are generally much flatter than in normal littermates, although there is marked variation in their appearance even between different lymph nodes from the same nude rat (Fossum et al. 1980). The flat-walled HEVs can be distinguished from other vessels of similar size because their nuclei remain more nearly round and therefore protrude more into the lumen than in other small veins. By electron microscopy the cytoplasm is seen to contain less mitochondria and endoplasmic reticulum and the Golgi complex is less obvious than normal (FOSSUM et al. 1980).

The high endothelial cells of normal HEVs actively synthesize a glycolipid in association with glycoprotein, originally believed to control the rate of influx of lymphocytes into lymph nodes from the blood; in nude rats this synthesis is diminished (reviewed in FORD et al. 1984). However, when syngeneic radiolabeled T and B cells were injected into nude and euthymic, control recipients, combined autoradiography and scintillation countings of the recipients' lymph nodes showed that the flattened nude HEVs were as efficient at capturing lymphocytes from the blood as were the high-walled euthymic HEVs (FOSSUM et al. 1983 a). The only difference found was that B and T lymphocytes took a longer time to cross the HEV wall while entering the nude lymph nodes. The number of recirculating lymphocytes, as measured by the thoracic duct output of lymphocytes, is only about one-third in nude compared with euthymic rats (FOSSUM et al. 1980). When nude rats were thymus transplanted or restored with syngeneic T cells, the number of recirculating cells soon rose to normal levels, and at the same time the endothelial cells of HEVs become more thick walled (FOSSUM and FORD, unpublished). These observations provide evidence that the plumpness of the endothelial cells is secondary to a high rate of lymphocyte traffic across the vessel wall.

3 Immunocytochemistry

3.1 T-like Cells

Just as in the nude mouse (RAFF 1973; LOOR and ROELANTS 1974; CHEN et al. 1984), lymphocytes with T markers are present in the nude rats. In the thoracic duct of young (<3 months old) nude PVG rats, FOSSUM et al. (1980) found 2.4% W3/13$^+$ cells (leucosialin, a pan-T cell marker) and 3.5% W3/25$^+$ cells (CD4) (figures are median values, ranges 1%–9% and 1.5%–5.2%, respectively). In nude lymph nodes many W3/13$^+$, OX19$^+$ (CD5), W3/25$^+$ (CD4), and OX8$^+$ (CD8) cells are found (FOSSUM 1983) (Fig. 1). However, none of these markers is specific for T cells; thus, leucosialin is present on activated B cells and plasma cells [and possibly also on monocytes (HEDLUND et al. 1986)], CD5 on a small subset of B cells, CD4 on monocytes and macrophages, and CD8 on NK cells. Nonetheless, there is no doubt that a large proportion of the cells binding W3/13, OX19, W3/25, or OX8 (Fig. 1) do not represent these other cell types, but belong to the T lineage.

Two questions then arise: Firstly, where do these nude T-like cells come from? Secondly, if they arise in the nude animal, to what extent do they share properties with genuine thymus-processed cells? As for the first question, it has been suggested that these cells are maternally derived T cells. Arguments against this hypothesis are that such cells are detected in nude mice born to nu/nu homozygous mothers (reviewed in Hünig 1983) and that small inocula of normal, syngeneic T cells are rapidly expanded in nude rat hosts (Bell et al. 1987). The alternative, favored view is that these cells are indeed derived from the nude animal. The question then arises whether they have developed under the hormonal influence of the maternal thymus or the thymic rudiment or whether there exist truly thymus-independent pathways for their maturation. This matter has not yet been settled, but is partly related to the second question.

The number of T-like cells is very low in young nude rats, but increases with age (Vaessen et al. 1986) (Table 3), just as in nude mice (MacDonald et al. 1981). Similarly, functional properties like mitogen responsiveness and IL-2 productions are barely detectable in the young animals, but are definitely present in older animals (Vaessen et al. 1986; Hünig 1983; Kung and Thomas 1988). The T-like cells express functional T-cell receptors (Kishihara et al. 1987; MacDonald et al. 1987; Lawetzky and Hünig 1988) but show poor immune responses to conventional antigens (reviewed in Hünig 1983, Vaessen et al. 1986; Harelbellan et al. 1987; Kung 1988) and fail to reject allografts where far smaller numbers of thymus-educated T cells would suffice (Ford et al. 1983). These shortcomings could reflect defects at the level of the whole population rather than at the level of individual cells, e.g., the poor responses could reflect lack of MHC-restriction, lack of subsets or imbalance between subsets (MacDonald et al. 1986), or a limited repertoire (MacDonald et al. 1987; Maleckar and Sherman 1987).

However, there is reason to believe that the T-like cells are qualitatively deficient as well: when serial sections of nude rat lymph nodes were stained with antibodies against CD5, CD4, CD8, and the rat α/β T-cell antigen receptor (TCR) (detected with the monoclonal antibody R73 – Hünig et al. 1989), the paracortex contained far fewer $CD5^+$ cells than either $CD4^+$, $CD8^+$, or α/β TCR^+ (Fossum, manuscript in preparation).

Table 3. Percentages of cells bearing "T-cell markers" in lymph node cell suspension from nude and euthymic rats (Vaessen et al. 1986)

Markers	Euthymic rats	rnu rats at age (months)			
		2	3	5	17
Leucosialin	57 (68[a])	25 (4[a])	24	37	46
CD5	61	2	14	18	34
CD4	45	14	14	17	31
CD8	18	12	10	13	27
Thy-1	16	23	15	13	15
B cells	29 (23[a])	51 (70[a])	53	49	30

[a] From Brooks et al. 1980.

For clarity, the figures are given here without SEM, which in the original table from Vaessen, et al. (1986) ranged from 1 to 4. The monoclonal antibodies used were: leucosialin (pan-T marker) – ER-1 (W3/13), CD5 – MRC OX19, CD4 – ER-2, CD8 – MRC OX8, Thy-1 – ER-4, B cells – MARK-1 all age groups

The T-like cells are interesting with respect to lymph node histophysiology for at least two different reasons. Firstly, the site of maturation of these cells has not yet been determined, but may well be the peripheral lymphoid tissues, including the lymph nodes. Secondly, the immune responsiveness of T cells is not only a question of possessing the relevant receptors and signal transduction structures; in vivo microenvironmental interactions are equally important, i.e., the cells must be able to recirculate and localize to their homing areas. It has not yet been studied whether the T-like cells recirculate, and the interpretation of the immunocytochemical studies has been complicated by the reactivity of the monoclonal antibodies with non-T cells. This cross-reactivity is usually not a problem in lymphoid tissues of euthymic animals, where the predominance of T cells renders their gross distribution patterns easily recognizable, but it calls for caution even in these animals when interpreting results from areas where T cells are few, such as in germinal centers. Bearing this complication in mind, the T-like cells seem to localize preferentially to the lymph node paracortex (Fossum 1983) (Fig. 1), permitting the conclusion that the T-like cells acquire the capacity to localize correctly in the lymphoid tissue. This conclusion has recently been corroborated by studies using the R73 antibody (Fossum, manuscript in preparation).

3.2 Nonlymphoid Cells

A large proportion of the $CD8^+$ cells in the nude rat are not T-like cells, but NK cells (Reynolds et al. 1981). These are operationally defined as non-T cells that without previous sensitization selectively kill particular target cells by a mechanism that does not require immunoglobulin, and they have been implicated in a variety of functions, such as defense against bacterial and viral infections, resistance to parasites, destruction of malignant cells, regulation of bone marrow derived cells, homeostasis of immune responses, and transplantation reactions against bone marrow derived cells. NK activity is preferentially associated with large lymphocyte-like cells with indented nuclei and prominent azurophilic granules – large granular lymphocytes or LGLs (Timonen et al. 1979). NK cells are thymus independent, as shown by normal or elevated numbers in nude mice and rats (Kiessling et al. 1975; Reynolds et al. 1982). These animals therefore offer clear advantages in the study of natural immunity, as it can be performed undisturbed by authentic T-cell responses, at least in young animals.

Normal lymph nodes are reported to contain relatively few NK cells, which appear to be situated predominantly within follicles (Banerjee and Thibert 1983; Pizzolo et al. 1984). In the nude rat most of the NK cells are localized within the paracortex, as shown by immunocytochemical staining with anti-CD8 and anti-asialo GM_1 and by morphological demonstration of LGLs by electron microscopy (Fossum and Rolstad 1986). There are also differences between lymph nodes in that nude cervical and other somatic lymph nodes have a much higher density of paracortical NK cells than do mesenteric nodes

(Fossum and Rolstad 1986). A particularly interesting example of graft rejection is the rapid elimination of transplanted allogenic lymphocytes – allogeneic lymphocyte cytotoxicity or ALC (reviewed in Heslop and McNeilage 1983; Rolstad and Ford 1983). ALC is T independent as it occurs with undiminished vigor in athymic rats (Tønnesen and Rolstad 1983). In vitro assays have shown that the effector cells copurify with LGLs and display similar surface markers (Rolstad and Fossum 1987). ALC is a heterodox example of natural immunity, but highly important for our understanding of the recognition mechanisms involved, as it is directed against resting mature normal cells with the target specificities coded for by the MHC region (Ager et al. 1988). Studies on nude rats have been instrumental in demonstrating that neither immunoglobulin nor T-cell receptors are involved in this recognition mechanism (Rolstad et al. 1985). ALC is relevant in the context of nude rat lymph nodes, because footpad injection of allogeneic T cells failed to elicit a local graft-versus-host (GvH) reaction in the draining popliteal lymph nodes, even though the three criteria for a GvH reaction apparently seemed to be fulfilled: MHC incompatibility, immunocompetent donor cells, and a host without T reactivity to the grafted cells. Subsequent autoradiographic studies revealed that allogeneic thoracic duct lymphocytes that had entered the lymph nodes were rapidly killed in the nude paracortex (Fossum and Rolstad 1986). Paracortical LGLs were probably responsible for the recognition and killing, while IDCs subsequently phagocytosed the allogeneic cells (Fossum and Rolstad 1986).

Nonlymphoid cells like IDCs, FDCs, and macrophages were described in Sect. 2, but they are particularly easily visualized by immunocytochemistry (Fig. 1). The figure illustrates that these nonlymphoid cells show normal regional distribution, but that in particular the density of IDCs is much higher than in euthymic nodes. The many labeled Thy-1$^+$ IDCs in Fig. 1 are also noteworthy. IDCs are derived from lymph-borne dendritic leukocytes (see Sect. 4.2) and a large proportion of these cells are also Thy-1$^+$ (Fossum 1984), but Thy-1$^+$ dendritic cells are less readily recognized in euthymic rat lymph nodes.

4 Cell Migration

4.1 Lymphocyte Migration

The first stage of lymphocyte recirculation is selective migration from the blood across vascular endothelium mainly into peripheral lymphatic tissues. As detailed above, this traffic proceeds normally across the HEVs in nude rat lymph nodes, despite the abnormally flattened appearance of the endothelium (see Sect. 2.2.3). The subsequent stages include the segregation of B and T cells into distinct compartments and their migration through interstitial and lymphatic channels, to return to the blood (Ford 1975). The recirculation of intravenously injected syngeneic T and B cells was studied by Fossum et al.

(1983a, b). In addition to the results referred to under Sect. 2.2.3, the most important findings were the following: Firstly, the routes of recirculation of B and T cells were similar in nude and euthymic rats, leading to the conclusion that neither a thymus nor a full complement of T cells is necessary for the passage of lymphocytes through the lymph nodes or for the follicular localization of B cells or paracortical localization of T cells. This finding counters the suggestion that different interaction modulation factors released by T and B cells, respectively, reduce the adhesiveness of the other cell type and thereby promote segregation (CURTIS and DE SOUSA 1975).

Secondly, the tempo of recirculation through the lymph nodes from blood to lymph was substantially slower in nude rats. The delay in recirculation was reversed by thymus grafting, showing that the abnormality was not permanent. The sluggish recirculation of lymphocytes in the nude rats could be due to a chronic state of antigen-induced shutdown or nonspecific retention of lymphocytes (HALL and MORRIS 1965) because of defective clearance of antigens from the nude rat lymph nodes. Another, not mutually exclusive possibility is that the recirculating lymphocytes take a longer time to negotiate a passage between the interdigitating processes of the densely packed IDCs.

4.2 Migration of Nonlymphoid Cells

Whereas most lymphocytes enter the lymph nodes from the blood, most nonlymphoid cells enter via afferent lymphatics. The influx of nonlymphoid cells is substantial; SMITH et al. (1970) measured flow rates of ca. 3×10^5, 4×10^5, and 9×10^5 in the peripheral lymph from sheep limbs, testis, and liver, respectively. Most of the nonlymphoid cells in peripheral lymph are veiled or dendritic cells (reviewed in FOSSUM 1989), i.e., irregularly shaped, constitutively MHC class II$^+$ cells that are believed to constitute a family of cells, the dendritic leukocytes or DLs, separate from the mononuclear phagocyte system (reviewed in STEINMAN 1981), which function primarily as antigen-presenting cells for resting T cells (reviewed in AUSTYN 1987). Once they have reached the marginal sinus the veiled cells adhere to and penetrate the lymphendothelium facing the underlying cortex (FOSSUM 1980). They then proceed to the paracortex where they transform into IDCs (FOSSUM 1988). There are few nonlymphoid cells in central lymph and no evidence that they leave with the blood, signifying that most are retained and die in the lymph nodes. After having entered the lymph nodes, IDCs survive for 1–2 weeks at most (unpublished). Taken together with a median transit time from their site of cell division, most probably the bone marrow, of only 4 days (unpublished), a picture materializes of a formidable migratory stream of cells proceeding from the bone marrow via nonlymphoid tissues into draining lymphatics to end in the lymph nodes (reviewed in FOSSUM 1989). The lymph node paracortex emerges as a crossing-point between two different streams of migratory cells, the immigrating DLs, vectorially transporting and presenting antigen, and the transmigrating T cells.

In nude rats the rate of immigration of DLs into draining lymph nodes seems to be even higher than in euthymic rats (Tønnesen and Fossum 1984), which would contribute to an apparently increased absolute number of IDCs within the nude as compared with the euthymic paracortex (Fossum et al. 1980). The transit time from bone marrow to lymph nodes is similar and there seems to be no major difference in intranodal life span of IDCs in nude and euthymic rats (unpublished results). Virtually nothing is yet known about the mechanisms of control of DL traffic apart from indications that it may be arrested by steroid administration (unpublished). The results from the work on nude rats show that the presence of T cells makes no difference; for instance, they do not inhibit DL migration.

5 Conclusions

Although older nude animals may be less T deficient than originally considered, young nude mice and rats should still provide valid animal models for the study of T deficiency. Despite the presence of numerous T-like cells, older animals are nonetheless clearly immunodeficient; they therefore provide exciting experimental models for the study of T-cell differentiation and maturation. The work presented here on nude rat lymph nodes demonstrates that although T cells are the predominant regulatory cell of the immune system, many aspects of lymph node histophysiology proceed apparently normally in the absence of T cells. To understand the factors regulating the organization, life history, and functional relationships of cell populations within lymphoid tissue, we must therefore turn our attention to other cell types, including the nonlymphoid cells.

References

Ager A, Fajumi J, Sparshott SM, Butcher GW, Ford WL (1988) Major histocompatibility complex antigens as targets for allogeneic lymphocyte cytotoxicity in rats: the contribution of strong and medial transplantation antigens. Transplantation 46:762

Austyn JM (1987) Lymphoid dendritic cells. Immunology 62:161–170

Banerjee D, Thibert RF (1983) Natural killer-like cells found in B-cell compartments of human lymphoid tissues. Nature 304:270–272

Bell EB, Sparshott SM, Drayson MT, Ford WL (1987) The stable and permanent expansion of functional T lymphocytes in athymic nude rats after a single injection of mature T cells. J Immunol 139:1379

Brooks CG, Webb PJ, Robins RA, Robinson RA, Baldwin RW, Festing MFW (1980) Studies on the immunobiology of rnu/rnu "nude" rats with congenital aplasia of the thymus. Eur J Immunol 10:58–65

Chen WF, Scollay R, Shortman K, Skinner M, Marbrook J (1984) T-cell development in the absence of a thymus: the number, the phenotype, and the functional capacity of T lymphocytes in nude mice. Am J Anat 170:339

Curtis ASG, de Sousa M (1975) Lymphocyte interactions and positioning. I. Adhesive interactions. Cell Immunol 19:282

de Sousa MAB, Pritchard H, Pantelouris EM (1969) The lymphoid tissues in mice with congenital aplasia of the thymus. Clin Exp Immunol 4:637
Festing MFW (1981) Athymic nude rats. In: Gershwin ME, Merchant B (eds) Immunologic defects in laboratory animals, vol 1. Plenum, New York, pp 267–283
Festing MFW, May D, Connors TA, Lovell D, Sparrow S (1978) An athymic nude mutation in the rat. Nature 274:365–366
Flanagan SP (1966) 'Nude', a new hairless gene with pleiotropic effects in the mouse. Genet Res 8:295
Ford WL (1975) Lymphocyte migration and immune responses. Prog Allergy 19:1–59
Ford WL, Sparshott SM, Rolstad B (1983) Do nude rats display any alloaggression? Transplant Proc 15:1658–1659
Ford WL, Allen TD, Pitt MA, Smith ME, Stoddart RW (1984) The migration of lymphocytes across specialized vascular endothelium: VIII. Physical and chemical conditions influencing the surface morphology of lymphocytes and their ability to enter lymph nodes. Am J Anat 170:377
Fossum S (1980) The architecture of rat lymph nodes. II. Lymph node compartments. Scand J Immunol 12:411–421
Fossum S (1983) The density and distribution of W3/13, OX19, W3/25, and OX8 positive cells in nude rat (rnu) lymph nodes. Transplant Proc 15:1638–1639
Fossum S (1984) Characterization of Ia^+ non-lymphoid cells in peripheral lymph from congenitally athymic nude rats. Scand J Immunol 19:49–61
Fossum S (1988) Lymph-bone dendritic leukocytes do not recirculate, but enter the lymph node paracortex to become interdigitating cells. Scand J Immunol 27:141–147
Fossum S (1989) The cellular kinetics of dendritic leukocytes. In: Iversen OH (ed) The cell kinetics of the inflammatory reaction. Springer, Berlin Heidelberg New York, pp 101–124
Fossum S, Ford WL (1985) The organization of cell populations within lymph nodes: their origin, life history and functional relationships. Histopathology 9:469–499
Fossum S, Rolstad B (1986) The roles of interdigitating cells (IDC) and natural killer (NK) cells in allogeneic lymphocyte cytotoxicity (ALC). Eur J Immunol 16:440–450
Fossum S, Smith ME, Bell EB, Ford WL (1980) The architecture of rat lymph nodes. III. The lymph nodes and lymph-borne cells of the congenitally athymic nude rat (rnu). Scand J Immunol 12:421–432
Fossum S, Smith ME, Ford WL (1983a) The migration of T and B lymphocytes across specialized vascular endothelium. VII. The migration of T and B lymphocytes from the blood of the athymic, nude rat. Scand J Immunol 17:539–550
Fossum S, Smith ME, Ford WL (1983b) The recirculation of T and B lymphocytes in the athymic, nude rat. Scand J Immunol 17:551–557
Fossum S, Ager A, Rolstad B (1987) Specific inhibition of natural killer (NK) activity against different alloantigens. Immunogenetics 26:329–338
Gowans JL, Knight EJ (1964) The route of recirculation in the rat. Proc R Soc Lond [Biol] 159:257–282
Gowans JL, McGregor DD (1965) The immunological activities of lymphocytes. Prog Allergy 9:1–78
Hall JG, Morris B (1965) The immediate effect of antigens on the cell output of a lymph node. Br J Exp Pathol 46:450
Harelbellan A, Fradelizi D, Gerard JP, Marchiol C, Quillet A (1987) Lack of reconstitution of nude mice alloreactivity by purified interleukin-2 and induction of non-H-2 specific effector-cells by crude supernatants. Cell Immunol 105:251–261
Hedlund G, Segrn S, Jansson B, Sjögren HO (1986) Evidence for the existence of $W3/13^+$ monocytes in the rat. Scand J Immunol 24:387–392
Heslop BF, McNeilage LJ (1983) Natural cytotoxicity: early killing of allogeneic lymphocytes in rats. Immunol Rev 73:35–51
Hünig T (1983) T-cell function and specificity in athymic mice. Immunol Today 4:84–87
Hünig T, Wallny H-J, Hartley JK, Lawetzky A, Tiefenthaler G (1989) A monoclonal antibody to a constant determinant of the rat T cell antigen receptor that induces T cell activation. J Exp Med 169:73–86
Ikehara S, Good RA, Hamashima Y et al. (1987) Thymic rudiments are responsible for induction of functional T-cells in nu/nu mice. Thymus 10:193–205

Kiessling R, Klein E, Wigzell H (1975) 'Natural' killer cells in the mouse. I. Cytotoxic cells with specificity of mouse Moloney leukemia cells. Specificity and distribution according to genotype. Eur J Immunol 5:112–117

Kindred B (1979) Nude mice in immunology. Prog Allergy 26:137–238

Kishihara K, Yoshikai Y, Matzukai G, Mak TW, Nomoto K (1987) Functional α/β T cell chain receptor messages can be detected in old but not in young athymic mice. Eur J Immunol 17:477

Klausen B, Hougen HP (1987) Quantitative studies of lymphoid organs, blood and lymph in inbred athymic and euthymic LEW rats under germfree and specified-pathogen-free conditions. Lab Anim 21:342–347

Kung JT (1988) Impaired clonal expansion in athymic nude $CD8^+$ $CD4^-$ T cells. J Immunol 140:3727

Kung JT, Thomas CA (1988) Athymic nude $CD4^+8^-$ T cells produce IL-2 but fail to proliferate in response to mitogenic stimuli. J Immunol 141:3691

Lawetzky A, Hünig T (1988) Analysis of CD3 and antigen receptor expression on T cell subpopulations of aged athymic mice. Eur J Immunol 18:409

Loor F, Roelants GE (1974) High frequency of T lineage lymphocytes in nude mouse spleen. Nature 251:229–230

MacDonald HR, Lees RK, Sordat B, Zaech P, Marganski JL, Bron C (1981) Age-associated increase in the expression of the T cell surface markers Thy-1, Lyt-1 and Lyt-2 in congenitally athymic (nu/nu) mice: analysis by flow microfluorometry. J Immunol 126:865

MacDonald HR, Blanc C, Lees RK, Sordat B (1986) Abnormal distribution of T cell subsets in athymic mice. J Immunol 136:4337

MacDonald HR, Lees RK, Bron C, Sordat B, Miescher G (1987) T cell antigen receptor expression in athymic (nu/nu) mice. Evidence for an oligoclonal chain repertoire. J Exp Med 166:195

Maleckar JR, Sherman LA (1987) The composition of the T cell receptor repertoire in nude mice. J Immunol 138:3873

Marchesi VT, Gowans JL (1964) The migration of lymphocytes through the endothelium of venules in lymph nodes: an electron microscopic study. Proc R Soc Lond [Biol] 159:283

Mason DW, Arthur RP, Dallman M, Green JR, Spickett GP, Thomas ML (1983) Functions of rat T-lymphocyte subsets isolated by means of monoclonal antibodies. Immunol Rev 74:57–82

Miller JFAP (1961) Immunological function of the thymus. Lancet II:748–749

Mjaaland S, Fossum S (1987) Follicular localization of antigen in congenitally athymic, nude rats. Scand J Immunol 26:141–147

Pantelouris EM (1968) Absence of thymus in a mouse mutant. Nature 20:247

Pizzolo G, Semenzato G, Chilosi M et al. (1984) Distribution and heterogeneity of cells detected by HNK-1 monoclonal antibody in blood and tissues in normal reactive and neoplastic conditions. Clin Exp Immunol 57:195–206

Pugh CW, MacPherson GG, Steer HW (1983) Characterisation of non-lymphoid cells derived from rat peripheral lymph. J Exp Med 157:1758–1779

Raff MC (1973) O-bearing lymphocytes in nude mice. Nature 246:350–351

Reynolds CW, Timonen T, Holden HT, Hansen CT, Herberman RB (1981) Natural killer activity in the rat. II. Analysis of surface antigens in LGL by flow cytometry. J Immunol 127:2204–2208

Reynolds CW, Timonen T, Holden HT, Hansen CT, Heberman RB (1982) Natural killer cell activity in the rat. Analysis of effector cell morphology and effects of interferon on natural killer cell functions in the athymic (nude) rat. Eur J Immunol 12:577–582

Rolstad B, Ford WL (1983) The rapid elimination of allogeneic lymphocytes: relationship to established mechanisms of immunity and to lymphocyte traffic. Immunol Rev 73:87–113

Rolstad B, Fossum S (1987) Allogeneic lymphocyte cytotoxicity (ALC) in rats: establishment of an in vitro assay, and direct evidence that cells with natural killer (NK) activity are involved in ALC. Immunology 60:151–157

Rolstad B, Fossum S, Bazin H, Kimber I, Marshall J, Sparshott SM, Ford WL (1985) The rapid rejection of allogeneic lymphocytes by a non-adaptive, cell mediated mechanism ("NK activity"). Immunology 54:127–138

Safieh B, Kendall MD (1988) Methods for assaying thymic hormones. In: Kendall MD, Ritter MA (eds) Thymus Update. 1. The microenvironment of the human thymus. Harwood Academic, Chur, Switzerland, pp 117–133
Smith JB, McIntosh GH, Morris B (1970) The traffic of cells through tissues: a study of peripheral lymph in sheep. J Anat 107:87–100
Sprent J, Miller JFAP (1972) Thoracic duct lymphocytes from nude mice: migratory properties and lifespan. Eur J Immunol 2:384
Steinman RM (1981) Dendritic cells. Transplantation 31:151–155
Tew J, Mandel TE, Phipps RP, Szakal AK (1984) Tissue localization and retention of antigen in relation to the immune response. Am J Anat 170:407–420
Tew J, Kosco MH, Szakal AK (1989) The alternative antigen pathway. Immunol Today 7:229–232
Timonen T, Saksela E, Ranki A, Häyry P (1979) Fractionation, morphological and functional characterization of effector cells responsible for human natural killer activity against cell-line targets. Cell Immunol 48:133–148
Timonen T, Ortaldo JR, Herberman RB (1981) Characteristics of human large granular lymphocytes and relationship to natural killer cells and K cells. J Exp Med 153:569–582
Tønnesen B, Fossum S (1984) Recovery of peripheral lymph cells from congenitally athymic, nude rats. Scand J Immunol 19:41–48
Tønnesen B, Rolstad B (1983) In vivo elimination of allogeneic lymphocytes in normal and T cell deficient rats. Elimination does not require T cells. Scand J Immunol 17:303–312
Vaessen LMB, Broekhuizen R, Rozing J, Vos JG, Schuurman H-J (1986) T-cell development during ageing in congenitally athymic (nude) rats. Scand J Immunol 24:223–235
Veerman AJP (1974) On the interdigitating cells in the thymus-dependent area of the rat spleen: a relation between the mononuclear phagocyte system and T lymphocytes. Cell Tissue Res 148:247–257
Veldman JE (1970) Histophysiology and electron microscopy of the immune response, N.V. Boekdrukkerij Dojkstra Niemeyer, Groningen
Warner NL, Szenberg A, Burnett FM (1962) The immunological role of different lymphoid organs in the chicken. I. Dissociation of immunological responsiveness. Aust J Exp Biol Med Sci 40:373
Yednock TA, Rosen SD (1989) Lymphocyte homing. Adv Immunol 44:313–378
Yoshikai Y, Reis MD, Mak TW (1986) Athymic mice express a high level of functional γ-chain but greatly reduced levels of α- and β-chain T-cell receptor messages. Nature 324:482

Structure and Function of High Endothelial Postcapillary Venules in Lymphocyte Circulation

P. P. H. DE BRUYN and Y. CHO

1 The Interorgan Lymphocyte Traffic

The interdependence of the tissue and organ components that constitute the immune system is maintained and controlled by continuous interorgan lymphocyte traffic via the circulation. This lymphocyte traffic is accompanied by differentiations of lymphocytes into lymphocytes with different qualities of immunocompetency and in this way determines the immune responses of the tissues and organs involved. This interorgan traffic is clearly not a random event. Specific and selective factors determine its high degree of organization. In their movement from one anatomical site to another, the lymphocytes cross endothelial barriers. The specificities involved in the interaction between lymphocytes and the endothelia concerned and which result in the selective lymphocyte transmural passage are the essential regulatory factors in the interorgan traffic of lymphocytes.

Studies on the factors regulating the interaction between lymphocytes and endothelium as well as studies on the mode of this transmural passage have so far largely been concerned with the circulatory component of interorgan lymphocyte traffic, i.e., their return to lymphatic tissues and organs. These studies have focused on the lymphocyte–endothelial interaction taking place in high endothelial postcapillary venules[1] of lymph nodes and mucosal lymphatic tissues such as Peyer's patches. These postcapillary venules are anatomically distinct. The lymphocyte traffic through their endothelial walls is massive as compared to that occurring through the squamous endothelia of other immune organs such as thymus, spleen, and bone marrow.

---

[1] These venules are usually termed either "high endothelial" or "postcapillary" venules. Neither term is adequately descriptive. We shall use both because of their general acceptance.

2 The Circulation of Lymphocytes

The site of transmural lymphocyte passage through the postcapillary venules of the lymphatic tissue is characterized by a marked structural alteration in the endothelial geometry as compared with the endothelium of larger venules and the postcapillary venules elsewhere. The peculiar structure of these venules was first observed by THOME (1898) in *Macacus cynomolgus*. He described these vessels as having a high, almost cylindrical endothelium of which the cells bulged into the vascular lumen. At first notice, he writes, one is inclined to think of the duct of a gland rather than that of a blood vessel. The larger venules in the medulla had no such high endothelium. The transition between the two venule types he found to be abrupt. VON SCHUMACHER (1899) confirmed these observations in other species, including human. In addition, VON SCHUMACHER described and depicted leukocytes (lymphocytes) migrating through the endothelium of these postcapillary venules. He postulated that lymphocytes entered the vascular lumen and concluded that there are two pathways by which the lymphocytes leave the lymph nodes, one via the efferent lymphatics and one by the small postcapillary venules. ZIMMERMANN (1923) fully confirmed these observations and concurred with VON SCHUMACHER regarding the direction of the movement of the lymphocytes through the postcapillary venule wall. SCHULTZE (1925) appeared to assume that the lymphocyte passage in these high endothelial postcapillary venules can take place in both directions and may be either through preformed stomata or through attentuated sites in the venule wall.

The functional significance of these early observations on the presence of lymphocytes in the walls of the high endothelial venules of lymphatic tissues was not fully realized until the question of the fate of the lymphocytes arose. Quantitative studies on the efflux of lymph, largely obtained through cannulization of the thoracic duct of various animals, revealed that very large numbers of lymphocytes daily entered the circulating blood. For comprehensive data on the magnitude of the lymphocyte output of various lymphatic organs of different species, we refer the reader to YOFFEY and COURTICE (1956). The number of lymphocytes in the peripheral blood remains, however, relatively constant under normal conditions. Therefore it follows that within a given time span as many lymphocytes leave the circulation as are entering it. Of the attempts to explain this disappearance of lymphocytes from the circulation we mention the supposition that they disappear by migration through the intestinal wall into the intestinal lumen (BUNTING and HUSTON 1921) and a possible disintegration in the peripheral blood (ERF 1940). SJOVALL (1936) postulated a lymphocyte circulation from the lymphatic tissue via the blood to the connective tissue spaces of the body and via the peripheral lymphatics to the blood and "back to the place of origin." Direct evidence for such a circulating pathway was, however, not provided. The first experimental evidence for a lymphocyte circulation was provided by R. S. FARR (1951). This investigator collected lymphocytes from the popliteal nodes of rabbits and labeled the lymphocytes with 3,6-diamino-10-methyl acridinium chloride. This fluorescent dye is a vital nuclear stain at nontoxic dose levels (De Bruyn et al. 1950). The labeled lymphocyte suspension was infused intravenously in the same rabbit and frozen-dried sections of tissues were examined at 2 and 12 h after the injection for the presence of labeled nuclei of which the cells were then identified by phase microscopy. Most of the labeled lymphocytes left the peripheral blood within 90 min. Labeled lymphocytes were found after 2 and 12 h in lymphatic tissues, including mesenteric lymph node, Peyer's patches, appendix, thymus, and white pulp of spleen. In the bone marrow lymphocytes were found after 2 h only. It was concluded that lymphocytes pass from the bloodstream directly to lymphatic tissues and also to the bone marrow. Thus the existence of a lymphocyte circulation was established. Farr (1951) mentioned the possibility that the lymphocyte entry into the lymphatic tissue may take place through the walls of small blood vessels in the lymph node but made no reference to the high endothelial venules.

In 1964, experiments to trace the fate of the lymphocytes were performed by labeling small and large lymphocytes with tritiated thymidine and tritiated adenosine and by determining the localization of infused lymphocytes in tissues by means of radioautography (Gowans and Knight 1964). These procedures allow semiquantitative estimates regarding the numbers of labeled lymphocytes in the various tissues involved. The autoradiographic localization showed that the transfused labeled small lymphocytes were present in large numbers in tissue sections of lymph nodes, white pulp of spleen, and Peyer's patches. Labeled lymphocytes were also found in the bone marrow, apparently in smaller numbers than in the lymphatic organs. Labeled cells penetrated the endothelia of the high endothelial venules and were seen in the immediate vicinity of lymph nodes perfused during a period of 12 min. Perfusions of longer duration (8 h) resulted in large accumulations of labeled lymphocytes in the lymphatic cortex. These experiments conclusively showed that circulating lymphocytes returned to the lymph nodes and Peyer's patches through the walls of the high endothelial postcapillary venules. It is to be noted, however, that in both sets of experiments, those with lymphocytes labeled with a fluorescent compound as well as those radioactively labeled, infused lymphocytes were found in organs not provided with high endothelial venules, such as bone marrow, thymus, and spleen. The migration of lymphocytes to these organs is generally not regarded as part of what is considered the circulation of lymphocytes – a process which involves massive numbers of cells. The interorgan movement of lymphocytes between these organs of the immune system involves fewer cells which are nevertheless also detected, though in smaller measure, by the labeling experiments cited above. Their interorgan traffic and intraorgan disposition are primarily associated with the differentiation of lymphocytes into specific types of immune response. The capture of these lymphocytes and their subsequent interparenchymal localization does not seem to require an affinity for the high endothelial postcapillary venules. It is, however, likely that also in these instances, a specific affintiy of lymphocytes for the endothelia of these organs is operative.

3 The Structure of the Wall of High Endothelial Postcapillary Venules

The unusual thickness of the endothelial components of the walls of the high endothelial venules has generally been attributed simply to a greater height of the endothelial cells as compared with those present in blood vessels elsewhere, and they have often been referred to as cuboidal or cylindrical in shape. Such designations, however, do not describe the unique geometrical arrangement of the cells of high endothelial postcapillary venules. Scanning electron microscopic micrographs make it immediately clear that this venule endothelium is distinctly different in its three-dimensional arrangement from other vascular endothelia and that it does not have the smooth adluminal surface of other vessels (CHO and DE BRUYN 1979). Two types of adluminal surface configuration can be distinguished by scanning electron microscopy (Figs. 1–3). One is best described as having a cobblestone pattern. The convex adluminal surfaces of the endothelial cells bulge deeply into the vascular lumen. The cells are separated by deep clefts of various widths. This form of surface relief occurs in the proximal section, i.e., the section immediately adjacent to the capillary supply of the postcapillary venule. The section with the cobblestone surface pattern is distally followed by a surface configuration resembling interlacing plates. Cytoplasmic processes in the form of flattened bands of plates arise from the endothelial cells and extend laterally, running generally parallel to the long axis of the venule. These endothelial plates overlap or intertwine with others so that the luminal aspect has the appearance of an interlacing network. These plates may disappear from view by penetrating adjacent ones or passing

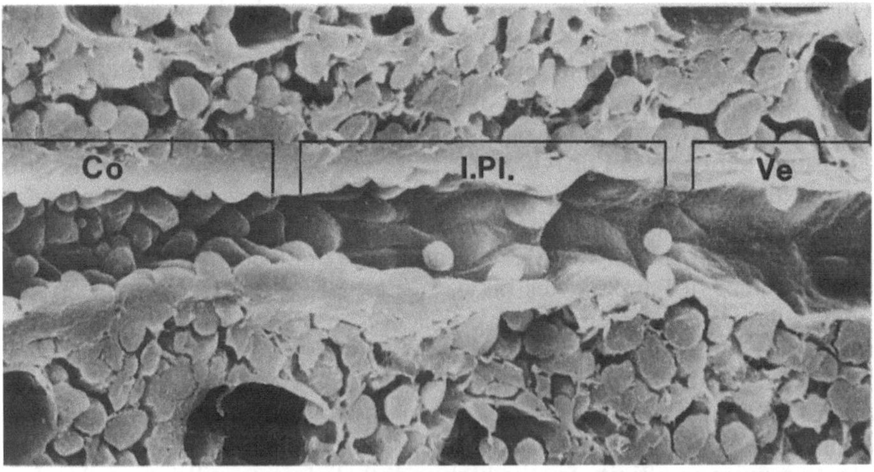

Fig. 1. Luminal view of the wall of a postcapillary venule of rat lymph node. A surface relief with a cobblestone pattern (*Co*) continues distally into a wall with a surface relief with a pattern of interlacing plates (*I.Pl.*) The latter continues into a smooth-walled squamous endothelial venule (*Ve*). ×840

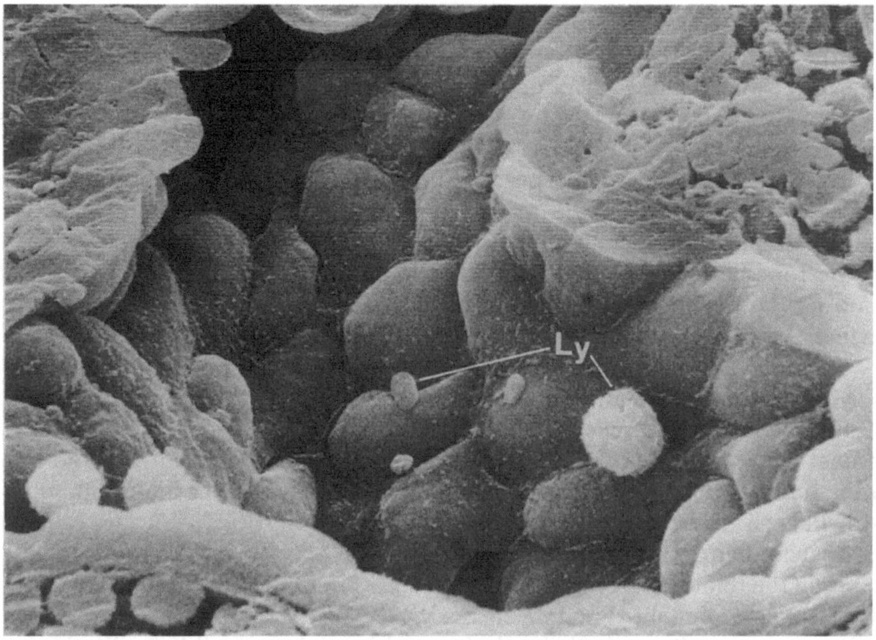

Fig. 2. Adluminal aspect of the wall of a postcapillary venule of rat lymph node. The surface relief is that of a cobblestone pattern. Lymphocytes (*Ly*) are captured in the crevices between the luminal protrusions of the endothelial cells. Some of these are only partially visible. Whether these lymphocytes are migrating through the endothelium cannot be determined from SEM images. × 2100

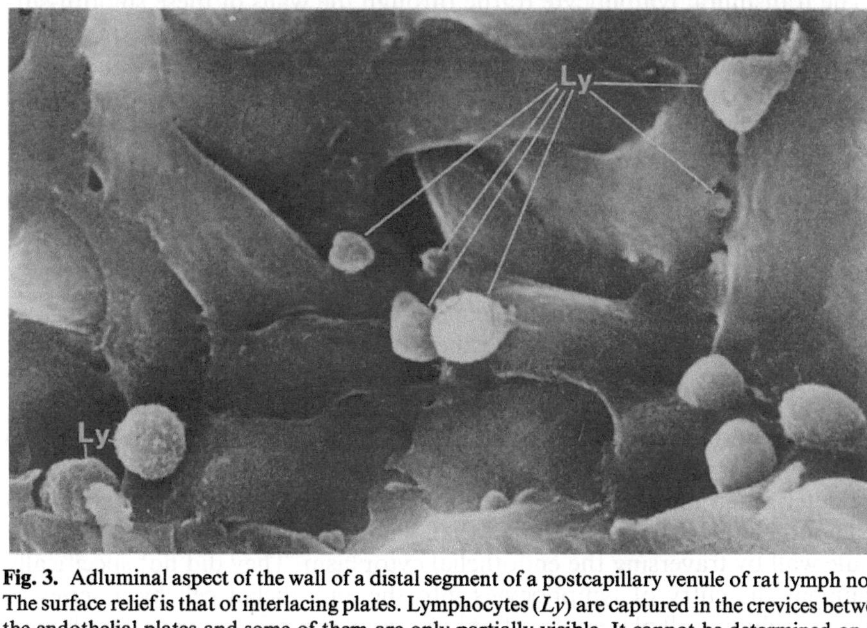

Fig. 3. Adluminal aspect of the wall of a distal segment of a postcapillary venule of rat lymph node. The surface relief is that of interlacing plates. Lymphocytes (*Ly*) are captured in the crevices between the endothelial plates and some of them are only partially visible. It cannot be determined on the basis of such SEM images whether the lymphocytes are migrating through the venule wall. × 2000

under others, or they may take a basal direction by entering junctions between endothelial cells (Fig. 3). Recesses of various depths are present underneath the cytoplasmic plates. Lymphocytes adhere to the walls of the venules of both surface types and are often lodged in the crevices between the endothelial cells and are then only partially visible.

Transmission electron microscopy shows that the interlacing of endothelial processes is also present in the interior of the endothelium (Cho and De Bruyn 1986). All endothelial cells of the postcapillary venules, those which form a cobblestone pattern as well as those forming an interlacing plate relief, rest upon the basement membrane and all endothelial cells reach the adluminal surface. In essence it is thus a single-layer endothelium.

These deviations from a smooth luminal vessel surface will modify a laminar flow into a turbulent one. As a consequence, this, as well as the increase in endothelial surface relief itself, will result in an increase in the chances of contact between circulating lymphocytes and the endothelial surface and thus in the number of "recognition events" between lymphocytes and luminal endothelial cell surface. It appears, then, that the peculiarities in surface relief of the postcapillary venules of the lymphatic tissue may have a functional significance in the removal of lymphocytes from the circulation at this particular site of the vascular system. The interlacing plates may well be in a dynamic state and may continually move their relative positions, thus possibly facilitating the movement of lymphocytes across the endothelium.

The section with the surface relief of interlacing plates changes distally into larger smooth-surfaced venules with a simple squamous endothelium (Figs. 1, 4). The transmural lymphocyte traffic through the walls of these smooth-surfaced venules is sharply diminished as compared with the massive lymphocyte traffic through the walls of the high endothelial venules. Fine structural images (Fig. 5) of the transmural lymphocytes in these particular venules favor the supposition that these lymphocytes are in direct entry into the circulation, bypassing the lymphatic channels (Cho and De Bruyn 1981).

4 The Transendothelial Pathway of the Lymphocytes

The uniqueness of the endothelial geometrical configuration of the postcapillary venules in lymphatic tissue and their being a site of selective removal of lymphocytes from the circulation has led to a number of studies regarding the structural relationship between the endothelium and the lymphocytes during their transmural passage. The first studies on the transmural lymphocyte pathway were reported by Marchesi and Gowans (1964). Using serial sections, they determined the position of the intraendothelial lymphocytes relative to the endothelial cells and concluded that the lymphocytes migrate across the venule wall by traversing the endothelial cytoplasm. They did not specifically document the entry of lymphocytes into the endothelial cell by a series of sections including all planes of sectioning at and around the site of lymphocyte penetration.

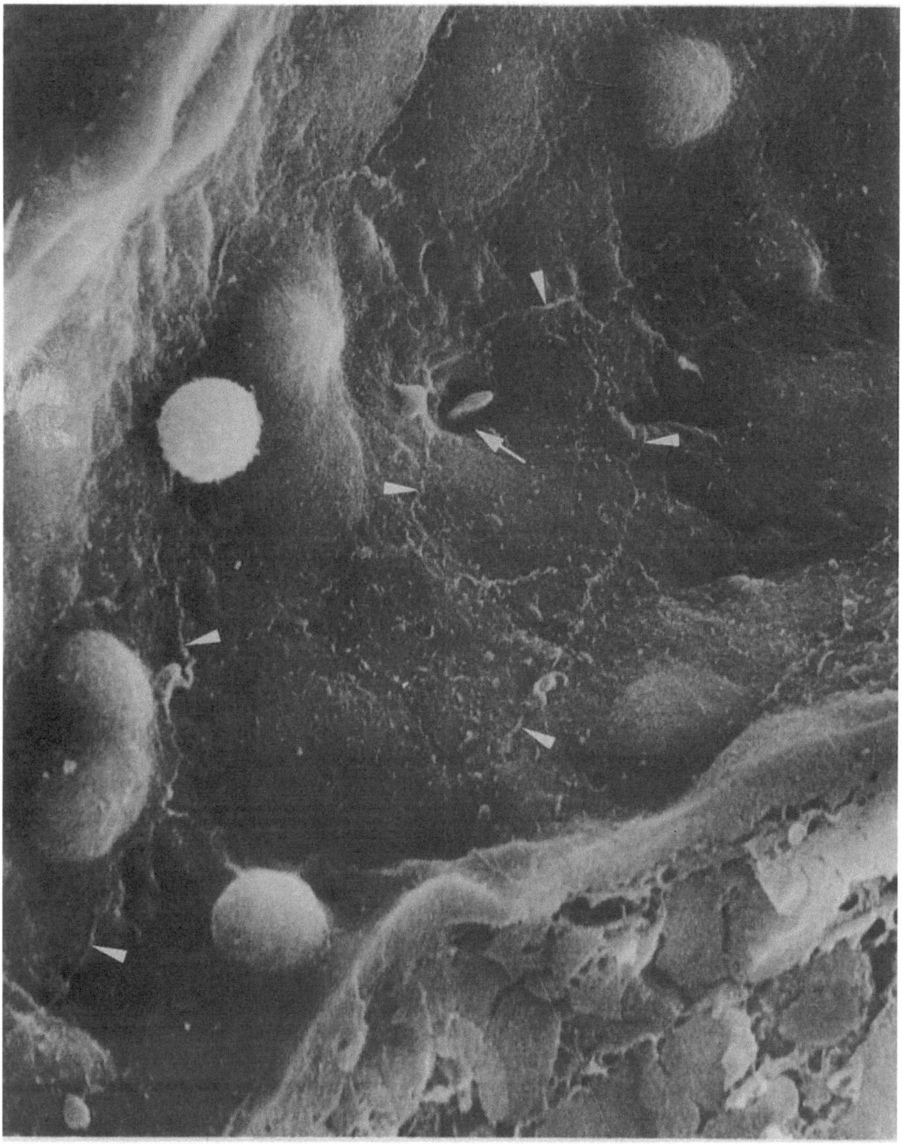

Fig. 4. Smooth-surfaced venule immediately distal to the high endothelial postcapillary venule. The *arrowheads* indicate the cell junctions. One cell is seen in transmural passage (*arrow*). The migration pore is independent from the intercellular junctions. Mouse lymph node. ×3000

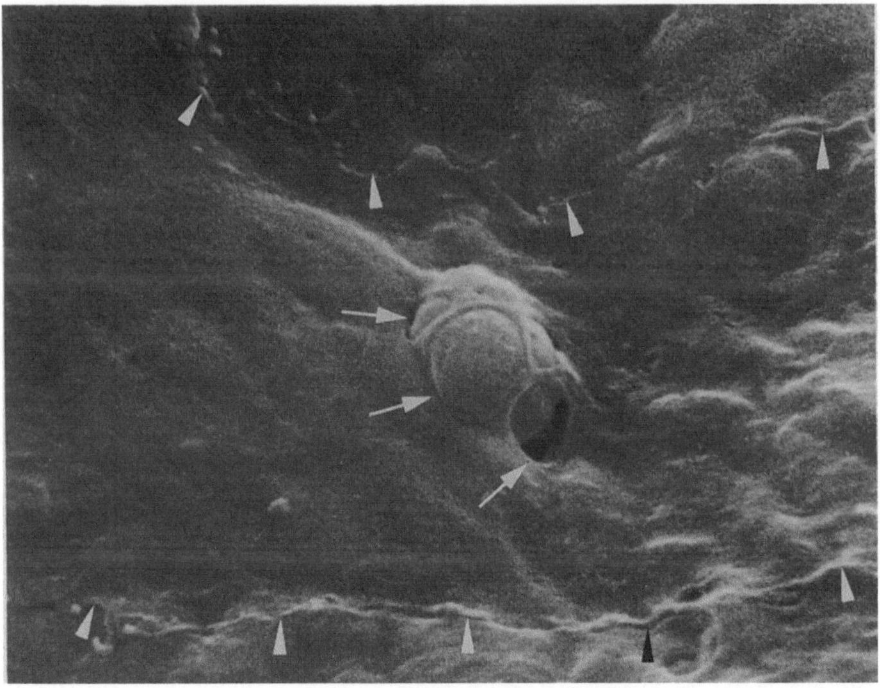

Fig. 5. Lymphocyte in transmural passage through the endothelium of a smooth-walled squamous venule. The migrating cell bulges into the lumen and there are multiple openings (*arrows*) in the overlying attenuated squamous endothelium. Cell junctions are indicated by *arrowheads*. This configuration is interpreted as lymphocyte entry into the vascular lumen. Mouse lymph node. × 12 600

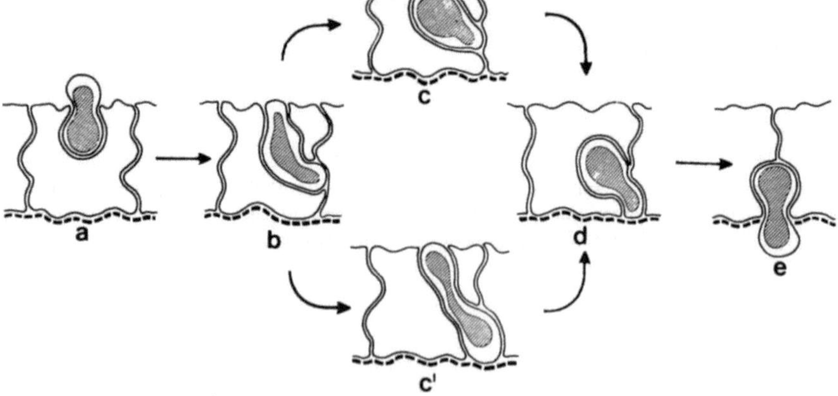

Fig. 6. Diagrammatic representation of the transmural pathway of lymphocytes through the endothelium of postcapillary venules

The transcellular mode of lymphocyte passage was subsequently questioned (CLAESSON et al. 1971; SCHOEFL 1972; WENK et al. 1974, ANDERSON and ANDERSON 1976; ANDERSON et al. 1976; UMETANI 1977; YAMAGUCHI and SCHOEFL 1983). An extracellular passage was proposed on the basis of images showing the presence of lymphocytes in an intraendothelial space connected with an intercellular endothelial space. It is to be noted that these investigators limited their observations to lymphocytes already encased in the endothelium. Clearly, the selective lymphocyte capture is determined by events at the adluminal endothelial–lymphocyte interface. Consequently, if the lymphocyte migration in the postcapillary high endothelial venule is determined at the adluminal endothelial face, then it is of importance to study the early contact of lymphocytes with endothelial cells rather than their subsequent travels within the endothelial layer. FARR and DE BRUYN (1975) reexamined the transvascular passage of lymphocytes in the postcapillary lymphatic venules with serial sections, paying particular attention to their mode of entry into the endothelial lining. Proceeding with this approach, they observed that the initial penetration by the lymphocytes is through the body of the endothelial cells. They did not observe diapedesing lymphocytes entering the endothelium through the intercellular spaces. Once the penetration of the endothelial cell body had been effected, the lymphocyte progressed through the cell body toward the intercellular spaces between the endothelial cells. Lymphocytes, while traversing the endothelial cells, were observed in part still in the vascular lumen, in part in the endothelial cell body, and in part in the intercellular space (Fig. 6). This position explains the presence of intravascularly administered tracer around lymphocytes seen inside the endothelium and which has been held to be evidence that the lymphocyte pathway is entirely through the extracellular spaces (ANDERSON and ANDERSON 1976).

Although FARR and DE BRUYN (1975) did not exclude the possibility that occasionally some lymphoctes traverse the endothelial cell through its entirety from the luminal surface to its base, they did not agree with MARCHESI and GOWANS' (1964) contention that this is the most common pathway. However, they did agree that there is a transcellular phase in the migration of lymphocytes across the endothelium of the postcapillary venules.

Scanning electron microscopy has been shown to be an important additional tool in examining the site of entry of lymphocytes into the venule endothelium. Relatively large endothelial surfaces can be examined and the relation between the site of lymphocyte entry and the endothelial intercellular junctions can be directly determined. Such studies (CHO and DE BRUYN 1979, 1986) show that the lymphocytes penetrate the luminally exposed endothelial surface of the venules in the segment with the cobblestone pattern as well as in that with the surface relief of interlacing plates at sites distant from the intercellular endothelial junctions (Fig. 7). Lymphocytes are present in the deep crevices of the endothelial surface relief (Figs. 2, 3). Serial sections show that their presence in these locations does not indicate an intercellular lymphocyte passage, but that these lymphocytes also migrate, deeper in the endothelium, in a transcellular fashion (Fig. 8).

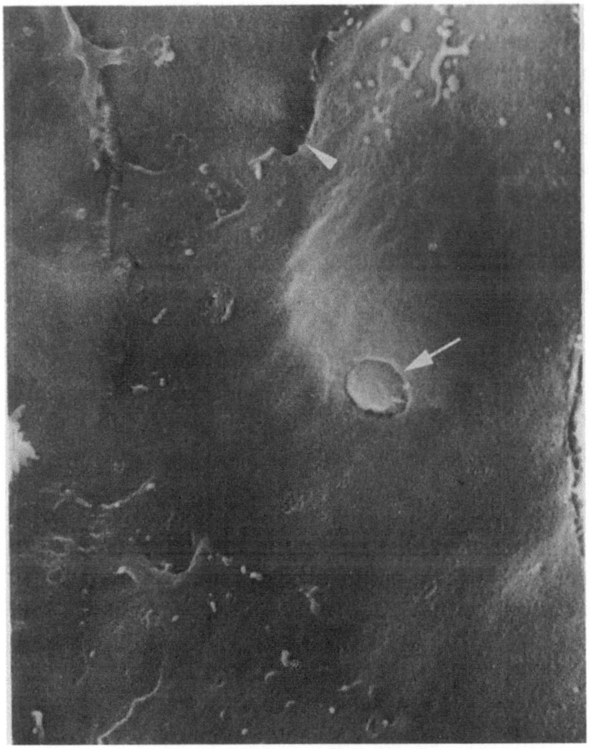

Fig. 7. Luminal view of a mouse postcapillary venule wall (interlacing plate pattern). A lymphocyte (*arrow*) has entered the body of an endothelial cell. The migration pore is independent of the endothelial cell junctions (*arrowhead*), indicating a transcellular pathway. ×7000

It is of interest to compare this selective process with the selective transvascular migration of blood cells in bone marrow (DE BRUYN et al. 1971; BECKER and DE BRUYN 1976) and embryonic rat liver (BANKSTON and PINO 1980). Here only mature cells pass through the sinusoidal endothelial lining, their immature precursors remaining in the extravascular locations. A corollary of this is the selective entry of malignant cells into the vascular lumen in the primary stage of metastasis formation (DE BRUYN and CHO 1979, 1982; DE BRUYN 1983) and the similarly selective entry into the extravascular parenchyma in the second stage of metastasis formation (DE BRUYN et al. 1989). This selective form of diapedesis is also a transcellular process. The similarities between these processes appear to strengthen the hypothesis that a transcellular entry and a transcellular route may be a characteristic of selective transvascular migration (DE BRUYN 1983).

The presence of lymphocytes inside other cells has been reported in cell cultures. By means of time cinemicrography of tissue cultures, living lymphocytes have been reported to be present in malignant cells (HUMBLE et al. 1958). This process has been termed "emperipolesis" – "inside round about

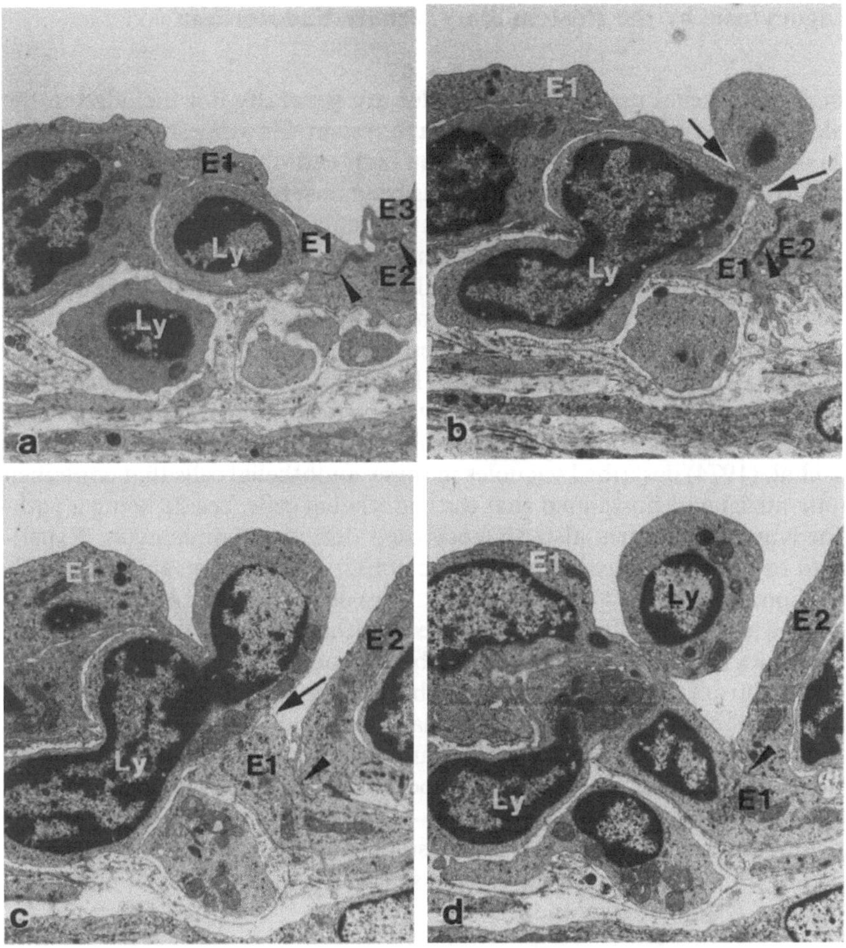

Fig. 8a–d. Four selections of a series of sections through the proximal (cobblestone) segment of a postcapillary venule of rat Peyer's patch showing that the partially visible lymphocytes in SEM, such as are seen in Figs. 3 and 4, migrate transcellularly through the endothelial wall. A lymphocyte (*Ly*) penetrates endothelial cell E1. The junction between E1 and E2 is marked by an *arrowhead*. **a** and **d** are from sections at opposite sites of the migration pore (*arrows* in **b** and **c**) and show that the cytoplasm of E1 is continuous at both sites. The migration pore is independent from the junction between E1 and E2. The intraluminal portion of the migrating lymphocyte (*Ly*) would in SEM be seen as a protrusion from the crevices between E1 and E2. The migrating lymphocyte is in part intravascular, in part transcellular, in part in the intercellular endothelial space, and in part extravascular. Other lymphocytes to the left and right of *Ly* are intraendothelial. × 6000

wandering." A functional significance for this was not proposed. Regarding the temporary presence of lymphocytes in the endothelium of the postcapillary venules, it has been suggested that this might provide a special opportunity for an interaction between small lymphocytes and an antigen passing from the blood into the lymph node (MARCHESI and GOWANS 1964).

5 Phagocytosis by the Postcapillary Venule Endothelium

The high endothelial postcapillary venules are generally not included in the so-called reticuloendothelial or macrophage system. However, marked phagocytosis of circulating leukemia cells by the high endothelial venules, resulting in the destruction of the leukemia cells, has been observed (Cho and De Bruyn 1978). In rats in which acute myelogenous leukemia (AML) was induced by the intravenous administration of a suspension of Shay AML cells, massive phagocytosis by macrophages in the circulatory circuit occurred. The endothelium of the postcapillary venules of the lymph nodes participated in the phagocytosis of circulating leukemia cells. These endothelail cells contained intact leukemia cells as well as their remnants (Fig. 9). It is particularly noteworthy that the endothelium of the postcapillary venules continued at the same time to be the site for the transcellular passage of normal lymphocytes (Fig. 9). Wenk et al. (1974) described vacuoles in these endothelial cells that contained pyknotic nuclei and postulated that the endothelial cells, beside being a pathway for lymphatic return, also phagocytosed defective lymphocytes. Experiments to examine the possible phagocytc activity of the postcapillary venule endothelium have yielded varying results. Hummel (1935) and Kruger (1968) did not find any phagocytic activity by the endothelial cells of the postcapillary venules. Mikata and Nikki (1971) described particulate transport by vacuoles that traveled from the luminal side to the base of the endothelial cell, where the vacuoles opened and released the particulate in the subendothelial space. They found that a few particles remained in multivascular bodies and phagosomes, thus providing evidence of some phagocytic and digestive function of the endothelium of the postcapillary venules. It would thus appear that while the high endothelial venules cannot be considered an active component of the macrophage system, they can nevertheless be markedly phagocytic under certain, not yet well defined, conditions.

6 Lymphocyte–High Endothelial Venule Interaction

The selective affinity of lymphocytes for high endothelial venules is of greater complexity than was first surmised and has been shown to involve interactions between functionally different sets of lymphocytes and the high endothelia of postcapillary venules of different lymphatic organs.

An important development in studies on the interaction between lymphocytes and the high endothelial venules was the in vitro model described by Stamper and Woodruff (1976). With this model, Stamper and Woodruff showed that lymphocytes display a specific adherence to the high endothelial venules present in fixed lymph node sections and not to endothelia of other vessels. They further reported that lymphocytes of the thoracic duct, lymph nodes, and spleen adhere to the high endothelial venules, while lymphocytes

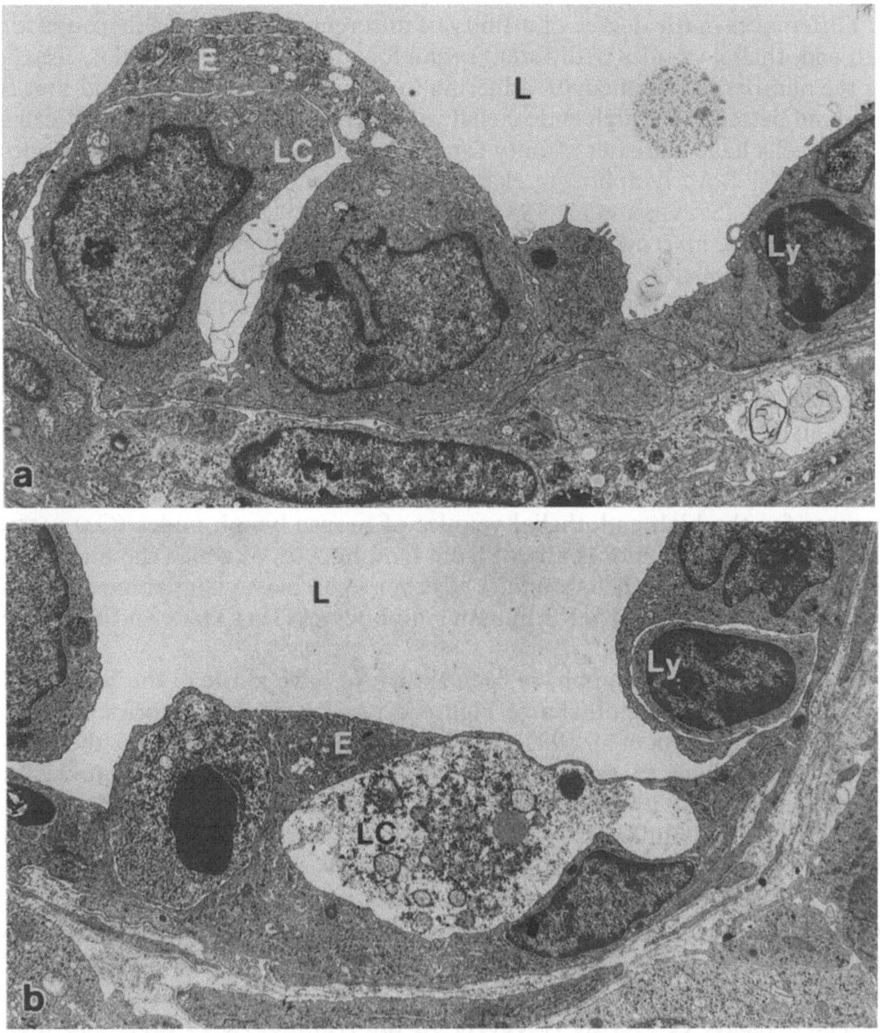

Fig. 9 a, b. Postcapillary venule of a rat with acute myelogenous leukemia (Shay). Leukemia cells (*LC*) as well as remnants of leukemia cells are present in the cytoplasm of the endothelium (*E*). Lymphocytes (*Ly*) are in transmural passage through the endothelium. *L*, lumen. ×4000

from thymus and bone marrow failed to bind to these venules in vitro. BUTCHER et al. (1979), using a modification of the Stamper-Woodruff model, showed that the affinity of lymphocytes to the high endothelial venules correlates to a high degree with the adherence of lymphocytes to high endothelial venules in vivo. The in vitro model gave rise to a series of studies further defining the specific interactions between lymphocytes and high endothelial venules and determining the affinities of functionally different sets of lymphocytes for high endothelial venules at different sites.

Differences in the degree of affinity of different lymphocyte subgroups for high endothelial venules in different organ locations were evaluated by assaying the number of lymphocytes adhering to these venules. It was found that B cells bind better to the high endothelial venules of Peyer's patches than T cells, while T cells have a greater affinity for the venules or peripheral lymph nodes than B cells. Both lymphocyte classes bind in equal measure to mesenteric lymph nodes (Stevens et al. 1982; Kraal et al. 1983). The low degree of binding of bone marrow and thymus lymphocytes to high endothelial venules described by Stamper and Woodruff (1976) was confirmed (Butcher et al. 1979). Activation of blast cells generally appears to depress the ability of these lymphocytes to bind to high endothelial venules (Daily et al. 1982). It is thus clear that specific lymphocyte surface receptors regulate the attachment of lymphocytes to the endothelium of postcapillary venules of different lymphatic organs and determine the interorgan distribution of the lymphocyte subtypes.

A monoclonal antibody has been described that recognizes a lymphocyte receptor for the high endothelial venules of mouse lymph nodes (Gallatin et al. 1983). This receptor is absent from lymphocytes of which the binding is restricted to high endothelial venules of Peyer's patches. A similar monoclonal antibody has been reported for human lymphocytes (Jalkanan and Butcher 1985).

Carbohydrate receptors have been shown to have a role in the binding of lymphocytes to the endothelia of high endothelial venules (Stoolman et al. 1984, 1987; Yednock et al. 1987a, b). Mannose-6-phosphate blocks the binding of lymphocytes to postcapillary venules of peripheral lymph nodes of rodents and humans and also binds to the endothelial surface of these venules. Apparently, the lymphocyte receptor behaves as a lectin in the binding of lymphocytes to the surfaces of high endothelial venules. This is in agreement with the observation that neuraminidase treatment prohibits lymphocyte attachment to the high endothelial venules of peripheral lymph nodes (Rosen et al. 1985). This carbohydrate receptor is probably identical to the receptors detected by monoclonal antibodies.

The presence of specific receptors on the lymphocyte surfaces and their being a part of the recognition system directing the movement of lymphocytes and their distribution to the various major lymphatic organs requires the presence of an appropriate tissue-specific ligand at the adluminal surface of the high endothelial venules. Such ligands have been identified on the postcapillary venules of the mucosal lymphatic tissue by means of monoclonal antibodies against high endothelial venules (Streeter et al. 1988a). They have also been reported to exist in the high endothelial venules of peripheral lymph node (Streeter et al. 1988b). The antibody that identifies the presence of such tissue-specific ligands on the high endothelial venules of peripheral lymph node also shows their presence in the abluminal territory of the high endothelial venules in Peyer's patches. It has been suggested that the function of these determinants at the abluminal perivascular areas may effect selective control of the transmural passage.

7 The Locomotor Force

The attachment of lymphocytes to the postcapillary venule endothelium is the first phase of the transmural passage of lymphocytes to the lymphatic parenchyma and determines its specificity. This is followed by the penetration of the lymphocytes into the endothelium, an event which per se is different from the lymphocyte-endothelial attachment at the lumen. It is worth considering that the transcellular movement by itself may well be initiated and effected by a lymphocyte–endothelial interaction different from that occurring during the attachment phase. The apposition of the plasmalemmas of the attached and subsequently migrating blood cell and the high endothelial cell is characterized by the presence of gap junctions (CAMPBELL 1983), which are generally held to be sites of intercellular communication. Gap junctions with intercellular bridges resembling conexons have been found at other sites of transcellular movement through endothelium (DE BRUYN et al. 1989). Transcellular movement does not require active locomotory properties of the cells in passage. Red blood cells which have no ability to move migrate in a transcellular fashion through endothelium (DE BRUYN et al. 1971; BECKER and DE BRUYN 1976). The transcellular transport of the lymphocyte might perhaps be described as follows: The lymphocyte, once attached to the endothelial surface, is transported through the endothelial cell body by an active change in the configuration of the internal cytoplasmic mass of the endothelial cell. Once the extraendothelial site is reached, the factors effecting the attachment to the endothelial cell cease to be operative and continuing changes in the endothelial cytoplasmic mass move the lymphocyte into the extracellular space. The transendothelial transport would thus not require locomotory activity by the transcellularly moving cell. It does require an intercellular interaction (or unilateral action), possibly mediated through the communicating gap junctions.

Acknowledgment. The research by the authors reported here has been supported by USPHS CA 05493.

References

Anderson AO, Anderson ND (1976) Lymphocyte emigration from high endothelial venules in rat lymph nodes. Immunology 31:731–747

Anderson ND, Anderson AO, Wyllie RR (1976) Specialized structure and metabolic activities of high endothelial venules in rat lymphatic tissues. Immunology 31:455–473

Bankston PW, Pino RM (1980) The development of the sinusoids of fetal rat liver: morphology of endothelial cells, Kupffer cells and transmural migration of blood cells into the sinusoids. Am J Anat 159:1–15

Becker RP, De Bruyn PPH (1976) The transmural passage of blood cells into myeloid sinusoids and the entry of platelets into the sinusoidal circulation; a scanning electron microscope investigation. Am J Anat 145:183–206

Bunting CH, Huston J (1921) Fate of lymphocyte. J Exp Med 23:593–600

Butcher EC, Scolley RG, Weissman IL (1979) Lymphocyte adherence to high endothelial venules: characterization of a modified in vitro assay, and examination of the binding of syngeneic and allogeneic lymphocyte populations. J Immunol 123:1996–2003
Campbell FR (1983) Intercellular contacts of lymphocytes during migration across high-endothelial venules of lymph nodes. An electron microscopic study. Anat Rec 207:643–652
Cho Y, De Bruyn PPH (1978) Destruction of circulating leukemia cells by phagocytosis in rats with myelogenous leukemia. J Natl Cancer Inst 60:185–195
Cho Y, De Bruyn PPH (1979) The endothelial structure of the postcapillary venules of lymph node and the passage of lymphocytes across the venule wall. J Ultrastruct Res 69:13–21
Cho Y, De Bruyn PPH (1981) Transcellular migration of lymphocytes through the walls of the smooth-surfaced squamous endothelial venules in the lymph node: evidence for the direct entry of lymphocytes into the blood circulation of the lymph node. J Ultrastruct Res 74:259–266
Cho Y, De Bruyn PPH (1986) Internal structure of the postcapillary high-endothelial venules of rodent lymph nodes and Peyer's patches and the transendothelial lymphocyte passage. Am J Anat 177:481–490
Claesson MH, Jorgensen O, Ropke C (1971) Light and electron microscopic studies of the paracortical post-capillary high-endothelial venules. Zellforschung 119:195–207
Daily MO, Fathman CG, Butcher EC, Pillemer F, Weissman IL (1982) Abnormal migration of T lymphocyte clones. J Immunol 128:2134–2136
De Bruyn PPH (1983) Transcellular cell movement and the formation of metastases. Perspect Biol Med 26:441–450
De Bruyn PPH, Cho Y (1979) The entry into the circulation of metastatic malignant cells from a subcutaneously growing tumor. J Natl Cancer Inst 62:1221–1227
De Bruyn PPH, Cho Y (1982) Vascular endothelial invasion via transcellular passage by malignant cells in the primary stage of metastasis formation. J Ultrastruct Res 81:189–201
De Bruyn PPH, Robertson RC, Farr RS (1950) In vivo affinity of diaminoacridines for nuclei. Anat Rec 108:279–308
De Bruyn PPH, Michelson S, Thomas TB (1971) The migration of blood cells of the bone marrow through the sinusoidal wall. J Morphol 133:417–438
De Bruyn PPH, Cho Y, Michelson S (1989) Endothelial attachment and plasmalemmal apposition in the transcellular movement of intravascular leukemic cells entering the myeloid parenchyma. Am J Anat
Erf AI (1940) The disappearance of intravenously injected lymphocytes in the absence of the gastrointestinal tract. Am J Med Sci 200:1–11
Farr AG, De Bruyn PPH (1975) The mode of lymphocyte migration through postcapillary venule endothelium in lymph node. Am J Anat 143:49–92
Farr RS (1951) Experiments on the fate of the lymphocyte. Anat Rec 109:515–534
Gallatin WM, Weissman IL, Butcher EC (1983) A cell surface molecule involved in organ-specific homing of lymphocytes. Nature 304:30–34
Gowans JL, Knight EJ (1964) The route of re-circulation of lymphocytes in the rat. Proc R Soc Lond [Biol] 159:257–282
Humble JG, Jayne WH, Pulvertaft RJ (1958) Biological interaction between lymphocytes and other cells. Int Rev Cytol 7:288–294
Hummel KP (1935) The structure and development of the lymphatic tissue in the intestine of the albino rat. Am J Anat 57:351–383
Jalkanen ST, Butcher EC (1985) In vitro analysis of the homing properties of human lymphocytes, developmental regulation of functional receptors for high endothelial venules. Blood 66:577–582
Kraal G, Weissman IL, Butcher EC (1983) Differences in in vivo distribution and homing of T cell subsets to mucosal vs non-mucosal lymphoid organs. J Immunol 1330:1097–1102
Kruger G (1968) Morphology of postcapillary venules under different experimental conditions. J Natl Cancer Inst 41:287–301
Marchesi VT, Gowans JL (1964) The migration of lymphocytes through the endothelium of venules in lymph nodes: an electron microscope study. Proc R Soc Lond [Biol] 159:283–290
Mikita A, Nikki R (1971) Permeability of postcapillary venules of the lymph node. An electron microscopic study. Exp Mol Pathol 14:289–305

Rosen SD, Singer MS, Yednock TA, Stoolman LM (1985) Involvement of sialic acid on endothelial cells in organ specific lymphocyte circulation. Science 228:1005–1007

Schoefl GI (1972) The migration of lymphocytes across the vascular endothelium in lymphoid tissue. J Exp Med 136:568–584

Schultze W (1925) Untersuchungen über die Capillaren und postcapillaren Venen lymphatischer Organe. Gesamte Anat 76:421–462

Sjovall H (1936) Experimentelle Untersuchungen über das Blut und die blutbildenden Organe – besonders das lymphatische Gewebe des Kaninchens bei wiederholten Aderlassen. Hakan Ohlssons Boktryckeri Lund

Stamper HB, Woodruff JJ (1976) Lymphocyte homing into lymph nodes: in vitro demonstration of the selective affinity of recirculating lymphocytes for high endothelial venules. J Exp Med 144:828–833

Stevens SK, Weissman IL, Butcher EC (1982) Differences in the migration of B and T lymphocytes, organ selectivity and the role of lymphocyte-endothelial cell recognition. J Immunol 128:844–851

Stoolman LM, Tendorde TS, Rosen SD (1984) Phosphomannosyl receptors may participate in the adhesive interaction between lymphocytes and high endothelial venules. J Cell Biol 99:1535–1540

Stoolman LM, Yednock TA, Rosen SD (1987) Homing receptors on human and rodent lymphocytes – evidence for a conserved carbohydrate-binding specificity. Blood 70:1842–1850

Streeter PR, Berg EL, Rouse BTN, Bargatze RF, Butcher EC (1988 a) A tissue-specific endothelial cell molecule involved in lymphocyte homing. Nature 331:41–46

Streeter PR, Rouse BTN, Butcher EC (1988 b) Immunohistologic and functional characterization of a vascular addressin involved in lymphocyte homing into peripheral lymph nodes. J Cell Biol 107:1853–1862

Thome R (1898) Endothelien als Phagocyten (auf den Lymphdrüsen von *Macacus cynomolgus*). Arch Mikrosk Anat 52:820–841

Umetani Y (1977) Postcapillary venule in rabbit tonsil and entry of lymphocytes into its endothelium. A scanning and transmission electron microscope study. Arch Histol Jpn 40:77–94

von Schumacher S (1899) Ueber Phagocytose und die Abfuhrwege der Leucocyten in den Lymphdrüsen. Arch Mikrosk Anat Entwickl Gesch 54:311–328

Wenk EJ, Orlic D, Reich EL, Rhodin JAG (1974) The ultrastructure of mouse lymph node venules and the passage of lymphocytes across their walls. J Ultrastruct Res 47:214–241

Yamaguchi K, Schoefl GI (1983) Blood vessels of the Peyer's patch in the mouse: III. High endothelial venules. Anat Rec 206:419–438

Yednock TA, Butcher EC, Stoolman LM, Rosen SD (1987 a) Lymphocyte homing receptors: relationships between the MEL-14 antigen and a carbohydrate receptor. J Cell Biol 104:725–734

Yednock TA, Stoolman LM, Rosen SD (1987 b) Phosphomannosyl derivatized beads detect a receptor involved in lymphocyte homing. J Cell Biol 1104:713–723

Yoffey J, Courtice F (1956) Lymphatics, lymph and lymphoid tissue. Harvard Press, Cambridge, Mass.

Zimmermann KW (1923) Der feinere Bau der Blutcapillaren. Z Anat Entwicklungsgesch 68:29–109

Rosen SD, Singer MS, Yednock TA, Stoolman LM (1985) Involvement of sialic acid on endothelial cells in organ-specific lymphocyte recirculation. Science 228:1005–1007
Schoefl GI (1972) The migration of lymphocytes across the vascular endothelium in lymphoid tissue. J Exp Med 136:568–588
Schulze E (1925) Untersuchungen über die Kapillaren und postkapillaren Venen lymphatischer Organe. Z Anat Entwickl Gesch 76:421–462
[illegible]

Germinal Center Reaction and B Lymphocytes: Morphology and Function

F. G. M. KROESE, W. TIMENS, and P. NIEUWENHUIS

1 Introduction

In peripheral lymphoid organs, B and T cells are predominantly, but not exclusively, located in different anatomical compartments: B cells are mainly observed in lymphoid follicles, whereas T cells constitute the so-called paracortical areas and interfollicular areas (e.g., lymph node and tonsil) or periarteriolar lymphocyte sheath (PALS) (spleen). In the spleen, but not in other lymphoid organs, an additional B-cell compartment associated with B-cell follicles can be found, i.e., the marginal zone. Marginal zone B cells are different from follicular B cells in several ways (e.g., phenotype, function, development), and it has been speculated that these B cells represent a distinct B-cell lineage (MACLENNAN et al. 1982).

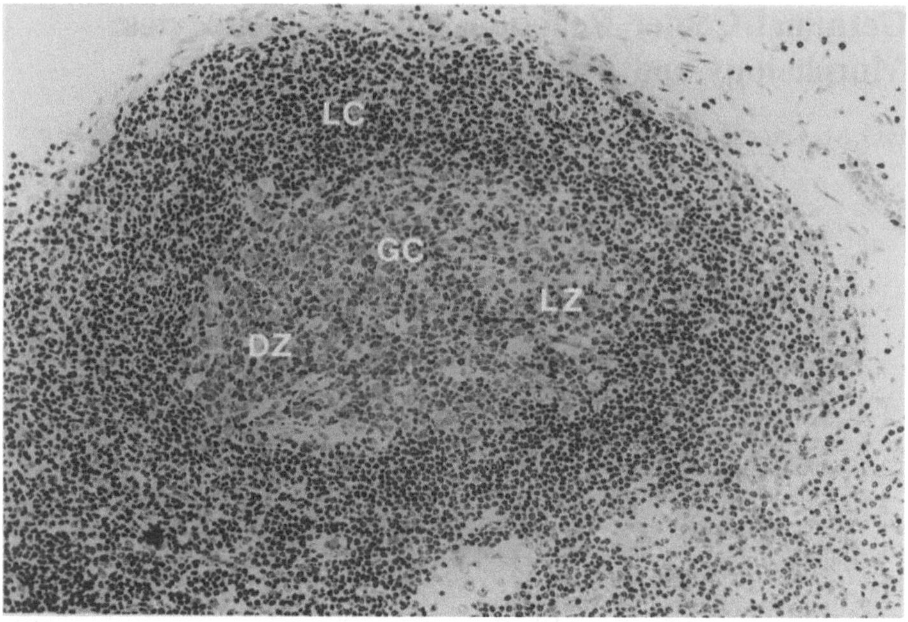

Fig. 1. Plastic (methyl methacrylate) section of a human lymph node stained with hematoxylin and eosin, showing a well-developed germinal center (*GC*) composed of a dark zone (*DZ*, centroblasts) and a light zone (*LZ*, centrocytes). The germinal center is surrounded by the lymphocyte corona (*LC*), composed of small B cells. × 140

After antigenic stimulation lymphoid organs undergo characteristic changes in their morphological appearance, depending upon the type of antigenic stimulation. One such pronounced feature often found in reactive peripheral lymphoid organs is the presence of large accumulations of actively dividing B-cell blasts in the center of the lymphoid follicles. These structures are called "germinal centers" and are surrounded by small follicular B cells constituting the lymphocyte corona or mantle zone (Figs. 1, 2).

Reviews on this subject from our group have appeared previously (Nieuwenhuis and Lennert 1980; Nieuwenhuis 1981; Nieuwenhuis and Opstelten 1984); the reader is referred to these papers especially for an overview of the history of germinal centers. The present chapter deals with an update on these structures and their possible function(s) in B cell related immunity.

Germinal centers are not exclusively found in lymph nodes but are structures that can be present in any peripheral lymphoid organ (Figs. 1, 2). To our knowledge, no fundamental differences are known to exist between germinal centers in lymph nodes and germinal centers in other peripheral lymphoid organs. Since many of the (experimental) data on germinal centers are from other lymphoid organs, we do not confine this review to germinal centers as found in lymph nodes only, but rather discuss them in a more general way, referring to germinal centers in other lymphoid organs as well in the explicit assumption that these data are also relevant for lymph node germinal centers.

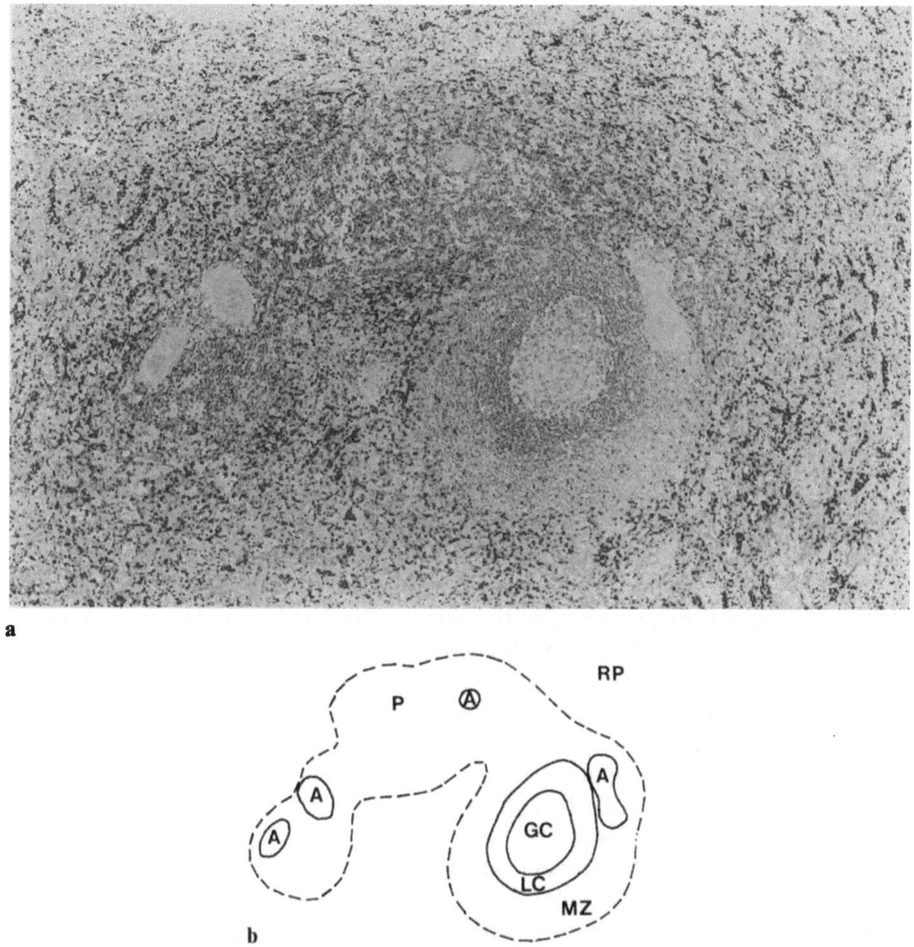

Fig. 2. a Giemsa-stained plastic (methyl methacrylate) section of a human spleen showing all lymphoid compartments, including a well-developed germinal center in a lymphoid follicle. **b** Schematic representation of the splenic lymphocyte compartments shown in **a**. *RP*, red pulp; *GC*, germinal center; *LC*, lymphocyte corona; *MZ*, marginal zone; *P*, periarteriolar lymphocyte sheath; *A*, arteriole. × 55. (From TIMENS and POPPEMA 1985; with permission of The American Journal of Anatomy

2 Germinal Centers and the B-Cell Immune Response

B cells can respond to antigen in two (different) ways (Fig. 3): (a) by the plasmacellular reaction and (b) by the germinal center reaction. In the plasmacellular reaction B lymphocytes proliferate to clones and differentiate into plasmablasts and plasma cells, secreting specific antibodies of various isotypes (for review see VAN ROOIJEN et al. 1986). In peripheral lymphoid organs, e.g.,

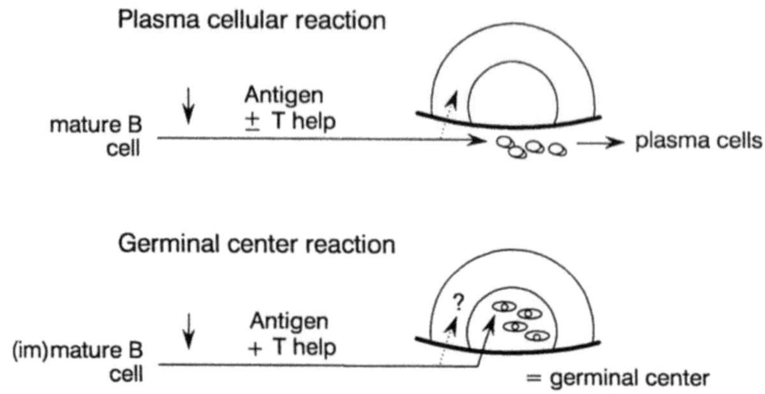

Fig. 3. In vivo responses of B cells to antigen (for explanation see text). The *dotted line* shows the normal migration pathway of the B cells

the spleen of rodents, upon antigenic stimulation the first cells containing high concentrations of immunoglobulin (Ig) are found by 2–3 days after primary immunization in the outer parts of the splenic T cell area, the PALS. To a lesser extent they can also be found in the lymphoid follicles. Somewhat later these cells are located around the terminal arterioles and eventually in the splenic red pulp. Elegant studies by VAN ROOIJEN and co-workers (as reviewed by VAN ROOIJEN et al. 1986) demonstrated clearly that these Ig-containing cells are specific for the stimulating antigen and they postulated that there is one final common "differentiation pathway" of B cells for both thymus-dependent and thymus-independent antigens.

During the second B-cell reaction to antigen, the so-called germinal center reaction, large clusters of B-cell blasts (intermediate to large cells) develop within the primary follicles of a peripheral lymphoid organ. For a detailed description of the germinal center reaction as seen in conventional histological sections the reader is referred to other review articles (e.g., NIEUWENHUIS and LENNERT 1980; STEIN et al. 1982). The first signs of germinal center formation as seen in histological sections occur 3–4 days after exposure to antigen, when a small group of pyroninophilic blast cells (centroblasts) appear centrally in primary follicles. Over the following days these clusters increase in size and many mitotic figures are seen. By day 5, a special type of macrophage, the "tingible body" macrophage, can be observed within the newly formed germinal center, resulting in a typical "starry sky" appearance. By day 7 medium-sized cells (centrocytes) start to develop within the germinal center, leading to the demarcation of two zones (Fig. 1): the dark zone consisting of actively dividing pyroninophilic centroblasts making up the lower part of the germinal center, and the light zone consisting of the smaller, less pyroninophilic centrocytes in the upper half. This picture of a germinal center remains the same for at least 2–3 weeks after antigenic stimulation. If there is no new antigenic stimulus the germinal center reaction stops and these structures will disappear.

3 Cells Observed Within a Germinal Center

Germinal centers are predominantly composed of B cells. However, in a typical well-developed germinal center other cell types are found as well, including T cells and at least two types of nonlymphoid cell, i.e., follicular dendritic cells and macrophages. In this section these four cell types will be considered in detail.

3.1 Germinal Center B Cells

In Table 1 the phenotype of germinal center B cells is compared with that of lymphocytes from the lymphocyte corona and splenic marginal zone (see also Fig. 2). The vast majority of germinal center B cells express Ig on their cell membrane (HOFFMAN-FEZER et al. 1976, 1981; STEIN et al. 1980; BHAN et al. 1981; BAILEY et al. 1982; OPSTELTEN et al. 1982, 1983; BUTCHER et al. 1982; KRAAL et al. 1982). In tissue sections this Ig is, however, difficult to detect due to the presence of immune complexes retained on the follicular dendritic cells (see below; Figs. 4, 5). Furthermore, the amount of Ig on the surface (sIg) of germinal center B cells is low. For example, flow cytometrical (fluorescence-activated cell sorter, FACS) analysis of cell suspensions prepared from mouse Peyer's patches showed that the modal fluorescence of germinal center cells stained for sIg is only 10%–15% of that of the small B cells from the lymphocyte corona (BUTCHER et al. 1982).

Germinal center cells may express sIgM, sIgG, or sIgA, but they are essentially negative for sIgD: immunohistological staining of tissue sections for IgD shows an IgD-negative germinal center, surrounded by intensely stained B cells of the lymphocyte corona (Figs. 4, 5). The isotype of the sIg expressed may depend on the immunization. After primary immunization of mice, lymph node germinal center B cells predominantly express IgM, whereas after secondary immunization they mainly express IgG (KRAAL et al. 1982). Germinal center cells isolated from mucosa-associated lymphoid tissues (which are continuously stimulated), like Peyer's patches, are predominantly sIgA^{+} (BUTCHER et al. 1982). In addition to the bulk of sIg^{+} germinal center cells, a few cells within the germinal center contain cytoplasmic Ig of any of the Ig heavy chain (sub-)classes, except for IgD (STEIN et al. 1980; BHAN et al. 1981; SMINIA and JANSE 1982; EIKELENBOOM et al. 1982). This Ig may be specific for the antigen that induced the germinal center reaction (SORDAT et al. 1970; TERASHIMA et al. 1977).

The B-cell nature of germinal center cells is further shown by their reactivity with monoclonal antibodies (mAbs) to pan-B lineage specific determinants such as CD19, CD20, and CD22 in man (e.g., BHAN et al. 1981; TIMENS and POPPEMA 1985). Germinal center cells also react with antibodies directed to the B-cell form(s) of the leukocyte common antigen (CD45R) as observed in man (POPPEMA et al. 1987), mice (BUTCHER et al. 1982), and rats (KROESE et al.

Table 1. Antigenic expression of lymphocyte compartments in human spleen

Monoclonal antibody[a]	Cluster of differentiation	PALS	Lymphocyte corona	Germinal centers	Marginal zone
Leu-6	CD1	–	–	–	–
Leu-5	CD2	++++	–	+	+
Leu-4	CD3	++++	–	+	+
Leu-3a	CD4	+++	–	+	+
Leu-1	CD5	++++	sp	+	+
Leu-9	CD7	++++	sp	+	+
T8	CD8	++	–	–	sp
CALLA	CD10	–	–	[++++]	–
Leu-12	CD19	sp	++++	++++	++++
B1	CD20	sp	++++	++++	++++
B2, HB5	CD21	sp	[++++]	–	++++
Leu-14	CD22	sp	++++	++++	++++
Anti IL2R	CD25	+	–	sp	–
Anti-CR1	CD35	sp	++++	++++	++++
T10	CD38	–	–	++++	–
MT1	CD43	++++	–	–	–
LCA	CD45	++++	++++	++++	++++
MT2	CD45R	++++	++++	–	++++
MB1	CD45R	++	++++	++++	++++
Leu-7	CD57	–	–	+	–
OKT9	CD71	–	–	++++	–
LN1	CDw75	–	–	++++	–
MB2		–	++++	++++	++++
MB3/LN2		–	++++	++++	++++
LN3		–	++++	++++	++++
OKIa		–	++++	++++	++++
Ki-67		–	–	++[+]	–
Anti-IgG		–	sp	sp	+
Anti-IgA		–	sp	–	+
Anti-IgM		sp	++++	+	++++
Anti-IgD		sp	++++	–	+[+]
Anti-κ		sp	+++	+	+++
Anti-λ		sp	++	+	++

+, 0%–25%; ++, 25%–50%; +++, 50%–75%; ++++, 75%–100% positive cells; sp, sporadically a reactive cell is seen, [ ], weak reactivity

[a] B1 and B2 were a gift from Dr. L. M. Nadler and HB5 from Dr. T. Tedder (both Dana Farber Cancer Institute, Harvard Medical School, Boston, Ma), and anti-immunoglobulin antibodies from Dr. J. Haaijman (R. I. V., Rijswijk, The Netherlands. Anti IL2R and Leu antibodies were from Becton-Dickinson (Mountain View, Ca), OK antibodies from Ortho Diagnostic Systems (Raritan, NJ), CALLA, anti-HLA-ABC, anti-CR1, DAKO-PC (Ki67), and DAKO-LCA from DAKO (Glostrup, Denmark), anti-IL2R and MT, MB, and LN antibodies from Biotest (Dreieich, West Germany)

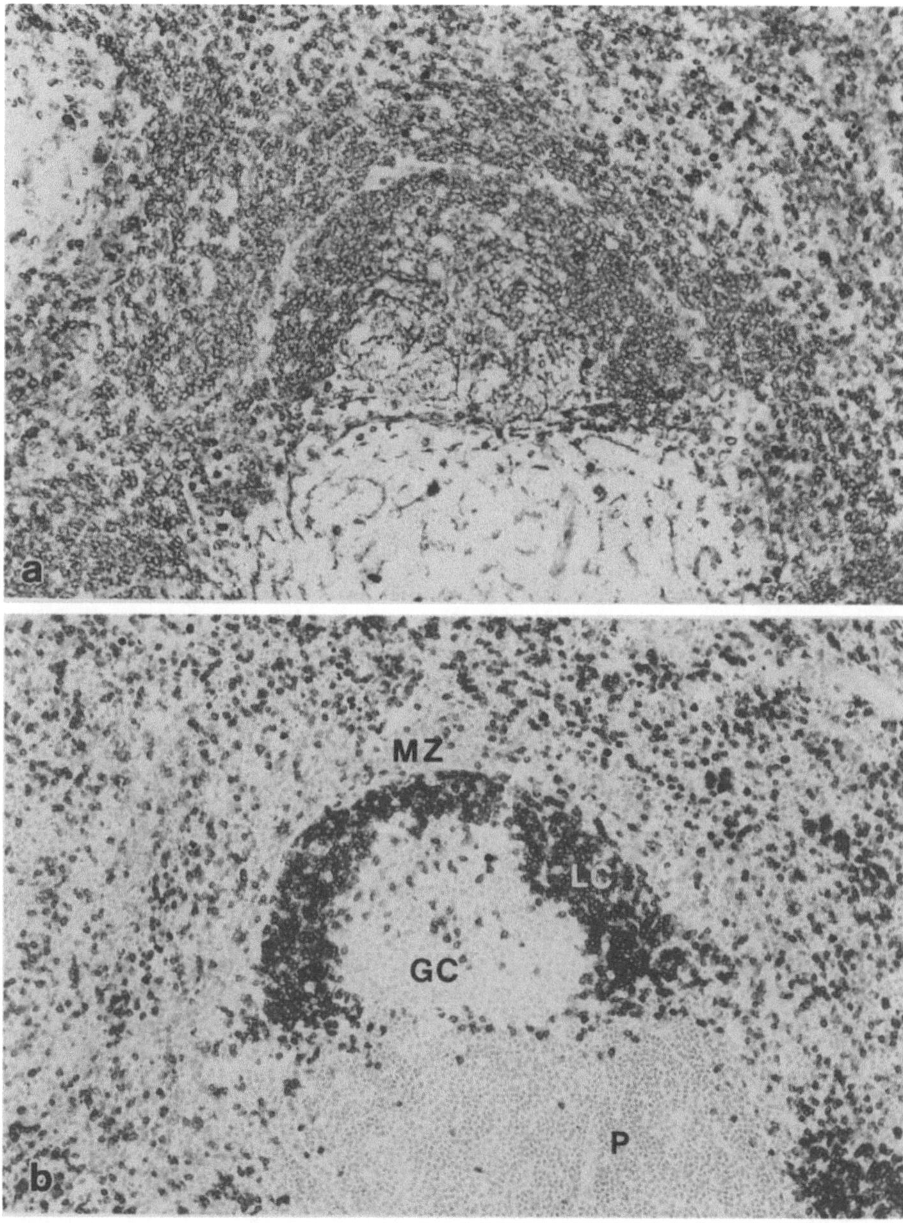

Fig. 4 a, b. Immunoperoxidase staining of serial frozen sections taken from a rat spleen, 7 days after immunization with SRBCs. Sections are stained with mAbs to **a** rat IgM or **b** rat IgD. Germinal center cells are clearly negative for IgD, whereas virtually all of the cells in the lymphocyte corona express high levels of IgM and IgD. The vast majority of marginal zone B cells express only very low amounts of IgD, but much IgM. Within the germinal center a dendritic staining pattern is seen with anti-IgM, due to immune complexes bound to FDCs. *GC*, germinal center; *LC*, lymphocyte corona; *MZ*, marginal zone; *P*, periarteriolar lymphocyte sheath. ×160

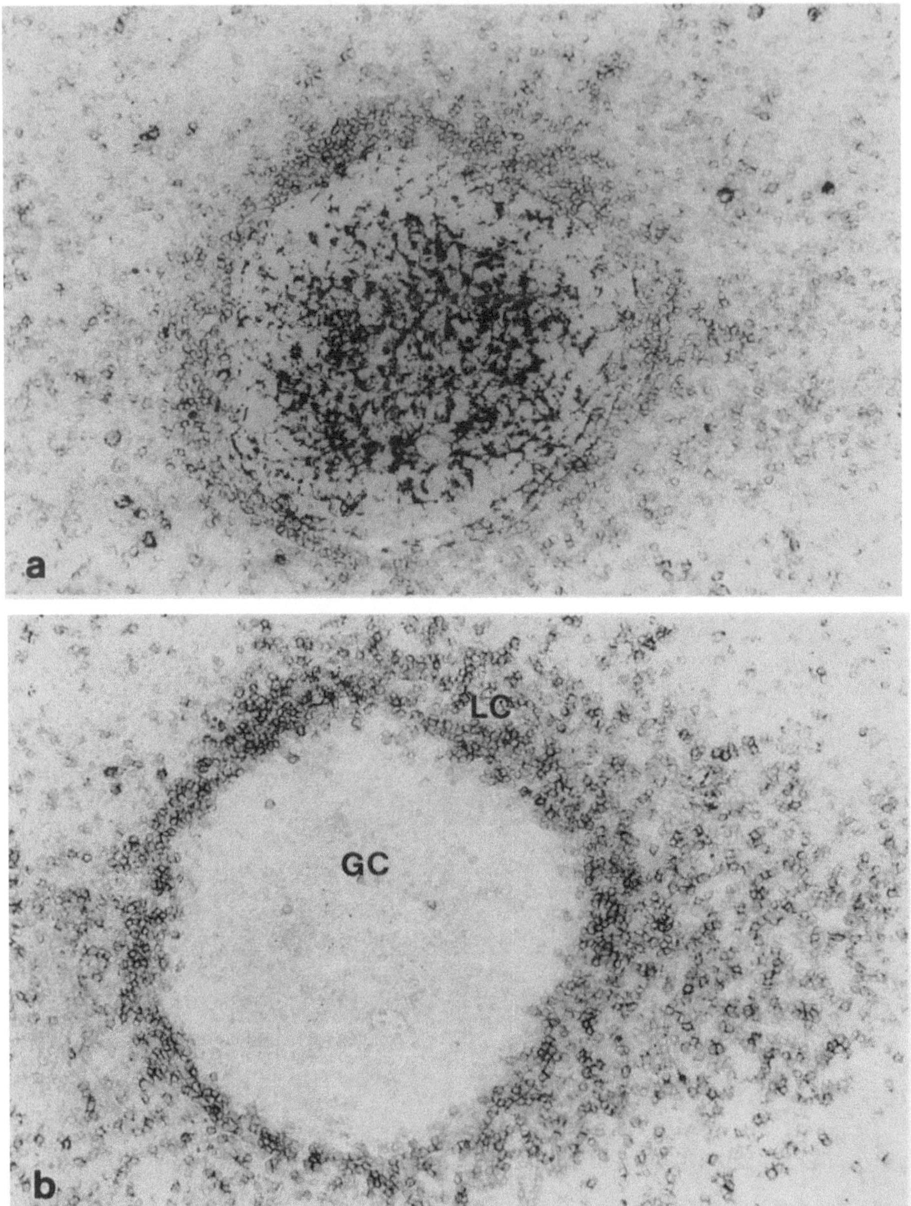

Fig. 5 a, b. Serial frozen sections taken from a human lymph node stained for **a** IgM and **b** IgD by immunoperoxidase. Germinal center cells are negative for IgD and almost all corona lymphocytes are positive for both IgM and IgD. In the germinal center intense dendritic staining is seen with anti-IgM, caused by localized immune complexes. *GC*, germinal center; *LC*, lymphocyte corona. ×140

1987a). In rats, germinal center B cells seem to express a unique set of B cell associated forms of the leukocyte common antigen (KROESE et al. 1987a).

Germinal center B cells react with antibodies specific for activated B cells, such as determinants recognized by the mAbs B-LAST 1 (THORLEY-LAWSON et al. 1982), B5 (FREEDMAN et al. 1985), and OKT10 (CD38) (TIMENS and POPPEMA 1985). Furthermore, germinal center B cells (but not B cells in the lymphocyte corona) weakly express the transferrin receptor (CD71) (MURRAY et al. 1984).

Germinal center cells also express determinants shared with other (non-B) cell types, like class I and II antigens of the major histocompatibility complex (MHC) and receptors for the Fc part of Ig and for the complement fragment C3b (CD35) (SEYMOUR et al. 1980; STEIN et al. 1980; TSUNODA et al. 1980; BARCLAY 1981; BHAN et al. 1981; BUTCHER et al. 1982; MAYRHOFER et al. 1983).

Although so far no mAb specific for germinal center B cells has been found, LN-1 (CDw75) almost exclusively labels human germinal center cells and no other (resting) B (or T) cells (EPSTEIN et al. 1984). In man and mice (but not in rats), the lectin peanut agglutinin (PNA) binds almost exclusively to germinal center cells (ROSE et al. 1980; ROSE and MALCHIODI 1981), allowing easy identification, isolation, and purification of germinal center B cells. The functional meaning (if any) of the intense binding capacity for PNA in certain species is not known; possibly it reflects the nonmigratory status of germinal center B cells (BUTCHER et al. 1982; REICHERT et al. 1983) or a relative immaturity (RAEDLER et al. 1981). The inability of germinal center B cells to migrate is also suggested by the absence of putative homing receptors for high endothelial venules on their cell membrane as recognized by the mAbs Hermes-1 and -3 (JALKANEN et al. 1986) and by MEL-14 in mice (REICHERT et al. 1983). These receptors are essential molecules involved in the homing of lymphocytes and other leukocytes to lymphoid organs through high endothelial venules.

3.2 Germinal Center T Cells

T cells are found in lymphoid follicles, including their germinal centers, as was first described by GUTMAN and WEISSMAN (1972) by immunohistological staining of murine lymph nodes with polyclonal anti-T-cell antisera. These observations have been confirmed and extended for mice, man, and rat, using mAbs to T-cell (sub-)populations (Figs. 6, 7) (WEISSMAN et al. 1976; HOFFMAN-FEZER et al. 1976, 1981; POPPEMA et al. 1981; BAILEY et al. 1982; ROUSE et al. 1982; KROESE et al. 1985a). Most of the T cells are located in the germinal center light zone (centrocytes); only a small number are found in the germinal center dark zone (centroblasts).

Analysis of the phenotype of T cells that are found within the germinal center clearly demonstrated a predominance of the $CD4^+$ T cells ("T helper cells") in all species investigated (Figs. 6, 7) (POPPEMA et al. 1981; BHAN et al. 1981; BAILEY et al. 1982; ROUSE et al. 1982; KROESE et al. 1985a; TIMENS and

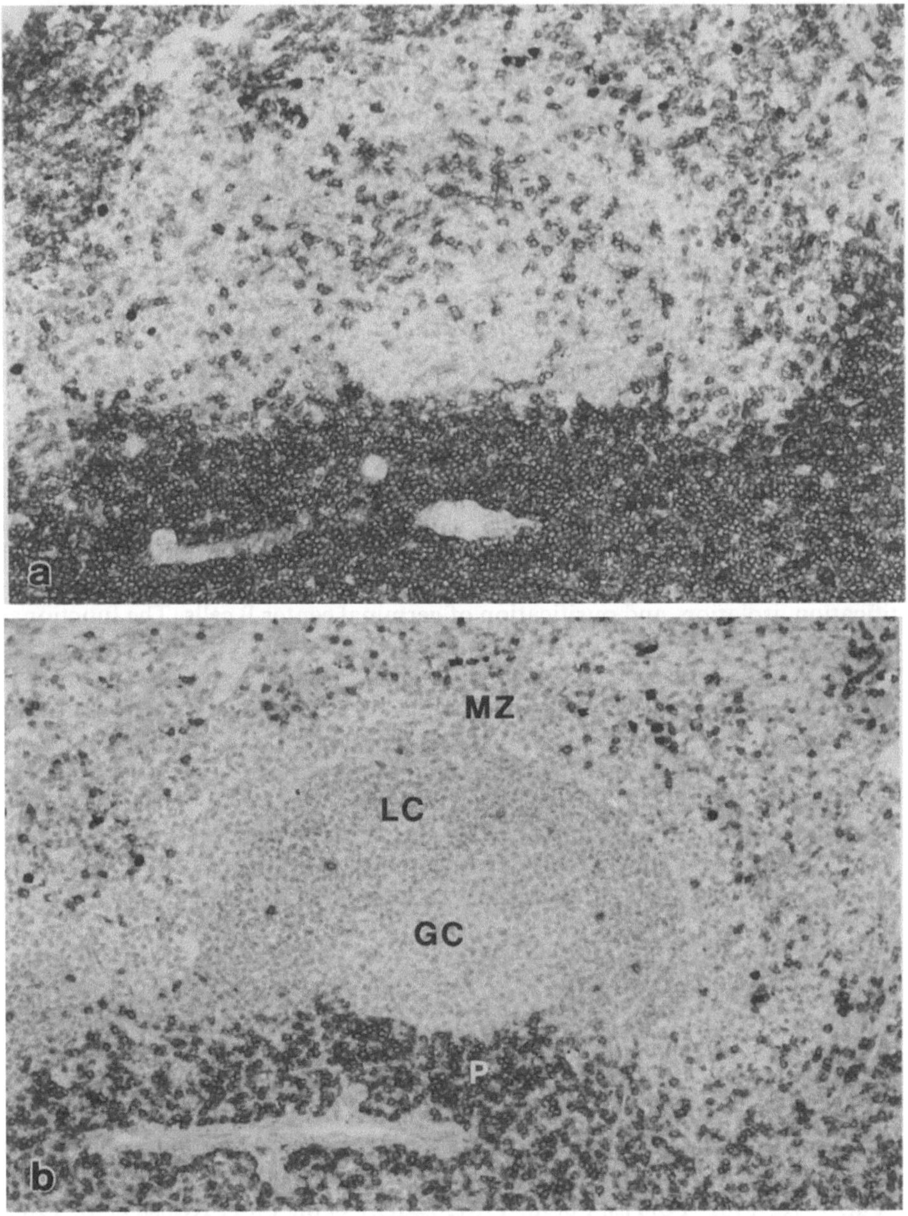

Fig. 6 a, b. Immunoperoxidase staining of spleen sections from an immunized rat using **a** anti-CD4 and **b** anti-CD8. The vast majority of T cells in the germinal center and lymphocyte corona are $CD4^+CD8^-$ cells. *GC*, germinal center; *LC*, lymphocyte corona; *MZ*, marginal zone; *P*, periarteriolar lymphocyte sheath. (From KROESE et al. 1985 a; with permission of Plenum Press, New York). ×160

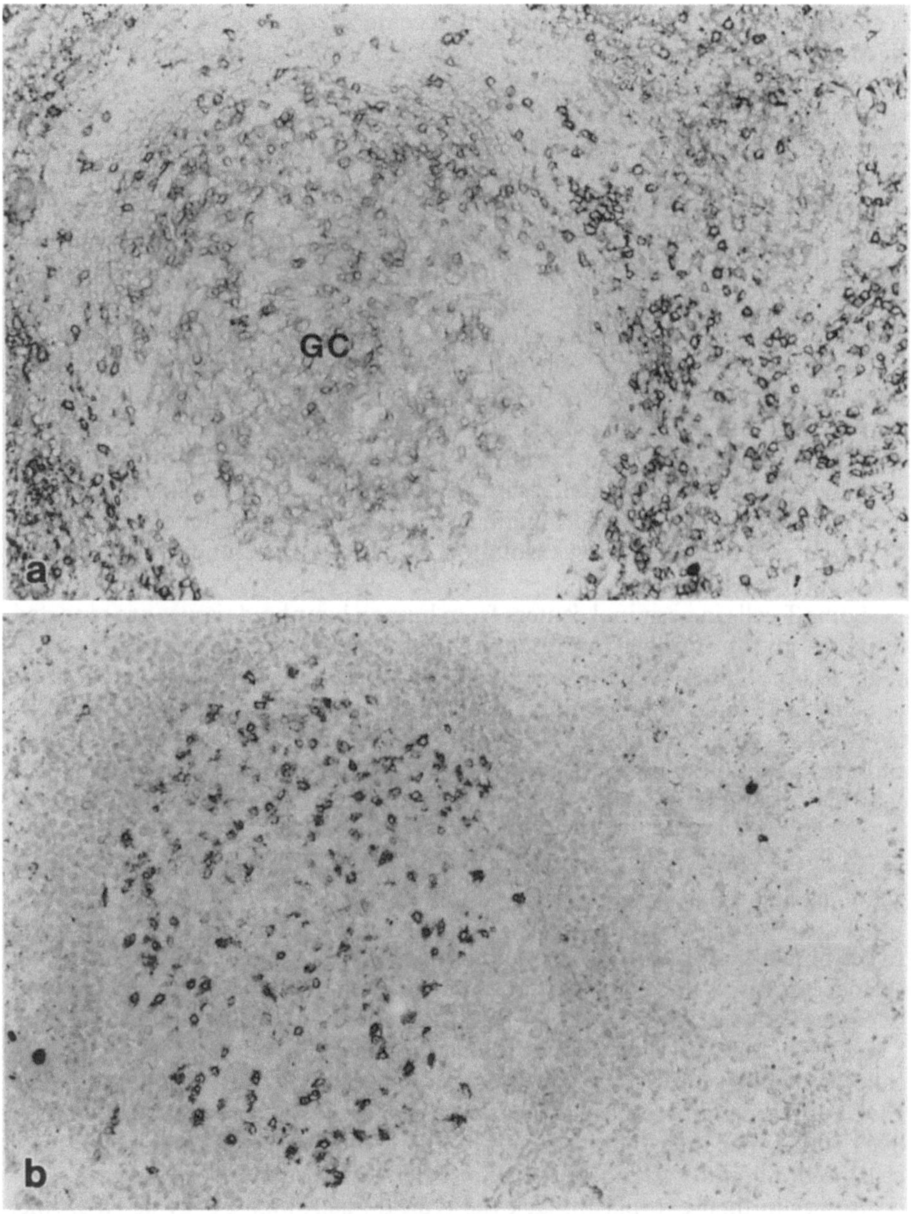

Fig. 7 a, b. Frozen sections from a human spleen stained by immunoperoxidase with **a** anti-CD4 and **b** CD57. These sections demonstrate that most human germinal center (*GC*) T cells are $CD4^+$ cells that coexpress the Leu-7 determinant. ×140

POPPEMA 1985). For example, in germinal centers from lymph nodes in immunized mice the ratio of $CD4^+$ to $CD8^+$ T cells is 12:1 (ROUSE et al. 1982). In the T-cell areas this ratio is approximately 2:1.

In man, a large proportion of the ($CD4^+$) T cells found within a germinal center express the determinant recognized by Leu-7 (CD57) (Fig. 7) (BANERJEE and THIBERT 1983; POPPEMA et al. 1983; PORWIT-KSIAZEK et al. 1983; PIZZOLO et al. 1984). This determinant is also expressed on killer cells and on natural killer cells (ABO and BALCH 1981), but its function is not clear. Furthermore, Leu-8, a determinant normally expressed by small (resting) B and T cells, is absent from human germinal center B and T cells (KANSAS et al. 1985). In rats, the majority of ($CD4^+$) T cells in follicles, including germinal centers, express a determinant recognized by the mAb ER3 (KROESE et al. 1985a). In suspensions from lymph nodes, this mAb detects all $CD8^+$ cells but only a low proportion (5%) of $CD4^+$ cells (JOLING et al. 1985). Thus, most T cells found in germinal centers seem to constitute a particular subpopulation of $CD4^+$ cells, by virtue of their reactivity with Leu-7 but not with Leu-8 in man and by their expression of ER3-determinant in rats. The specific phenotype of these T cells in rats and man allows isolation of these cells to study their possible function(s) in vitro.

Some T cells in germinal centers from human lymphoid tissues are reported to express the Tac antigen (representing the interleukin-2 receptor) (MIYAWAKI et al. 1984). This may indicate that these T cells are in an activated state, possibly instrumental in germinal center B-cell activation. Like germinal center B cells, the germinal center T cells also lack homing receptors for high endothelial venules (JALKANEN et al. 1986), suggesting that germinal center T cells too, are nonmigratory and do not belong to the recirculating pool of T cells.

3.3 Follicular Dendritic Cells

In germinal centers a special nonlymphoid cell type is observed which has long slender processes that are closely intermingled with the surrounding lymphocytes (NOSSAL and ADA 1971; MANDEL et al. 1980; SCHRIEVER et al. 1989). These cells, unique for lymphoid follicles (primary as well as secondary), are called follicular dendritic cells (FDCs) or sometimes dendritic reticulum cells. FDCs differ in many respects from macrophages and other dendritic cell types, like the so-called interdigitating cells found in T-cell areas and the Langerhans cells predominantly found in the skin. FDCs are nonphagocytotic cells, lack lysosomes in their cytoplasm, lack the typical macrophage enzyme lysozyme, and do not have typical Birbeck granules in their cytoplasm. Furthermore they do not react with the vast majority of mAbs to monocytes/macrophages and dendritic cells (HUMPHREY and GRENNAN 1982; FRANKLIN et al. 1986; KOSCO et al. 1986; BUCKLEY et al. 1987; SCHRIEVER et al. 1989).

Characteristically, FDCs are able to trap and retain antigen–antibody complexes for long periods on their cell membrane (reviews by NOSSAL and ADA 1971; KLAUS et al. 1980; TEW et al. 1980; VAN ROOIJEN 1980). Binding of immune complexes on the surface of FDCs is probably complement (C3) mediated (PAPAMICHAIL et al. 1975; KLAUS and HUMPHREY 1977), although the Fc part of the Ig might also be involved (HERD and ADA 1969; RADOUX et al. 1985). These findings are consistent with the presence of all three receptors for the third complement component (CR1, CR2, and CR3) and of Fc receptors on the surface membrane of FDCs (GERDES and STEIN 1982; GERDES et al. 1983; HEINEN et al. 1984; 1985; SCHNIZLEIN et al. 1985; BUCKLEY et al. 1987). FDCs also express the low affinity Fc IgE receptor (CD23) (SCHRIEVER et al. 1989; GORDON et al. 1989), which not only is important for binding of IgE but also seems to be involved in B-cell regulation processes (for review see GORDON et al. 1989). This suggests a CD23-mediated role for FDCs in germinal center B-cell development. Specific mAbs directed against human and rat FDCs have been developed (R4/23 and ED5, respectively) (NAIEM et al. 1983; JEURISSEN and DIJKSTRA 1986).

Analysis of the expression of determinants on FDCs, like MHC class II antigens, that are known to be present on follicular B cells (including germinal center cells) is hardly possible because FDC staining cannot be unequivocally distinguished from the staining of surrounding B cells in immunohistology. Proper evaluation of the presence of such determinants requires isolation of FDCs or immunoelectron microscopy. Initially, HUMPHREY and GRENNAN (1982) were unable to detect MHC class II antigens on the surface of FDCs isolated from mice and rats, whereas RALFKIAER et al. (1985) failed to show these antigens on FDCs in situ in human lymph nodes. However, all other studies could demonstrate expression of MHC class II antigens by FDCs isolated from human tonsils and adenoids (GERDES et al. 1983; HEINEN et al. 1984; SCHRIEVER et al. 1989) or from murine and rat lymph nodes (SCHNIZLEIN et al. 1985; KOSCO et al. 1986). Furthermore, expression of MHC class II antigens on FDCs was demonstrated in situ by electron microscopy of lymph nodes from mice and rats (KOSCO et al. 1986). The reason for the possible discrepancy in the expression of MHC class II antigens found by different groups is not known. Apart from methodological differences and differences in organs used (spleen vs lymph nodes and tonsils), it is possible that the expression of MHC class II antigens is not permanent, but is induced after antigenic stimulation. Alternatively, FDCs themselves do not express MHC class II antigens but passively acquire these molecules, e.g., from surrounding B cells.

Scanning electron microscopy revealed two different forms of FDC: one with filiform dendrites and the other with "beaded" dendrites (SZAKAL et al. 1985). Intermediate forms are found as well, suggesting that they can transform into each other. The "beads" are coated with immune complexes and are therefore called iccosomes ("immune complex coated bodies"). Iccosomes are produced by FDCs early after secondary immunization and are endocytosed by germinal center B cells (SZAKAL et al. 1988). The role of this phenomenon in the germinal center reaction is unclear but it is suggested that germinal center B cells, upon endocytosis, process the antigen and present it on their cell membrane to (germinal center) T cells (KOSCO et al. 1988).

The origin of FDCs has not yet unequivocally been elucidated. Since human FDCs react with some mAbs directed to macrophages (GERDES et al. 1983; PARWARESCH et al. 1983; HEINEN et al. 1984; FRANKLIN et al. 1986), these authors speculate that FDCs may originate from monocytes/macrophages. Expression of the leukocyte common antigen (CD45) (a marker for most hemopoietic cells) by human and mouse FDCs (KOSCO et al. 1986; RALFKIAER et al. 1985; SCHNIZLEIN et al. 1985) also suggests a relationship with the hemopoietic system. However, most other data indicate that FDCs do not originate from bone marrow derived myeloid cells. First, as noted before, FDCs are totally different from macrophages in many respects, including phenotype and function. Second, in contrast with the above-mentioned findings recent data on isolated and highly purified human FDCs or FDCs in situ indicate that these cells do not express CD45 (SCHRIEVER et al. 1989; TIMENS, unpublished observations). Finally, transfer experiments of bone marrow cells to lethally X-irradiated recipient mice show that in these bone marrow chimeras, even one year after transfer, FDCs are not derived from transferred bone marrow cells (HUMPHREY et al. 1984), and thus may not be derived from stem cells in the bone marrow. In these experiments, however, the possibility cannot be excluded that FDCs are very long lived cells, with extremely low turnover rates. Indeed, it is known that FDCs are relatively radioresistant (HUNTER et al. 1969; NETTESHEIM and HANNA 1969; BROWN et al. 1973; KROESE et al. 1986). The data thus suggest that FDCs are not related to bone marrow derived monocytes/macrophages. The presence of transitional forms between reticulum cells and FDCs during the postnatal development of peripheral lymphoid organs of rodents (GROSCURTH 1980; VILLENA et al. 1983; DIJKSTRA et al. 1984) and during the primary immune response in adult rats and rabbits (KAMPERDIJK et al. 1978; HEUSERMANN et al. 1980) indicates that FDCs might be related to reticulum cells.

The (ultra)structure of FDCs with their many processes extending between surrounding lymphocytes, does not make it likely that FDCs are actively migrating cells. Consistent herewith is the fact that (human) FDCs express the majority of adhesion molecules that belong to the VLA family (VLA-3,-4,-5,-6, and their common β-chain) (SCHRIEVER et al. 1989) which are involved in adhesion of cells to the extracellular matrix. While FDC lack LFA-1 (CD11 a/CD18), they express its natural ligand, ICAM-1 (DUSTIN et al. 1986; SCHRIEVER et al. 1989). As these molecules play an important role in cell–cell adhesion events, this suggests that LFA^+ cells (expressed by most lymphoid cells) may adhere to the ICAM-1^+ FDCs which is probably of significance for germinal center formation (see below).

3.4 Tingible Body Macrophages

Another nonlymphoid cell type found in germinal centers is the macrophage. These cells, which are predominantly found later on during the germinal center reaction, are responsible for the typical "starry sky" appearance of germinal centers. Most of these macrophages are characterized by the presence of many "tingible bodies" in their cytoplasm, which give them their name (tingible body macrophages, TBMs). Tingible bodies are phagolysosomes, which can also be detected by light microscopy and are probably derived from ingested centroblasts (FLIEDNER et al. 1964). These phagocytosed centroblasts seem to have died just before or at mitosis (ODARTCHENKO et al. 1967). TBMs also exhibit the characteristic phenotype of other macrophages: they contain the enzymes lysozyme, α_1-chymotrypsin, nonspecific esterase and acid phosphatase (see STEIN et al. 1982) and react, for example, with antimacrophage antibodies OKM1 (CD11b), Leu-M5 (CD11c), Leu-M2, T9 (CD71), for about 50% with Leu-M3 (CD14), and with mAb to HLA-DR (HOFMAN et al. 1984; FRANKLIN et al. 1986; BARONI et al. 1987; BUCKLEY et al. 1987). However, in man not all mAbs to macrophages also react with TBMs (BUCKLEY et al. 1987), indicating that TBMs are a distinct subpopulation of macrophages. In lymph nodes TBMs are derived from macrophages present in the afferent lymph (HOEFSMIT et al. 1980; KOTANI et al. 1982). Like other cells within the germinal centers, TBMs may have lost their migratory capacity, since they lack the microfilaments needed for this migration (HOEFSMIT et al. 1980).

4 Histophysiological Aspects of the Germinal Center Reaction

4.1 Antigen Dependency of Germinal Centers

It is well known that the development of germinal centers requires stimulation with antigen. This is well illustrated by the virtual absence of germinal centers in peripheral lymphoid organs of animals reared under germ-free conditions (e.g., THORBECKE 1959; POLLARD 1967; KIM and WATSON 1971). Furthermore, there is a close correlation between the time of antigen administration and the appearance of germinal centers in lymphoid organs and between the antigen dose and the extent of germinal center reactivity (HANNA et al. 1966). Surprisingly little, however, is known with respect to the nature of antigens that can induce a germinal center reaction. It seems that in particular T cells dependent antigens are capable of inducing a germinal center reaction; the sparse data on T cell independent antigens suggest that these antigens only poorly lead to the formation of germinal centers (WEISSMAN et al. 1976; EIKELENBOOM et al. 1982).

4.2 Germinal Center Precursor Cells

B lineage cells from which germinal centers develop directly are called germinal center precursor cells (GCPCs) (NIEUWENHUIS and LENNERT 1980; GASTKEMPER et al. 1981; NIEUWENHUIS and OPSTELTEN 1984). By definition, GCPCs transform directly into the large centroblasts. Like (most) other B cells,

GCPCs derive from precursor cells in the bone marrow: germinal centers reappear in lethally X-irradiated animals reconstituted with bone marrow cells (KOTANI et al. 1974; ROZING et al. 1978). It is currently not known whether B cells that belong to the Ly-1 (CD5) B lineage also can give rise to germinal centers. These Ly-1 B cells constitute a second lineage of B cells consisting of self-replenishing cells which in adult mice develop independently from the bone marrow (HERZENBERG et al. 1986).

With respect to the GCPCs, the question is whether precursor cells for germinal centers are different from precursor cells that are involved in the generation of plasma cells (the ultimate fate of probably every mature B cell). In other words, are GCPCs a particular subpopulation of B cells, or can any B cell give rise to germinal centers? In our department GCPCs are characterized by transfer of cells from various sources [usually thoracic duct lymphocytes (TDLs)] to lethally X-irradiated rats, immediately followed by antigenic (sheep red blood cells, SRBCs) stimulation to induce germinal center formation in recipient spleens (GASTKEMPER et al. 1981). In this assay system, phenotypically normal germinal centers can be observed in recipient spleens from 4 days after antigenic stimulation and transfer of lymphocytes (KROESE et al. 1986). Since TDLs are clearly capable of germinal center formation, it is suggested that GCPCs are – at least to some extent – recirculating cells. Using this germinal center formation assay in conjunction with panning procedures to isolate subpopulations of B cells, we are analyzing the phenotype of GCPCs. Recent experiments show that GCPCs present in thoracic duct lymph express both sIgM and sIgD; sIg^+ but not $sIgM^-$ or $sIgD^-$ cells isolated from thoracic duct lymph are unable to give rise to germinal centers in recipient spleens (SEIJEN et al. 1988). The $sIgM^+sIgD^+$ are thought to belong to the circulating B-cell pool (GRAY et al. 1982) and in situ they are predominantly located in primary follicles and the lymphocyte coronas of secondary follicles (STEIN et al. 1980; BAZIN et al. 1982; BUTCHER et al. 1982; KRAAL et al. 1982). Support for the $sIgM^+$ character of GCPCs comes from experiments in which animals are treated from birth with anti-IgM antisera. In these experiments, anti-IgM treatment totally prevents the development of germinal centers in their lymphoid organs (ENRIQUEZ-RINCON and KLAUS 1984; BAZIN et al. 1985). However, mice treated from birth with anti-IgD antibodies are still able to generate germinal centers in their lymphoid organs, although primary follicles and lymphocyte coronas are virtually absent (JACOBSON et al. 1981; FINKELMAN et al. 1983). Assuming that the anti-IgD treatment is really 100% effective in killing $sIgD^+$ cells, these findings may suggest that, essentially, GCPCs do not need to express sIgD.

4.3 T-Cell Dependency of Germinal Centers

Germinal centers are clearly T cell dependent structures. In (immunized) athymic (T-cell-less) "nude" mice and rats, and in patients with complete T-cell defects, germinal centers are virtually absent (DE SOUSA et al. 1969;

MITCHELL et al. 1972; KLAUS and KUNKL 1982; PARADINAS 1985). Furthermore, injection of nude mice with thymocytes restores the capability for germinal center formation in athymic animals (JACOBSON et al. 1974; DE SOUSA and PRITCHARD 1974). Also, lethally X-irradiated animals require reconstitution with both T and B cells for germinal centers to develop (KOTANI et al. 1974; GASTKEMPER et al. 1981). Selective depletion of $CD4^+$ or $CD8^+$ T cells in vivo by treating animals with mAbs indicates that predominantly the $CD4^+$ cells are involved in germinal center formation (ERMAK et al. 1988; SEIJEN et al., manuscript in preparation). These data are consistent with the observed predominance of $CD4^+CD8^-$ T cells in germinal centers. The unique phenotype of (human) germinal center T cells (i.e., $CD4^+CD8^-$Leu-7^+Leu-8^-) suggests a selective function. Indeed, cloned human $CD4^+$Leu-7^+ T cells seem to be unable to produce IL-2 after CD3 or PHA stimulation (VELARDI et al. 1988). Furthermore, Leu-8^- Th cells seem to be important for B-cell differentiation events whereas Leu-8^+ T cells are more important for *inducer* functions (KANSAS et al. 1985). Probably part of their function is mediated through the production and secretion of lymphokines. Indeed, experiments by KELLY and WOLSTENCROFT (1974) show that an intralymphatic injection of guinea pigs with a crude lymphokine preparation leads to a marked increase of the germinal center area in the draining lymph nodes. Furthermore in preliminary experiments in our department, we found that (germ-free) mice injected intravenously with SRBCs together with a crude IL-2 preparation (probably containing other lymphokines as well) showed enhanced germinal center reactivity, compared with antigen or IL-2 extract alone (KROESE, WUBBENA, and NIEUWENHUIS, unpublished observations).

4.4 Immune Complex Trapping and the Germinal Center Reaction

Some time after antigenic stimulation, antigens localize on the surface of FDCs (reviews by NOSSAL and ADA 1971, KLAUS et al. 1980; TEW et al. 1980; VAN ROOIJEN 1980). These antigens are trapped and retained for very long periods (months) by the FDCs in the form of antigen-antibody immune complexes, and in fact this is the only site in the animal where antigens can be detected for prolonged periods after their administration. During an immune response, these immune complexes bind to FDCs as soon as they are formed in the circulation.

As mentioned before, the trapping of immune complexes is complement dependent: depletion of complement (C3) using cobra venom factor abrogates the trapping of immune complexes completely (PARAMICHAIL et al. 1975; KLAUS and HUMPHREY 1977). Furthermore, antigens like aggregated Ig or levan, which can activate complement immediately, localize in follicles directly, i.e., in the absence of specific Ig.

The follicular localization of immune complexes strongly suggests that "immune complex trapping" plays an important role in germinal center formation. Indeed, in the absence of follicular localization of immune complexes, as is the case after complement depletion with cobra venom factor, the production of B memory cells by germinal centers (see below) is severely impaired (KLAUS and HUMPHREY 1977). A direct influence of immune complexes on the germinal center reaction was demonstrated by LAISSUE et al. (1971) and KUNKL and KLAUS (1981), who have shown that (preformed) immune complexes are far more effective in the generation of germinal centers (and B memory cells) compared with antigen alone. Based upon these findings, KLAUS et al. (1980) postulated that it is the (C3-mediated) localization of antigen-antibody complexes in primary follicles which initiates the germinal center reaction. These immune complexes would be formed using preexisting antibody in the serum and/or antibody produced during the plasmacellular reaction of the (primary) immune response.

Although immune complexes certainly may play an important role in germinal center formation, in our opinion the notion that they are involved in the initiation of the germinal center reaction, i.e., the activation of GCPCs, is questionable. Following the fate of an antigen during a primary immune response, follicular localization of the antigen is only found when germinal centers are already present (VAN ROOIJEN 1972). Accordingly, newly developing germinal centers do not contain extracellular antibody bound to FDCs (VAN EWIJK et al. 1977; OPSTELTEN et al. 1982) and extracellular antibody, specific for the immunizing antigen, is detected on FDCs only after the onset of the germinal center reaction (TERASHIMA et al. 1977).

Lethal X-irradiation effectively impairs the follicular antigen trapping mechanism (HUNTER et al. 1969; NETTESHEIM and HANNA 1969; BROWN et al. 1973). We have studied the germinal center formation and follicular antigen trapping capacity in spleen of irradiated rats after reconstitution with TDLs and stimulation with SRBCs (KROESE et al. 1986). In these experiments, SRBC-induced germinal centers can be found about 2 days before the follicular antigen trapping mechanism, as assessed by peroxidase-antiperoxidase immune complexes, is restored. These data clearly show that even in the absence of an intact follicular antigen trapping mechanism, germinal centers still can be induced.

All these findings indicate that young germinal centers can be formed in the absence of immune complexes trapped by FDCs. Therefore it is highly unlikely that follicular localization of immune complexes on these FDCs plays a crucial role in the early phases (including initiation) of the germinal center reaction. This might also imply that activation of the GCPCs does not occur in situ at the site of the future germinal center. Only some time after the development of a young germinal center is follicular immune complex trapping demonstrated, pointing to a role for follicular immune complexes during later phases of the germinal center reaction, e.g., by providing an essential stimulus for the continuation of the germinal center reaction (see below). Indeed, preliminary experiments by one of us show that depletion of complement by cobra venom factor treatment to prevent follicular immune complex trapping does not prevent the generation of germinal centers after antigenic stimulation but seems to abort the germinal centers a few days after their induction (NIEUWENHUIS, unpublished observations).

4.5 The Germinal Center Microenvironment

Germinal centers develop in B-cell follicles as present in peripheral lymphoid organs. As such, these follicles provide the appropriate "microenvironment" which allows germinal center formation. The microenvironment is constituted by both lymphoid (B and T cells) and nonlymphoid cells, including FDCs, macrophages, and possibly other less well characterized cell types (JEURISSEN and DIJKSTRA 1986).

As noted before, in germinal centers proper, none of the cell types present appear to migrate actively. This is illustrated by the phenotype of the germinal center B cells (and T cells) since both lack putative homing receptor(s) for high endothelial venules as recognized by mAbs (REICHERT et al. 1983; JALKANEN et al. 1986). These receptors are essential for the homing of lymphocytes and other leukocytes in lymphoid organs like lymph nodes and Peyer's patches by virtue of binding of these receptors to molecules (called addresins) on the surface of high endothelial venules (for review see, e.g., LAKEY-BERG et al. 1989). Indeed, isolated germinal center cells are unable to bind in vitro to high endothelial venules, in marked contrast to other B cells, and they do not home into lymph nodes or Peyer's patches after intravenous inoculation (OPSTELTEN et al. 1981, 1983; REICHERT et al. 1983). However, experiments in rabbits clearly demonstrated that germinal center cells, when injected directly into the afferent lymph, can localize immediately (within 3 h after injection) in germinal centers of draining lymph nodes (DEENEN et al. 1984; NIEUWENHUIS and OPSTELTEN 1984). Although it is not known whether germinal center cells also can migrate under physiological circumstances, these experiments indicate that the injected cells have a selective affinity for the germinal center microenvironment. Virtually nothing is known about possible receptors and ligands involved in the formation of such a microenvironment. Interestingly, however, FDCs express the molecules ICAM-1 and CD11b (CR3 = C3bi-receptor) (GERDES et al. 1983; DUSTIN et al. 1986; SCHRIEVER et al. 1989). These molecules are involved in cell–cell adhesion events, and LFA-1$^+$ lymphocytes bind to ICAM-1 (MARLIN and SPRINGER 1987). ICAM-1 expression by FDCs might therefore be a factor involved in the adhesion of (LFA-1$^+$) germinal center B cells to these FDCs, thereby immobilizing these cells and leading to local accumulation of germinal center blast cells. ICAM-1 is clearly not the only factor involved since injected small B lymphocytes, the majority of which, as we now know, express LFA-1, do not have direct access to germinal centers (PARROTT 1967; NIEUWENHUIS and FORD 1976; DEENEN et al. 1984). As we suppose that activated B cells (GCPCs) constitute the primordial germinal center it might be that these GCPCs somehow have a higher affinity binding to FDCs compared with other B cells (see also "centron" theory of MENZIES 1965).

4.6 Dynamics of the Germinal Center Reaction

Germinal center B cells are mitotically very active and many mitotic figures can be seen, in particular among centroblasts. Indeed the majority of human germinal center B cells, but not corona B cells, are stained in situ with the mAb Ki-67 reactive with cycling (i.e., non-G_0) cells (Fig. 8a) (GERDES et al. 1984). Furthermore, FACS analysis of tonsil cell suspensions, which were stained with propidium iodide to measure the amount of DNA in combination with PNA, indicates that almost all of the cells that are in $S+G_2/M$ phase are PNA^+ cells (germinal center cells) (WEINBERG et al. 1986). This high proliferative activity of germinal center B cells can also be demonstrated after a single injection of ^3H-thymidine or BrdU (Fig. 8b) followed by autoradiography or immunohistology, respectively. In these experiments, germinal center cells are almost exclusively labeled (NIEUWENHUIS and KEUNING 1974; HARMS et al. 1986).

Clearly, germinal centers are major sites where B cells can expand to form clones in response to antigenic stimulation. To understand the physiology of the germinal center reaction it is of crucial importance to know how these germinal center B cells actually do expand. In other words, does each germinal center develop from only one precursor cell (monoclonal development), from a few precursor cells (oligoclonal development), or from many precursor cells (polyclonal development)? We have addressed this question in short-term reconstitution experiments involving lethally X-irradiated rats (KROESE et al. 1987b, 1988). Basically, X-irradiated rats were reconstituted with mixtures of TDLs collected from two different donors and subsequently stimulated with SRBCs. Donor cells could be discriminated by using TDLs from rats differing in allotype for either MHC class II, the leukocyte common antigen (RT7), or Ig $\varkappa$ light chain in combination with allotype-specific mAbs. As is shown in Fig. 9, after reconstitution with mixtures of TDLs (in different ratios), three types of germinal center could be found up to 10 days after stimulation: germinal centers entirely composed of cells derived from one of the donors, or germinal centers composed of a mixture of the two donor populations. The relative frequencies of these three germinal center types indicate that under these experimental conditions, de novo generated germinal centers develop oligoclonally, involving up to three precursor cells per germinal center, on average.

Whether this postulated oligoclonal development of germinal centers also holds for more physiological situations needs further investigation. Some support for an (oligo-)clonal germinal center development comes from data by RAZZECA et al. (1986), who studied the distribution of phosphorylcholine idiotype (PC-Id) expressing cells in situ after immunization with PC in the mouse. The vast majority of germinal center cells in suspension (defined as PNA^{high} cells) and in tissue sections did not express PC-Id, indicating that PC-Id GCPCs occur in these mice only at very low frequencies. The presence of occasional but confluently $PC\text{-}Id^+$ staining germinal centers in these animals

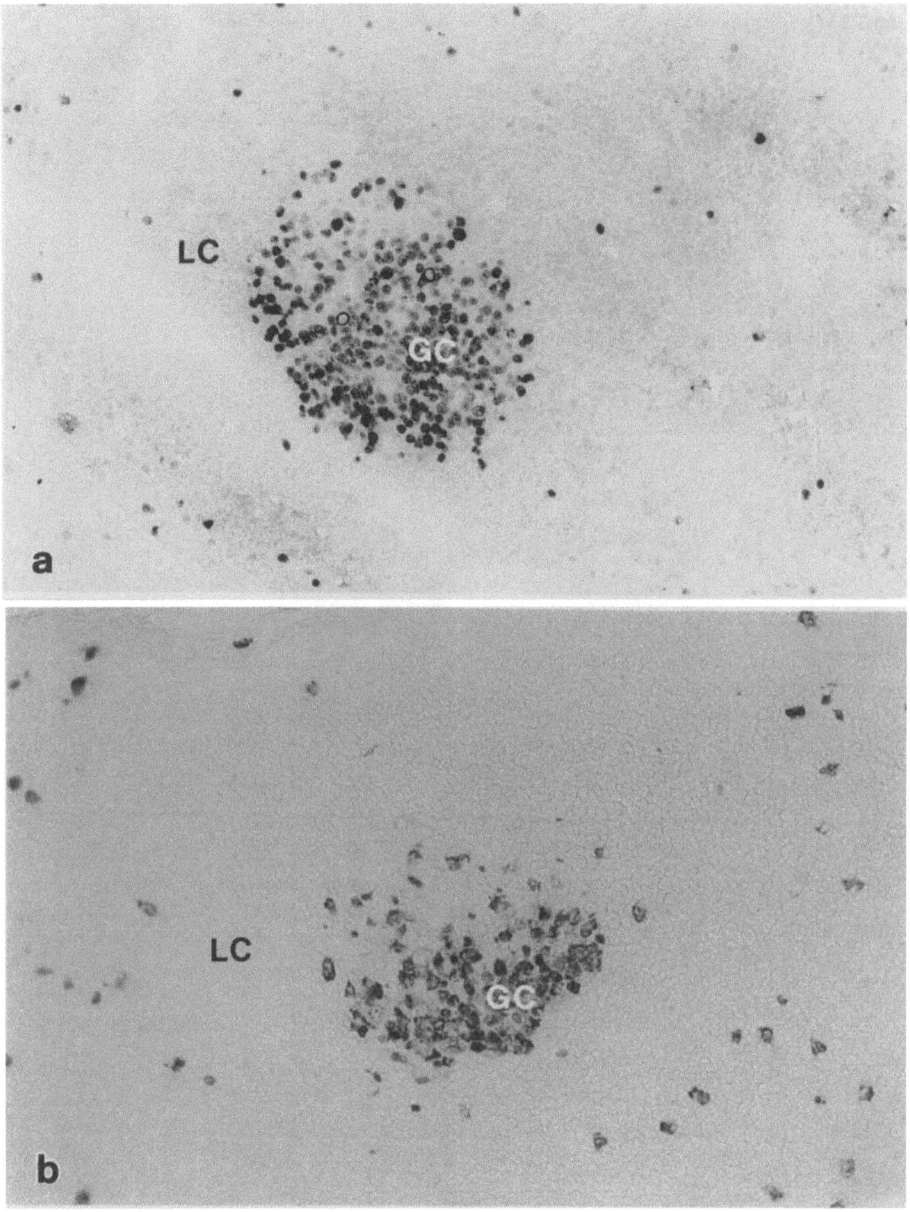

Fig. 8. **a** Human lymph node stained with the mAb Ki-67 directed to non-G_0 cells. Germinal center (*GC*) cells (centroblasts) show strong staining, whereas cells in the lymphocyte corona (*LC*) are clearly negative. ×140. **b** Peripheral lymph node taken from a rat 2 h after intravenous injection of BrdU. Sections, stained with an mAb to BrdU, demonstrate intense labeling of germinal centers (centroblasts) but not of small B cells in the lymphocyte corona. (Courtesy of G. Harms, Department of Pathology). ×160

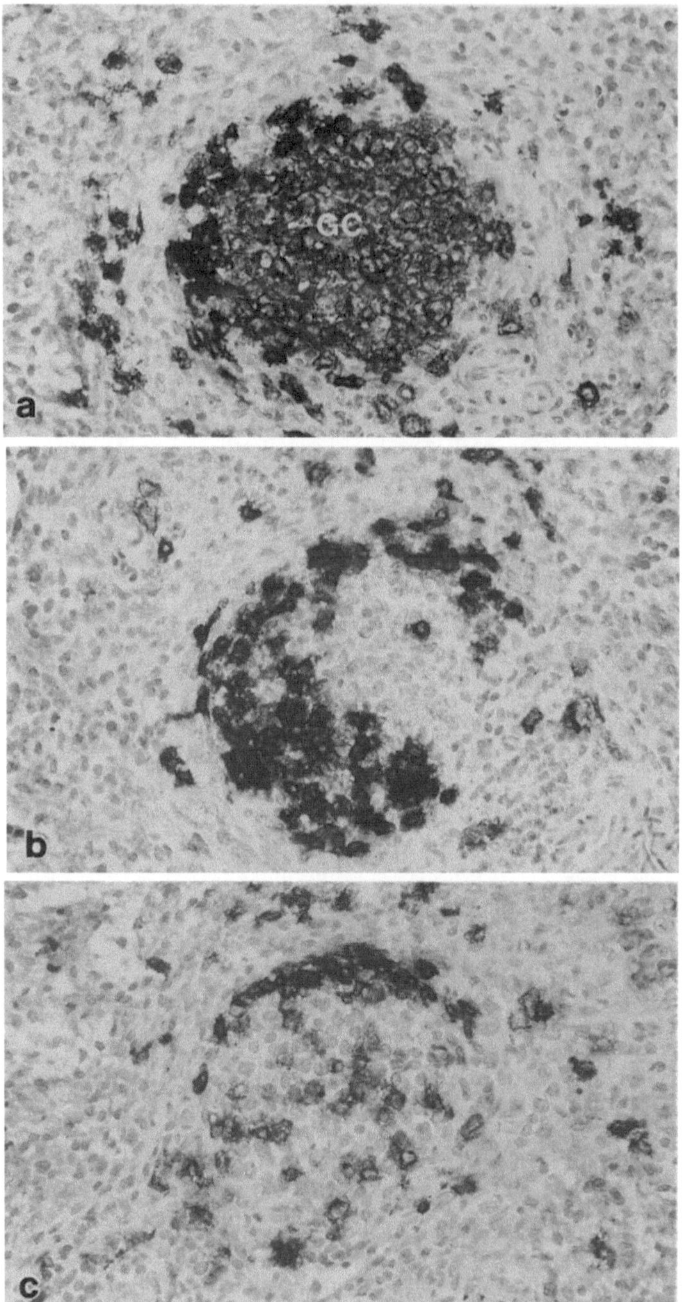
GC
a
b
c

therefore suggests that also under these physiological circumstances, individual germinal centers may develop from very few or even a single precursor cell.

Calculations on the exact numbers of cells produced during the germinal center reaction are difficult to make, since several factors are difficult to estimate, such as how many cells leave the germinal center or die within the germinal center. Furthermore, experiments carried out in our laboratory (NIEUWENHUIS et al. 1974; OPSTELTEN et al. 1980) suggest that during the germinal center reaction to a particular antigen, both antigen-specific and antigen-unspecific B cells are recruited to participate in the germinal center reaction (NIEUWENHUIS 1981). In the experiments described above (KROESE et al. 1987b, 1988), germinal center formation was studied in recipient spleens 5 days after antigenic challenge. At that time cell death is not observed and since germinal center formation is almost clonal under these conditions (even up to 10 days after stimulation, KROESE et al. 1988), recruitment of cells during this early phase of germinal center formation does not seem to take place to any significant extent. In similar experiments, the total number of germinal centers in spleens of reconstituted rats 7 days after stimulation with SRBCs has been estimated at 800 ± 100, with a total volume of 4.4 ± 0.4 mm^3 (SEIJEN et al. unpublished observation). Assuming that germinal center blasts cells have a diameter of 14 µm and that as yet no cells have left the germinal center (and no cells have died or been recruited), this means that at 7 days after immunization, each germinal center contains about 4000 cells. With a cell cycle time for germinal center cells of 12–14 h (FLIEDNER et al. 1964; ZAITOUN 1980), and an oligoclonal development of germinal centers, this implies that GCPCs are already triggered to divide within the first 24 h after antigenic stimulation. It also illustrates the enormous expansion potential of B-cell clones that may exist in germinal centers.

5 Functional Aspects of Germinal Center Formation

A close correlation between the formation of germinal centers and the development of B memory cells has been demonstrated in several earlier studies using experimental animals (THORBECKE et al. 1974; KLAUS et al. 1980). These B memory cells are responsible for the accelerated and elevated responses of high

◄ **Fig. 9a–c.** Immunoperoxidase staining of frozen sections from the spleen of a chimeric rat, 5 days after reconstitution and immunization with SRBCs. Chimeric rats were constructed by lethal X-irradiation, followed by reconstitution with a mixture of TDLs derived from (AO × BN) F_1 hybrid rats (65%) and from AO TDLs that were rendered tolerant for the BN haplotype (35%) (for details see KROESE et al. 1987b). Sections were stained with an mAb directed to MHC class II antigens of the BN haplotype (unreactive with the AO haplotype). In spleens of these chimeras three types of germinal center could be identified: **a** germinal centers entirely composed of AO × BN cells, **b** germinal centers entirely composed of AO cells, and **c** germinal centers containing a mixture of both. ×250. (From KROESE et al. 1987b; with permission of VCH Verlagsgesellschaft mbH)

affinity antibodies, especially of the advanced isotypes (IgG and IgA), upon renewed contact with the same antigen (see, e.g., KLAUS 1977). The extensive antigen-specific proliferation of B-cell clones within a germinal center thus simply leads to more antigen-specific B cells that now have acquired properties to assure a long life time (memory B cells). Upon renewed contact with the same antigen, this situation obviously may lead to triggering of more antibody-forming cell precursors, which results directly in an elevated and earlier antibody response.

More direct proof for a role of germinal centers in the generation of B memory cells was obtained more recently when PNA became available as a marker for germinal center B cells in mice (ROSE et al. 1980). Lymph node B cells were taken at the peak of germinal center formation during a primary immune response (i.e., 7–10 days after antigenic stimulation), separated into PNA^{high} cells and PNA^{low} cells, and transferred into lethally X-irradiated recipient mice (COICO et al. 1983; KRAAL et al. 1985, 1988). Especially in mice that had received PNA^{high} cells, well-developed B memory responses (to the same antigen used to induce germinal centers in donor mice) could be demonstrated. If in similar experiments lymph node cells are taken several weeks to months after priming (i.e., presumably after cessation of the immune response), then memory B cells are found in the PNA^{low} fraction (COICO et al. 1983) and now (re-)express the putative homing receptor for lymph node high endothelial venules recognized by MEL-14 (KRAAL et al. 1985, 1988). Furthermore, findings of HOBBS and FELDBUSH (1980) demonstrate that with increasing time after immunization B memory is carried by smaller cells and not by lymphoblasts. Taken together these data indicate, as expected, that after a sessile phase within the germinal center, the (memory) B cells derived from the germinal centers enter the recirculating B-cell pool.

Another characteristic feature of B memory responses is that the isotype of the antibody formed changes from a predominant IgM response after primary immunization to a predominant IgG (or IgA) response after secondary challenge. This IgG is produced by plasma cells that derive from precursor cells (probably memory cells) that express surface IgG (OKUMURA et al. 1976; MASON 1976). Possibly germinal centers play a role in this switch of isotype usage seen after secondary immunization. After primary immunization of mice, the vast majority of (antigen-specific) germinal center cells (defined as PNA^{bright} cells) in lymph nodes express sIgM, but after secondary immunization with the same antigen most germinal center B cells now express sIgG (KRAAL et al. 1982). Germinal center B cells obtained from a continuously stimulated organ like the Peyer's patch predominantly express sIgA (BUTCHER et al. 1982). Since, at least during primary immune responses, GCPCs are thought to express sIgM (see above), these findings suggest that isotype switching from sIgM to sIgG (in lymph nodes) or to sIgA (in Peyer's patches) may occur within the germinal center microenvironment (KRAAL et al. 1982). After switching, germinal center cells that express sIgG (or sIgA) may leave the germinal center as memory B cells, being responsible for the predominant IgG (or IgA) character of secondary antibody responses. T cells and T cell derived factors have been shown to be involved in isotype switching (e.g., ISAKSON et al. 1982; KAWANISHI et al. 1983; MAYER et al. 1985), and it is therefore possible that the typical germinal center T cells play a role in this process.

In ongoing primary immune responses and in secondary immune responses the average affinity of the produced antibodies, specific for a particular antigen, is higher than that of antibodies found immediately after immunization (see, e.g., SISKIND and BENACERRAF 1969). A major contribution to this so-called affinity maturation of the immune response is the introduction of somatic mutations in the Ig heavy and light chain V (variable) gene regions (reviews by BEREK and MILSTEIN 1988, KOCKS and RAJEWSKY 1989). Somatic mutations occur at a high frequency in V regions, as witnessed by their high estimated mutation rate of 10^{-3} per base pair per cell division (MCKEAN et al. 1984).

In a series of experiments, MILSTEIN and co-workers (as reviewed by BEREK and MILSTEIN 1987, 1988) extensively studied the V genes involved in the immune response to oxazolone in mice by fusion of spleen cells from immunized mice with a myeloma cell line. Shortly (i.e., 7 days) after primary immunization of mice with oxazolone, only very rare somatic mutations were detected in the V genes of oxazolone-specific hybridomas, whereas at 14 days after immunization or after secondary immunization accumulated numbers of somatic mutations were seen. Importantly, the presence of these somatic mutations corresponded with an increase in affinity of the antibodies to oxazolone. Hypermutation is not continuously operating after antigenic stimulation; only for a brief period (i.e., 1 or 2 weeks after immunization does the hypermutation machinery seem to be switched on leading to accumulated numbers of somatic mutations during clonal expansion of B cells (BEREK and MILSTEIN 1988; LEVY et al. 1989).

Germinal centers are sites of an enormous clonal expansion of (antigen-specific) B cells and they are therefore likely candidates for the anatomical sites where somatic hypermutation of the V region may take place, as speculated by several authors (e.g., ROUSE et al. 1984; MACLENNAN and GRAY 1986; BEREK and MILSTEIN 1988; KOCKS and RAJEWSKY 1989). Indeed, somatic mutations are found in V genes from hybridoma cell lines prepared from germinal center B cells (defined by their strong binding to Peanut agglutinin) 10–14 days after immunization with oxazolone (BEREK and APEL 1989).

In germinal centers, antigen is present in the form of immune complexes at the surface of FDcs. It is therefore possible that, in addition to this hypermutation, antigen-induced selection is involved in the generation of clones with high affinity Ig: mutated germinal center B cells with increased affinity for the immunizing antigen are selectively stimulated over cells with lower affinity (or even defective Ig), thus possibly leading to an accumulated number of mutations in responding cells. This selective stimulation could be due to competition of B cells for antigen (SISKIND and BENACERRAF 1969). A relationship between the presence of antigen on FDCs, i.e., within germinal centers, and affinity maturation follows from experiments by KLAUS et al. (1980). These experiments demonstrate that, compared with antigen alone, immunization of mice with immune complexes (that are known to bind exclusively to FDCs) not only leads to enhancement of the germinal center reaction but also accelerates the development of memory cells which can produce antibodies with higher affinity.

Taken together, the data presented in this section indicate that germinal centers may be involved in all three characteristic events of the production of memory cells, namely: (a) amplification of the number of plasma cell precursors, (b) switching of the isotype, and (c) production of B cells with higher affinity for a given antigen, resulting in more antigen-specific B cells with a repertoire skewed to higher affinity.

6 Phylogeny of the Germinal Center

Germinal centers are not only found in peripheral lymphoid organs of mammals, but also in those of birds. Despite differences in morphology of lymphoid organs, the features of avian germinal centers are very similar to those of mammalian germinal centers (Cooper et al. 1965; Hoshi 1972; White et al. 1975; Hoffman-Fezer et al. 1977; Eikelenboom et al. 1983). Germinal centers in chicken spleen express only low amounts of sIg, are T cell dependent, do contain some T cells, and are able to trap and to retain immune complexes on the surface of a dendritic cell type. In contrast to the situation in mammals, however, germinal centers in chicken spleen are not surrounded by a lymphocyte corona but by a thin layer of fibrous tissue.

Germinal centers (and lymphoid follicles) are absent from lymphoid organs of "lower" poikilothermic vertebrates (i.e., fishes, amphibians, and reptiles) (Murata 1959; Good and Finstad 1967; Cohen 1977; Pitchappan 1980; Kroese and van Rooijen 1982; Kroese et al. 1985b). A very characteristic property of germinal centers (lymphoid follicles) as found in mammals and birds is the capability of retaining immune complexes for long periods on the surface of FDCs. Despite the apparent absence of germinal centers (and lymphoid follicles) in lymphoid organs of lower vertebrates, immune complex trapping could be demonstrated in the spleens of different species, including fishes, amphibians, and reptiles (Collie 1974; Secombes and Manning 1980; Kroese et al. 1982; Kroese and van Rooijen 1983; Kroese et al. 1985b). Retention of immune complexes in the spleens of poikilothermic vertebrates occurs in well-defined splenic areas on the surface of nonphagocytic, dendritic cells, thus resembling the mammalian and avian FDCs.

Although germinal centers are absent in poikilothermic vertebrates, these animals are able to elicit anamnestic responses to certain antigens (see, e.g., Manning and Turner 1976; Manning 1980). However, these secondary responses do not seem to be as vigorous as in mammals and birds. This indicates that germinal centers are not per se essential for the generation of B memory cells. Immune complex trapping may, however, be a prerequisite for B memory cell production. The presence of germinal centers in mammals and birds might be the result of the anatomical arrangement of immune complex trapping cells in groups. In these germinal centers, activated B cells expand into very large clones, probably leading to a more effective generation of B memory compared with the lower vertebrates, which do not possess germinal centers.

7 Ontogeny of the Germinal Center

In neonates, human as well as rodent, the first "spontaneous" germinal centers can be observed by 2–4 weeks after birth (VEERMAN 1975; BARZANJI and EMERY 1978; DIJKSTRA and DÖPP 1983; SMINIA et al. 1983; VILLENA et al. 1983; VAN REES et al. 1985; KROESE et al. 1987). The absence of germinal centers in neonates is not due to an absence of appropriate antigenic stimulation only. In human fetuses and neonates, normal as well as in the case of sepsis, no germinal centers are present in lymphoid tissues until about 3 weeks after birth (TIMENS et al. 1989). In rats bred under conventional conditions but not deliberately immunized, the first germinal centers are detected in the spleen by 3 weeks after birth (VEERMAN 1975; DIJKSTRA and DÖPP 1983; KROESE et al. 1987c). Deliberate antigenic stimulation was found by KROESE et al. (1987c) to lead to germinal center formation in neonatal rat spleen after immunization of 7-day-old rats but not after immunization of 3-day-old rats. However, transfer experiments using neonatal spleen cells to X-irradiated adult recipient rats have shown that even spleen cells taken from 3-day-old rats are able to give rise to germinal center formation upon antigenic stimulation (KROESE et al. 1987c). Apparently, 3-day-old rat spleens contain all the essential lymphoid elements (GCPCs and T cells) needed for germinal center development in an adult "microenvironment." In neonates this microenvironment is probably as yet too immature to allow germinal center formation.

In adults, the germinal center microenvironment is created by the lymphoid follicles and one could easily envisage that when follicles are not yet formed during the development of a peripheral lymphoid organ, germinal centers cannot develop either. Indeed, our studies in rats show that as soon as primary follicles can be found (by 14 days after birth), spontaneous germinal centers may be present (KROESE et al. 1987c). In man, too, formation of germinal centers is preceded by the development of primary follicles (TIMENS et al. 1987, 1988, 1989; WESTERGA and TIMENS 1989). Both in man and in rats, the development of primary follicles in lymphoid organs coincides with the appearance of FDCs in these organs: as soon as primary follicles are present, FDCs can be detected (KROESE et al. 1987c; TIMENS et al. 1987; WESTERGA and TIMENS 1989). As a working hypothesis we would like to speculate here that when precursor-FDCs mature (or FDCs are formed), these cells form clusters at certain locations ("centron" theory according to MENZIES 1965) in lymphoid organs where follicles (and germinal centers) now can develop. Possibly, cell–cell adhesion molecules like ICAM-1 expressed by FDCs play a key role in such follicle formation during the ontogenetic development of lymphoid organs.

8 Pathology of the Germinal Center Reaction

Apart from a role of the germinal center in the normal immune system, there are also several pathological conditions associated with these structures. The germinal center reaction itself could be impaired by certain pathological conditions, like immune deficiencies, and in some diseases the appearance of the germinal center is abnormal. Finally, neoplastic transformation of the germinal center cells generally results in the development of malignant (B-cell) lymphomas of which various subtypes are known.

8.1 The Germinal Center Reaction and Immunological Deficiencies

Generally, in cases of defects in humoral immunity, such as congenital sex-linked recessive agammaglobulinemia, acquired primary hypogammaglobulinemia, and variable immune deficiency, not only are primary lymphoid follicles absent or highly atrophic but germinal centers are also lacking. This indicates that the development of primary follicles and germinal centers probably is dependent on a common B-cell precursor.

In cellular immune deficiencies a more variable histological picture is observed, but in general the generation of germinal centers is impaired, illustrating once more the T-cell dependency of germinal center formation.

In DiGeorge's syndrome structures derived from the third and fourth pharyngeal pouch are congenitally lacking or defective, including the thymus, which is hypoplastic or absent. Many endocrine disorders can be observed and cellular immunity is deficient. Lymph nodes are characterized by a depletion of paracortical areas, while follicles with germinal centers are mostly present (except for the rare cases of total thymic aplasia).

Ataxia-telangiectasia is characterized by neurological problems, telangiectases, and immunological defects. The latter mainly relate to deficient cellular immunity but often there is also a lack of secretory IgA and IgE. The thymus is hypoplastic lacking lymphoid cells. Lymph nodes generally show a depletion of the paracortex, poorly developed follicles, and absence of germinal centers.

In the acquired immunodeficiency syndrome (AIDS) and AIDS-related complex (ARC) an immune defect is present, mainly affecting the cellular immune system, caused by infection (and destruction) of $CD4^+$ cells (mainly T helper cells) by the human immunodeficiency virus (HIV). However, before the stage of full-blown AIDS is reached, the disease is characterized by persistent generalized lymphadenopathy (PGL), in which alteration of the germinal center is one of the most prominent features. These alterations will be discussed briefly here. Other features of the lymphoid system in patients with full-blown AIDS or ARC are discussed more extensively in other chapters of this book. At present different stages of PGL are recognized by their histological picture. Recently, a histological classification of HIV-related lymphadenopathy has been proposed which is reported to be reproducible and to have clinical significance (Öst et al. 1989). The basic features of this classification are: follicular hyperplasia without (1) or with (2) severe fragmentation, follicular involution (3), and diffuse pattern (4). In the early stages there are numerous irregularly shaped follicles with activated centers. In subsequent stages an increasing fragmentation of germinal centers is observed, characterized by multifocal invasion of germinal centers by small lymphocytes and blood vessels. This is accompanied by an increasing attenuation or loss of the mantle zone. In the final stages there is a picture of small-sized follicles, lacking normal germinal center cells, which in the end are absent, leaving only small follicular remnants. In these remnants fibrosis and amorphous PAS-positive material may be present. Lymph nodes in these final stages may be lymphocytopenic or may be infiltrated by immunoblasts, plasma cells, mast cells, macrophages, and even numerous lymphocytes. Pronounced angiogenesis can be present.

8.2 Abnormal Germinal Centers

8.2.1 Reactive Disorders Affecting the Germinal Center

The most basic reaction pattern commonly observed in the lymph node in the event of a predominantly B-lmyphocyte response is reactive follicular hyperplasia, which is characterized by the presence of enlarged lymphoid follicles with prominent germinal centers and by the appearance of plasma cells. Reactive follicular hyperplasia is commonly seen in relation to all kinds of infections, together with other more or less specific features, but should not be considered abnormal. It is particularly characteristic in children and young adults but is less often observed in the elderly.

This picture of histologically normal germinal centers may sometimes become aberrant (Ioachim 1982; Stansfeld 1985). First, most often observed in lymph nodes from children is a progressive expansion of the germinal center, until the mantle zone (lymphocyte corona) is completely absent. In this situation the expanding germinal centers sometimes appear to fuse with each other, leading to the formation of tumor-like masses, which may result in the erroneous diagnosis of malignancy.

The second type of alteration has been described as "progressively transformed germinal centers" (PTGCs). This entity is characterized by a general lymphadenopathy with an aberrant lymphoid tissue architecture (Poppema et al. 1979). The changes are marked by irregular follicles consisting of an FDC meshwork with small B cells and irregularly scattered germinal center B cells (centrocytes and centroblasts). Characteristic in these lesions is the presence of scattered $CD4^{+}CD57^{+}$ T cells. As mentioned before, this subpopulation of T cells is highly characteristic for germinal centers and is not found in other lymphoid compartments.

A third type of abnormal germinal center raction pattern is presented by germinal centers that are almost exclusively composed of cells with epithelioid cell morphology (Paradinas 1985; Severson et al. 1988). These so-called epithelioid germinal centers can be found in some cases of angioimmunoblastic lymphadenopathy, and in the multicentric variant of Castleman's disease, but also sometimes in lymph nodes from young children who have succumbed as a result of fulminating infections. A considerable number of these epithelioid cells react with the mAb R4/23 (anti-FDC) and are negative for macrophage markers like Leu-M1 (Cd15), Leu-M3 (CD14), and lysozyme. It was concluded that the dominant cells constituting the epithelioid germinal centers are (residual) FDCs rather than macrophages/histiocytes (SEVERSON et al. 1988). At present it is not known whether the marked histological picture is caused by an underlying immune defect or by overwhelming infection.

8.2.2 Disorders of the Germinal Center with Unknown Etiology

8.2.2.1 Castleman's Disease

Besides the above-described reactive changes involving germinal centers, other disorders are known of which the etiology is as yet unclear. One such disorder is "giant lymph node hyperplasia" or Castleman's disease proper, subdivided into the plasma cell type and the hyaline vascular type (reviewed by FRIZZERIA 1985). These two types probably represent two distinct disease entities. The plasma cell type generally shows no germinal center abnormalities and will not be discussed here. The hyaline vascular type is characterized histologically by lymphoid follicle hyperplasia with a typical concentric layering of FDCs and marked proliferation of capillaries with endothelial hyperplasia and effacement of normal lymph node sinuses. The lymphoid follicles show hypervascular hyaline germinal centers sometimes containing concentrically layered and flattened germinal center cells. Mostly, the centers of these structures consist of a blood vessel with often proliferated endothelial cells, arranged concentrically with interposed hyaline material. In these follicles the remainder ("expanded" mantle zone) is made up of closely packed, also concentrically arranged, small lymphocytes. Although in most cases the disease is localized, systemic (multicentric) forms are known. The pathogenesis of the hyaline vascular type of Castleman's disease is not known. An abnormal reaction to certain (microbial) antigens or a defect in regulatory mechanisms of the immune system has been suggested (PARADINAS 1985). Other speculations include lymphoid tissue hamartoma and benign lymphoid tumor (FRIZZERA 1985).

8.2.2.2 Nodular Lymphocyte Predominant Type of Hodgkin's Disease

Progressively transformed germinal centers (PTGCs) (see above) and the nodular lymphocyte predominant type of Hodgkin's disease (NLPHD), formerly called nodular paragranuloma, are closely related disease entities (POPPEMA et al. 1979; TIMENS et al. 1986). In NLPHD follicular changes are similar to those observed in PTGCs, but it is differentiated from PTGCs by the presence of a diagnostic cell type, namely the L&H type (referring to the original morphological designation: "lymphocytic and histiocytic") Reed-

Sternberg cell (POPPEMA et al. 1979). In patients in whom the diagnosis NLPHD has been made the histopathological picture of PTGCs is also frequently observed, sometimes preceding the disease by several years. In the course of NLPHD, PTGCs are observed both in lymph nodes where NLPHD nodules are present and in other "unaffected" lymph nodes.

The L&H type Reed-Sternberg cell has been demonstrated to be of B-cell origin by the cytoplasmic presence of J chain (POPPEMA et al. 1979; TIMENS et al. 1986) and supposedly represents a germinal center derived cell. Whereas PTGCs are considered to represent a reactive process, NLPHD is considered to be neoplastic in nature. Taking all features of NLPHD together, this entity can be designated a germinal center lymphoma (TIMENS et al. 1986). Despite the supposed neoplastic origin of NLPHD, a truly malignant character is doubtful. For example, clonal expansion could not be demonstrated in NLPHD (LINDEN et al. 1988). Furthermore clinically this disease generally has a very protracted, often benign course although the development of malignant non-Hodgkin's lymphomas in patients with NLPHD has been described (MIETTINEN et al. 1983). Since in NLPHD several immune defects are clinically observed, it can be speculated that NLPHD represents (one feature of) an abnormal reaction of the immune system.

8.3 Malignant Germinal Center Lymphomas

Malignant B-cell lymphomas are supposed to represent a more or less "frozen stage" of normal B-lymphocyte development. Malignant lymphomas are characterized by proliferation of a cell population that phenotypically resembles a cell subset normally observed. An extensive review of germinal center cell lymphomas has been given by STEIN et al. (1982). Therefore in this section just a brief outline will be given of the malignant germinal center.

In the normal germinal center reaction different B-cell subtypes (centroblasts, centrocytes) can be recognized. Consequently, neoplastic changes of germinal center cells result in at least three different types of germinal center lymphoma (STEIN et al. 1982), which in their follicular form resemble different stages in the normal germinal center reaction:

1. Centroblastic (CB) type lymphoma, predominantly consisting of centroblasts
2. Centroblastic-centrocytic (CB-CC) type lymphoma, which closely resembles the normal reactive germinal center, although the malignant cells are arranged in a more disorderly fashion
3. Centrocytic (CC) lymphoma, putatively consisting of a pure population of centrocytes

The relationship between non-Hodgkin's lymphoma of centrocytic subtype and normal germinal center cells has for a long time not been as evident as in the case of the other subtypes. Whereas the centrocytes in CB-CC lymphomas are phenotypically comparable to the centrocytes observed in the normal germinal center, the phenotype of purely CC lymphomas could not be related to that of the normal germinal center centrocytes. In a recent immunohistological study of CB-CC and CC lymphomas, the centrocytic cells in these lymphoma subtypes showed distinct phenotypes (Hollema and Poppema 1988). The centrocytes in CB-CC lymphomas would represent the "malignant centrocyte proper," bearing a resemblance to normal centrocytes. The centrocytes in CC lymphomas, however, seem to represent a centrocyte-like precursor of the centroblasts (i.e., the GCPCs). For example, these CC lymphomas are $sIgM^{+}IgD^{+}$, like GCPCs (see above), and they may constitute a new subtype in their own right (Hollema and Poppema 1988).

In the CB-CC and CC, and in some of the CB lymphoma subtypes, an extensive meshwork of FDCs is observed between the tumor cells expanding along with the proliferating malignant germinal center cells. As there are no arguments that these FDCs are also neoplastic in nature, this expansion of the FDC meshwork seems most probably induced by the germinal center tumor cells. The immunophenotype of FDCs in germinal center lymphomas resembles that seen in normal germinal centers, including the expression of receptors for complement fragments and for the Fc portion of Ig. Moreover, in contrast to the normal situation, in neoplastic follicular lesions generally no immune complexes or complement factors can be demonstrated on the surface of these FDCs (Stein et al. 1982).

9 A Model for the Development of Germinal Centers

In adult life, bone marrow has been postulated to be the major site for the production of B cells directly from hemopoietic stem cells (Osmond and Nossal 1974). In this central lymphoid organ, pre-B cells containing free μ chains (cμ) in their cytoplasm give rise to B cells expressing sIgM. Possibly, $c\mu^{+}$ cells are derived from μ^{-} cells containing the nuclear enzyme terminal deoynucleotidyl transferase (Janossy et al. 1979; Opstelten et al. 1986). Many B cells are formed in the bone marrow every day. In the mouse about 5×10^{7} cells are produced per day by the pre-B cell compartment (Opstelten and Osmond 1983), whereas in the rat the number of B cells produced by the pre-B cells is approximately 10 times higher (Deenen et al. 1987). This high number of newly generated B cells in the bone marrow appears to be sufficient to supply the animal continuously with enough (virgin) B cells expressing Ig V region genes specific for a wide range of antigens (the "naive repertoire," Berek and Milstein 1988). The generation of B cells in the bone marrow is largely independent both of T cells and of antigenic stimulation.

In this chapter we have described another major site for production of B cells, i.e., the germinal center, which occurs in peripheral lymphoid organs as a consequence of antigenic stimulation and is regulated by T cells. Within the germinal center, B cells expand to very large clones of B memory cells, thereby adding to the "available repertoire" (Jerne 1971; Freitas et al. 1986) of the

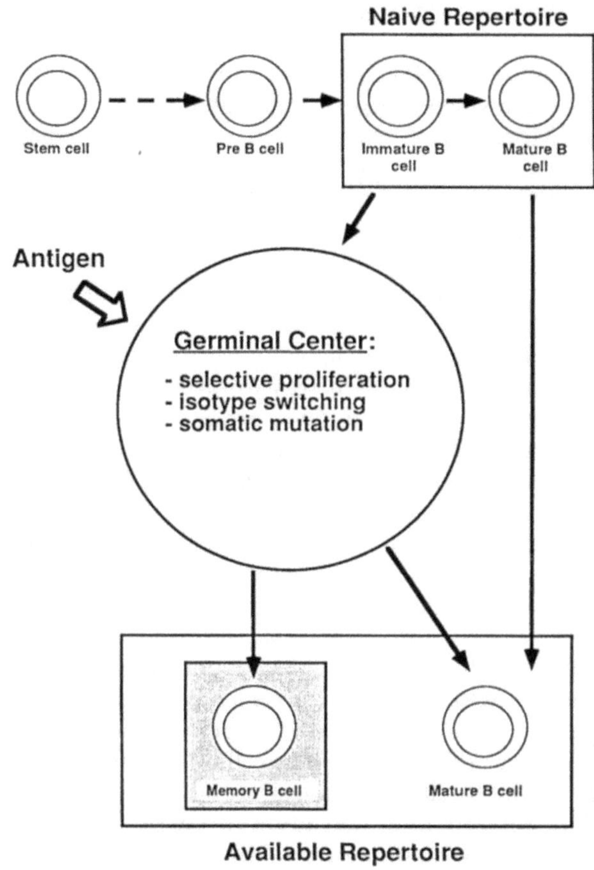

Fig. 10. The generation of germinal centers and their role in B cell differentiation: a model. For explanation see text

peripheral B cell pool. In Fig. 10 a model for the generation of germinal centers is given, which summarizes some of the data discussed in this chapter.

Two phases of the germinal center reaction can be distinguished: (a) the actual induction of germinal center formation by triggering or activation of GCPCs and (b) the local expansion of thus activated B cells in primary follicles, which will lead to visible germinal centers. Activation of B cells by antigen (in vitro) requires specific interaction between B cells, antigen-presenting cells, and T cells (for review see, e.g., MELCHERS and ANDERSSON 1984). By this activation B cells transit from the G_0 to the G_1 phase of the cell cycle. The interaction of B, T, and antigen-presenting cells is restricted by MHC class II antigens, which are present on both B cells and the antigen-presenting cells. T helper cells recognize antigen in the context of these MHC class II antigens. We assume that similar requirements are also needed for the activation of GCPCs. When and where in situ the actual initiation of the germinal center reaction starts is largely unknown. It has been speculated previously that antigen trapped in the form of immune complexes by the FDCs initiates the germinal center reaction (KLAUS et al. 1980). However, as discussed above, several data do not fit this hypothesis. For one thing, it is highly unlikely that during a primary immune response, immune complexes localize on FDCs within 1 day after immunization, i.e., at a time when the germinal center reaction might start (KROESE et al. 1987b). Moreover, T cells do not seem to recirculate through follicles (NIEUWENHUIS and FORD 1976), which makes it rather unlikely that an antigen-specific GCPC will encounter the right T cell in the follicle. We therefore speculate that the initiation of the germinal center reaction in general may take place outside the lymphoid follicle, e.g., at the periphery of the T-cell areas in lymphoid organs where the plasmacellular reaction also starts (reviewed by VAN ROOIJEN et al. 1986). In these regions all elements essential for the activation of B cells are present: high numbers of (recirculating inducer-type T cells, recirculating B cells on their way towards the lymphoid follicles (NIEUWENHUIS and FORD 1976), and antigen-presenting cells in the form of MHC class II expressing interdigitating cells and macrophages (VEERMAN and VAN EWIJK 1975; HOEFSMIT et al. 1980). Alternatively, GCPCs are not activated in peripheral lymphoid organs but at the primary sites of antigenic penetration (e.g., skin or gut), and activated B blasts may enter the draining lymph nodes by afferent lymph (KELLY 1970), to localize in germinal centers (DEENEN et al. 1984). These two possibilities, however, do not need to be mutually exclusive.

After the initial activation of GCPCs, these cells may migrate onwards into follicles, where they subsequently expand to become visible germinal centers. After activation of B cells (in vitro), these cells become susceptible to lymphokines produced by T helper cells and accessory cells. These factors are required for the proliferation of the B cells (MELCHERS and ANDERSSON 1984). It is therefore very likely that similarly after activation of GCPCs, lymphokines, presumably produced within the confinement of the microenvironment of the germinal center, are essential for their further proliferation. Indeed, as noted above, injection of lymphokines (crude preparations) stimulates the germinal center reaction. A role for CD23, as a B-cell differentiation factor, in germinal center formation has been suggested (GORDON et al. 1989). Obvious candidates for lymphokine production during the germinal center reaction are the unique subset of T cells present in germinal centers and the FDCs.

An important question that still remains is why – in vivo – activated B cells either expand to form germinal centers inside follicles or differentiate to plasma cells outside follicular structures. One explanation could be that GCPCs differ from plasma cell precursors. As noted above, some evidence for this was obtained by SEIJEN et al. (1988), who showed that only $sIgM^+IgD^+$ cells from rat thoracic duct lymph are capable of germinal center formation in spleen. Furthermore, these data indicate that memory cells (as present in TDLs), once they have switched their isotype to IgG or IgA (and lack IgM and/or IgD), possibly are unable to reenter a germinal center reaction.

Another explanation could be that most activated B cells become plasma cells and only a very few (one or two) that accidentally (?) enter the follicle expand locally to form a germinal center. The follicular microenvironment may favor proliferation of activated B cells and inhibit (or prevent) massive plasma cell formation. It is possible that special lymphokines essential for differentiation to plasma cells are not produced by germinal center T cells or FDCs. In this context it should be noted here that isolated FDCs do not express IL-6 mRNA (Schriever et al. 1989), a lymphokine important in terminal B-cell differentiation.

Although activated B cells can divide several times even when antigen is not specifically bound to sIg, specific antigen is required to continue the proliferation of these B cells (Melchers and Andersson 1984). Some time after the start of the germinal center reaction, the continuing antigenic stimulus needed for the proliferation of the germinal center B cells (centroblasts) might be provided by immune complexes trapped and retained by the FDCs at a time when the primary antibody response is well on its way. In addition to providing a proliferative signal to the B cells, immune complexes simultaneously may inhibit differentiation of germinal center B cells to plasma cells by cross-linking the antigen receptor and the Fc receptor on the B cell. In this way, blocking of differentiation to plasma cells may direct development of B cells to memory cells, as suggested previously (Kölsch et al. 1980). Consistent herewith are observations that injection of immune complexes (unknown ratio of antibody to antigen) can suppress the humoral immune response (Sinclair et al. 1974; Oberbarnscheidt and Kölsch 1978) and stimulate (immune complexes prepared at equivalence) the formation of germinal centers (Kunkl and Klaus 1981).

While germinal center cells are expanding dramatically to very large clones, germinal center B cells may undergo important molecular changes, especially at the level of the Ig (genes). First, they seem to lose their sIgD. Second, somatic mutations may be introduced in the V region genes of the mitotically very active centroblasts, resulting in an increase in the affinity of the Ig for the stimulating antigen. As a by-product, however, (many?) mutations will not lead to an increase in the affinity for that particular antigen but to a decrease in affinity or even to defective Ig. Germinal center B cells with mutations that have resulted in increased affinity Ig might be selected and be preferentially stimulated further, at the expense of germinal center B cells with lower affinity (or defective) Ig. This antigen-driven selection of mutated B cells can be achieved by competititon for (complexed) antigen bound to the FDCs. Unselected germinal center B cells may die by apoptosis (Liu et al. 1989). Alternatively, these cells leave the germinal center. Dead germinal center cells can be phagocytosed by the tingible body macrophages found in germinal centers (Fliedner et al. 1964). The introduction of somatic mutations in germinal center B cells leading to low affinity Ig may be an alternative explanation for the suggested additional role of germinal centers, i.e., the production of virgin (antigen-inexperienced) B cells as against high affinity (antigen-experienced) B memory cells (Nieuwenhuis et al. 1974; Opstelten et al. 1980; Nieuwenhuis and Opstelten 1984).

Another molecular event associated with germinal centers is the switch in isotype expression. Germinal center B cells may switch from sIgM to sIgG (or sIgA) (KRAAL et al. 1982; BUTCHER et al. 1982), and it is speculated that isotype switching stops the hypermutation mechanism (RAJEWSKY et al. 1987). It is possible that germinal center T cells are somehow involved in this postulated switch (ISAKSON et al. 1982; KAWANISHI et al. 1983; MAYER et al. 1985). Finally, germinal center B cells that are "functionally ready" (centrocytes?) will again acquire receptors needed for homing into lymphoid organs when they leave the germinal center as memory cells (KRAAL et al. 1988). From ^{3}H-thymidine labeling studies it is known that cells derived from the germinal center leave through the lymphocyte corona in the spleen to reach the marginal zone (KOBURG 1967; NIEUWENHUIS and KEUNING 1974; NIEUWENHUIS 1981).

As antibody production proceeds during the plasmacellular reaction of the immune response, eventually all possible sites of the antigen component of immune complexes trapped by FDCs will be occupied by antibody. This may block the proliferative effect of the immunizing antigen on germinal center cells and cause the termination of the germinal center reaction (see also VAN ROOIJEN 1980). In this model of germinal center formation, immune complexes play a key role in the germinal center reaction, both by sustaining the proliferative stimulus and by participating in the selection of high affinity B memory cells as well as in the eventual termination of the reaction.

To conclude, germinal centers are histologically defined, unique structures found in peripheral lymphoid organs as a response to antigenic stimulation, as a corollary to the formation of plasma cells. Within germinal centers B cells expand to very large clones of B memory cells. This proliferation affects the B-cell pool not only quantitatively by adding more antigen-specific B cells but also qualitatively by skewing the available repertoire as well as by producing (possibly mutated) B memory cells of higher affinity. We wish to emphasize here that germinal centers have a significant role in the antigen response of B cells in vivo and that so far, but for one possible exception (KOSCO et al. 1989), these structures have not been mimicked in vitro. Thus, when studying B-cell differentiation in vitro one may be studying only part of the story.

Acknowledgments. The authors would like to thank Gerry Hoogenberg, Doete Niermeijer, Peter van der Sijde, and Hilbrand Wierenga for their help in preparing the manuscript.

References

Abo T, Balch CM (1981) A differentiation antigen of human NK and K cells identified by a monoclonal antibody (HNK-1). J Immunol 127:1024–1029

Bailey DJ, Rainey M, Habeshaw JA (1982) Immunoperoxidase analysis of B and T cell populations in human lymphoid follicles. Adv Exp Med Biol 149:809–816

Banerjee D, Thibert R (1983) Natural killer-like cells found in B-cell compartments of human lymphoid tissues. Nature 304:270–272

Barclay AN (1981) Different reticular elements in rat lymphoid tissue identified by localization of Ia, Thy-1 and MRC OX-2 antigens. Immunology 44:727–736

Baroni CD, Vitolo P, Remotti D, Biondi A, Pezella F, Ruco LP, Uccini S (1987) Immunohistochemical heterogeneity of macrophage subpopulations in human lymphoid tissues. Histopathology 11:1029–1042

Barzanji AJ, Emery JL (1978) Germinal centres in the spleens of neonates and stillbirths. Early Human Dev 1:363–369

Bazin H, Gray D, Platteau B, MacLennan ICM (1982) Distinct δ^+ and δ^- B lymphocyte lineages in the rat. Ann N Acad Sci 399:157–173

Bazin H, Platteau B, MacLennan ICM, Johnson GD (1985) B-cell production and differentiation in adult rats. Immunology 54:79–88

Berek C, Apel M (1989) Somatic changes in the immune response to the hapten 2-phenyloxazolone. In: Melchers et al. (eds) Progress in Immunology Vol. VII. Springer-Verlag, Berlin, pp 99–105

Berek C, Milstein C (1987) Mutation drift and repertoire shift in the maturation of the immune response. Immunol Rev 96:23–41

Berek C, Milstein C (1988) The dynamic nature of the antibody repertoire. Immunol Rev 105:5–26

Bhan AK, Nadler LM, Stashenko P, McCluskey RT, Schlossman SF (1981) Stages of B cell differentiation in human lymphoid tissue. J Exp Med 154:737–749

Brown JC, Harris G, Papamichail M, Sljivic VS, Holborow EJ (1973) The localization of aggregated human γ-globulin in the spleens of normal mice. Immunology 24:955–968

Buckley PJ, Smith MR, Braverman MF, Dickson SA (1987) Human spleen contains phenotypic subsets of macrophages and dendritic cells that occupy discrete microanatomic locations. Am J Pathol 128:505–520

Butcher EC, Rouse RV, Coffman RL, Nottenburg CN, Hardy RR, Weissman IL (1982) Surface phenotype of Peyer's patch germinal center cells: implications for the role of germinal centers in B cell differentiation. J Immunol 129:2698–2707

Cohen N (1977) Phylogenetic emergence of lymphoid tissue and cells. In: The lymphocyte structure and function, part I. (ed. J. J. Marchalonis), Marcel Dekker, New York, p 149–202

Coico RF, Bhogal BS, Thorbecke GJ (1983) Relationship of germinal centers in lymphoid tissue to immunologic memory. IV. Transfer of B cell memory with lymph node cells fractioned according to their receptors for peanut agglutinin. J Immunol 131:2254–2257

Collie MH (1974) The location of soluble antigen in the spleen of *Xenopus laevis*. Experientia 30:1205–1206

Cooper MD, Peterson RDA, Good RA (1965) Delineation of the thymic and bursal lymphoid systems in the chicken. Nature 205:143–146

Deenen GJ, Opstelten D, Nieuwenhuis P (1984) Homing of germinal center cells into germinal centers of lymph node via afferent lymphatics. An autoradiographic study. Cell Tissue Res 238:183–189

Deenen GJ, Hunt SV, Opstelten D (1987) A stathmokinetic study of B lymphocytopoiesis in rat bone marrow: proliferation of cells containing cytoplasmic μ-chains, terminal deoxy-nucleotidyl transferase and carrying HIS24 antigen. J Immunol 139:702–710

de Sousa M, Pritchard H (1974) The cellular basis of immunological recovery in nude mice after thymus grafting. Immunology 26:769–776

de Sousa MAB, Parrot DMV, Pantelouris EM (1969) The lymphoid tissues in mice with congenital aplasia of the thymus. Clin Exp Med 4:637

Dijkstra CD, Döpp EA (1983) Ontogenetic development of T and B lymphocytes and non-lymphoid cells in the white pulp of the rat spleen. Cell Tissue Res 229:351–363

Dijkstra CD, Kamperdijk EWA, Döpp EA (1984) The ontogenetic development of the follicular dendritic cell. An ultrastructural study by means of intravenously injected horseradish peroxidase (HRP)-anti-HRP complexes as marker. Cell Tissue Res 236:203–206

Dustin ML, Rohlein R, Bhan AK, Dinarello CA, Springer TA (1986) Induction by IL-1 and interferon-γ: tissue distribution, biochemistry, and function of natural adherence molecule (ICAM-1). J Immunol 137:245–254

Eikelenboom P, Boorsma DM, Rooijen N van (1982) The development of IgM- and IgG-containing plasmablast in the white pulp of the spleen after stimulation with a thymus-independent antigen (LPS) and a thymus-dependent antigen (SRBC). An immunohistoperoxidase study. Cell Tissue Res 229:83–93

Eikelenboom P, Kroese FGM, van Rooijen N (1983) Immune complex-trapping cells in the spleen of the chicken. Cell Tissue Res 231:377–386

Enriquez-Rincon F, Klaus GGB (1984) Follicular trapping of hapten-erythrocyte-antibody complexes in mouse spleen. Immunology 52:107–116

Epstein AL, Marder RJ, Winter JN, Fox RI (1984) Two new monoclonal antibodies (LN-1, LN-2) reactive in B5 formalin-fixed, paraffin-embedded tissues with follicular center and mantle zone human B lymphocytes and derived tumors. J Immunol 133:1028–1036
Ermak TH, Steger HJ, Owen RL, Heyworth MF (1988) Modulation of lymphocyte subsets in Peyer's patches of mice treated with monoclonal antibody against helper T cells. J Histochem Cytochem 36:417–423
Finkelman FD, Mond JJ, Metcalf ES (1983) Effects of neonatal anti-antibody treatment on the murine immune system. I. Suppression of development of surface IgD^+ B cells and expansion of a surface IgM^+ IgD^- B lymphocyte population. J Immunol 131:593–600
Fliedner TM, Kesse M, Cronkite EP, Robertson JS (1964) Cell proliferation in germinal centers of the rat spleen. Ann NY Acad Sci 113:578–594
Franklin WA, Mason DY, Pulford K et al. (1986) Immunohistological analysis of human mononuclear phagocytes and dendritic cells by using monoclonal antibodies. Lab Invest 54:322–335
Freedman AS, Boyd AW, Anderson KC, Fisher DC, Schlossman SF, Nadler LM (1985) B5, a new B cell restricted activation antigen. J Immunol 134:2228–2235
Freitas AA, Rocha B, Coutinho AA (1986) Lymphocyte population kinetics in the mouse. Immunol Rev 91:5–37
Friedman S, Sillcocks D, Rao A, Faas S, Cantor H (1985) A subset of Ly-1 inducer T cell clones activates B cell proliferation but directly inhibits subsequent IgG secretion. J Exp Med 161:785–804
Frizzeria G (1985) Castleman's disease: more questions than answers. Hum Pathol 16:202–205
Gastkemper NA, Wubbena AS, Gimbrère FJH, de Graaf A, Nieuwenhuis P (1981) Germinal centres and the B cell system. V. Presence of germinal centre-precursor cells among lymphocytes of the thoracic duct in the rat. Cell Tissue Res 219:281–289
Gerdes J, Stein H (1982) Complement (C3) receptors on dendritic reticulum cells of normal and malignant lymphoid tissue. J Clin Exp Immunol 48:348–352
Gerdes J, Stein H, Mason DY, Ziegler A (1983) Human dendritic reticulum cells of lymphoid follicles: their antigenic profile and their identification as multinucleated giant cells. Virchows Arch [B] 42:161–172
Gerdes J, Lemke H, Balsch H, Wacker HH, Schwab U, Stein H (1984) Cell cycle analysis of a cell proliferation-associated human nuclear antigen defined by the monoclonal antibody Ki-67. J Immunol 133:1710–1715
Good RA, Finstad J (1967) The phylogenetic development of immune responses and the germinal center system. In: Cottier H, Odartchenko N, Schindler R, Congdon CC (eds) Germinal centers in immune responses. Springer, Berlin Heidelberg New York, pp 4–27
Gordon J, Flores-Romo L, Cairns JA, Millsum MJ, Lane PJ, Johnson GD, MacLennan ICM (1989) CD23: a multifunctional receptor/lymphokine. Immunol Today 10:153–157
Gray D, MacLennan ICM, Bazin H, Khan M (1982) Migrant $\mu^+ \delta^+$ and static $\mu^+ \delta^-$ B lymphocyte subsets. Eur J Immunol 12:564–569
Groscurth P (1980) Non-lymphatic cells in the lymph node cortex of the mouse. II. Postnatal development of the interdigitating cells and the dendritic reticular cells. Pathol Res Pract 169:235–254
Gutman GA, Weissman IL (1972) Lymphoid tissue architecture. Experimental analysis of the origin and distribution of T-cells and B-cells. Immunology 23:465–479
Hanna MG Jr, Congdon CC, Wust CJ (1966) Effect of antigen dose on lymphatic tissue germinal centers. Proc Soc Exp Biol Med 121:286–291
Harms G, van Goor H, Koudstaal J, de Ley L, Hardonk MJ (1986) Immunohistochemical demonstration of DNA-incorporated 5-bromodeoxyuridine in frozen and plastic embedded sections. Histochemistry 85:139–143
Heinen E, Lilet-Leclerq C, Mason DY et al. (1984) Isolation of follicular dendritic cells from human tonsils and adenoids. II. Immunocytochemical characterization. Eur J Immunol 14:267–273
Heinen E, Radoux D, Kinet-Denoël C, Moeremans M, de Mey J, Simar LJ (1985) Isolation of follicular dendritic cells from human tonsils and adenoids. III. Analysis of their Fc receptors. Immunology 54:777–784
Herd ZL, Ada GL (1969) The retention of ^{125}I-immunoglobulins, IgG subunits and antigen-antibody complexes in rat footpads and draining lymph. Aust J Exp Biol Med Sci 47:63

Herzenberg LA, Stall AM, Lalor PA, Sidman C, Moore WA, Parks DR, Herzenberg LA (1986) The Ly-1 B cell lineage. Immunol Rev 93:81–102

Heusermann U, Zurborn UH, Schroeder L, Stutte HJ (1980) The origin of the DRC. An experimental enzymehistochemical and EM study in the rabbit spleen. Cell Tissue Res 209:279–294

Hobbs MV, Feldbush TL (1980) Antigen modulation of the immue response. VI. Rate of large memory cell appearance in lymph nodes and thoracic duct lymph. Cell Immunol 50:30–40

Hoefsmit ECM, Kamperdijk EWA, Hendriks HR, Beelen RHJ, Balfour BM (1980) Lymph node macrophages. Morphology. In: Carr I, Daems WT (eds) The reticuloendothelial system, vol I. Plenum, New York, pp 417–468

Hoffman-Fezer G, Rodt H, Eulitz M, Thierfelder S (1976) Immunohistochemical identification of T- and B-lymphocytes delineated by the unlabeled antibody enzyme method. I. Anatomical distribution of θ-positive and Ig-positive cells in lymphoid organs of mice. J Immunol Methods 13:261–270

Hoffman-Fezer G, Rodt H, Götze D, Thierfelder S (1977) Anatomical distribution of T and B lymphocytes identified by immunohistochemistry in the chicken spleen. Int Arch Allergy Appl Immunol 55:86–95

Hoffman-Fezer G, Löhrs U, Rodt HV, Thierfelder S (1981) Immunohistochemical identification of T- and B-lymphocytes. Delineated by the unlabeled antibody enzyme method. III. Topographical and quantitative distribution of T- and B-cells in human palatine tonsils. Cell Tissue Res 216:361–375

Hofman FM, Lopez D, Husmann L, Meyer PR, Taylor CR (1984) Heterogeneity of macrophage populations in human lymphoid tissue and peripheral blood. Cell Immunol 88:61–74

Hollema H, Poppema S (1988) Immunophenotypes of malignant lymphoma centroblastic-centrocytic and malignant lymphoma centrocytic: an immunohistologc study indicating a derivation from different stages of B cell differentiation. Hum Pathol 19:1053–1059

Hoshi H (1972) On the nature of the periellipsoidal lymphoid tissue of chick spleen. Tohoku J Exp Med 106:285–305

Humphrey JH, Grennan D (1982) Isolation and properties of spleen follicular dendritic cells. Adv Exp Med Biol 149:823–827

Humphrey JH, Grennan D, Sundaram V (1984) The origin of follicular dendritic cells in the mouse and the mechanism of immune complexes on them. Eur J Immunol 14:859–864

Hunter RL, Wissler RW, Fitch FW (1969) Studies on the kinetics and radiosensitivity of dendritic macrophages. Adv Exp Med Biol 5:101–111

Ioachim HL (1982) Lymph node biopsy. JB Lippincott, Philadelphia

Isakson PC, Puré E, Vitetta ES, Krammer PH (1982) T cell-derived B cell differentiation factor(s). Effect on the isotype switch of murine B cells. J Exp Med 155:734–748

Jacobson EB, Caporale LH, Thorbecke GJ (1974) Effect of thymus cell injections on germinal center formation in lymphoid tissue of nude (thymusless) mice. Cell Immunol 13:416–430

Jacobson EB, Baine Y, Chen YW et al. (1981) Physiology of IgD. I. Compensatory phenomena in B lymphocyte activation in mice treated with anti-IgD antibodies. J Exp Med 154:318–332

Jalkanen S, Reichert RA, Gallatin WM, Weissman IL, Butcher EC (1986) Homing receptors and the control of lymphocyte migration. Immunol Rev 91:39–60

Janossy G, Bollum FJ, Bradstock KF, McMichael A, Rapson N, Reaves MF (1979) Terminal transferase positive human bone marrow cells exhibit the antigenic phenotype of common acute leukemia. J Immunol 123:1525–1529

Jerne NK (1971) What precedes clonal selection? In: Ontogeny of acquired immunity. A Ciba Foundation Symposium. Elsevier, Amsterdam, pp 1–15

Jeurissen SHM, Dijkstra CD (1986) Characteristics and functional aspects of non-lymphoid cells in rat germinal centers, recognized by two monoclonal antibodies ED 5 and ED 6. Eur J Immunol 16:562–568

Joling P, Tielen FJ, Vaessen LMB, Hesse CJ, Rozing J (1985) Intrathymic differentiation in the rat. Adv Exp Med Biol 186:235–244

Kamperdijk EWA, Raaymakers EM, de Leeuw JHS, Hoefsmit ECM (1978) Lymph node macrophages and reticulum cells in the immune response. I. The primary response to parathyphoid vaccine. Cell Tissue Res 192:1–23

Kansas GS, Wood GS, Fishwild DM, Engleman EG (1985) Functional characterization of human T lymphocyte subsets distinguished by monoclonal anti-Leu-8. J Immunol 134:2995–3002

Kawanishi H, Saltzman LE, Strober W (1983) Mechanisms regulating IgA class-specific immunoglobulin production in murine gut-associated lymphoid tissues. I. T cells derived from Peyer's patches that switch sIgM B cells to sIgA B cells in vitro. J Exp Med 157:433–450

Kelly RH (1970) Localization of afferent lymph cells within the draining lymph node during a primary response. Nature 227:510–513

Kelly RH, Wolstencroft RA (1974) Germinal centre proliferation in response to mitogenic lymphokines. Clin Exp Immunol 18:321–336

Kim YB, Watson DW (1971) Histological changes of lymphoid tissues in relation to the ontogeny of the immune response in germfree piglets. Adv Exp Med Biol 12:169–177

Klaus GGB (1977) B cell maturation: its relationship to immune induction and tolerance. In: Loor F, Roelants GE (eds) B and T cells in immune recognition. John Wiley, London, pp 235–260

Klaus GGB, Humphrey JH (1977) The generation of memory cells. I. The role of C3 in the generation of B memory cells. Immunology 33:31–40

Klaus GGB, Kunkl A (1982) The role of T cells in B cell priming and germinal centre development. Adv Exp Med Biol 149:743–749

Klaus GGB, Humphrey JH, Kunkl A, Dongworth DW (1980) The follicular dendritic cell: its role in antigen presentation in the generation of immunological memory. Immunol Rev 53:3–28

Koburg E (1967) Cell production and cell migration in the tonsil. In: Cottier H, Odartschenko N, Schindler R, Congdon CC (eds) Germinal centers in immune responses. Springer, Berlin Heidelberg New York, pp 176–182

Kocks C, Rajewsky K (1989) Stable expression and somatic hypermutation of antibody V regions in B cell differentiation pathways. Ann Rev Immunol 7:537–560

Kölsch E, Oberbarnscheidt J, Brüner K, Heuer J (1980) The Fc-receptor: its role in the transmission of differentiation signals. Immunol Rev 49:61–78

Kosco MH, Szakal AK, Tew JG (1980) In vivo obtained antigen presented by germinal center B cells to T cells in vitro. J Immunol 140:354–360

Kosco MH, Tew JG, Szakal AK (1986) Antigenic phenotyping of isolated and in situ rodent follicular dendritic cells (FDC) with emphasis on the ultrastructural demonstration of Ia antigens. Anat Rec 215:201–213

Kosco MH, Gray D, Burton GF, Szakal AK, Tew JG (1989) Germinal center formation in vitro: requirement for follicular dendritic cells (FDC). In: Abstracts 7th International Congress of Immunology: Berlin (West). Gustav Fischer Verlag, Stuttgart. Abstract number 30-11, p 164

Kotani M, Nawa Y, Fujii H, Fukumoto T, Miyamoto M, Yamashita A (1974) Involvement of thymus cells in the formation of germinal centers. Acta Anat (Basel) 90:585–590

Kotani M, Ezaki T, Ekino S, Matsuno K, Fudjii H, Nawa Y (1982) Lymph macrophages enter the germinal center of regional lymph nodes. Adv Exp Med Biol 149:837–841

Kraal G, Weissman IL, Butcher EC (1982) Germinal centre B cells: antigen specificity and changes in heavy chain class expression. Nature 298:377–379

Kraal G, Weissman IL, Butcher EC (1985) Germinal center cells: antigen specificity, heavy chain class expression and evidence of memory. Adv Exp Med Biol 186:145–151

Kraal G, Hardy RR, Gallatin WM, Weissman IL, Butcher EC (1986) Antigen-induced changes in B cell subsets in lymph nodes: analysis by dual fluorescence flow cytometry. Eur J Immunol 16:829–834

Kraal G, Weissman IL, Butcher EC (1988) Memory B cells express a phenotype consistent with migratory competence after secondary but not short-term primary immunization. Cell Immunol 15:78–87

Kroese FGM (1983) Antigen trapping in the spleen of the red-eared turtle. Dev Comp Immunol 7:711–712

Kroese FGM, van Rooijen N (1982) The architecture of the spleen of the red-eared slider, *Chrysemys scripta elegans* (Reptilia, Testudines). J Morphol 173:279–284

Kroese FGM, Rooijen N van (1983) Antigen trapping in the spleen of the turtle, *Chrysemys scripta elegans*. Immunology 49:61–68

Kroese FGM, Eikelenboom P, van Rooijen N (1982) Electron-microscopical and enzymehistochemical characterization of immune complex trapping cells in the spleen of different vertebrate species. Dev Comp Immunol [Suppl 2]:69–74

Kroese FGM, Wubbena AS, Joling P, Nieuwenhuis P (1985a) T lymphocytes in rat lymphoid follicles are a subset of T helper cells. Adv Exp Med Biol 186:442–450

Kroese FGM, Leceta J, Döpp EA, Herraez MP, Nieuwenhuis P, Zapata A (1985b) Dendritic immune complex cells in the spleen of the snake, *Python reticulatus*. Dev Comp Immunol 9:641–652

Kroese FGM, Wubbena AS, Nieuwenhuis P (1986) Germinal centre formation and follicular antigen trapping in the spleen of lethally X-irradiated and reconstituted rats. Immunology 57:99–104

Kroese FGM, Wubbena AS, Opstelten D et al. (1987a) B lymphocyte differentiation in the rat: production and characterization of monoclonal antibodies to B lineage-associated antigens. Eur J Immunol 17:921–928

Kroese FGM, Wubbena AS, Seijen HG, Nieuwenhuis P (1987b) Germinal centres develop oligoclonally. Eur J Immunol 17:1069–1072

Kroese FGM, Wubbena AS, Kuijpers KC, Nieuwenhuis P (1987c) The ontogeny of germinal centre forming capacity of neonatal rat spleen. Immunology 60:597–602

Kroese FGM, Wubbena AS, Seijen HG, Nieuwenhuis P (1988) The de novo generation of germinal centers is an oligoclonal process. Adv Exp Med Biol 237:245–250

Kunkl A, Klaus GGB (1981) The generation of memory cells. IV. Immunization with antigen-antibody complexes accelerates the development of B memory cells, the formation of germinal centres and the maturation of antibody affinity in the secondary response. Immunology 43:371–378

Laissue J, Cottier H, Hess MW, Stoner RD (1971) Early and enhanced germinal center formation and antibody responses in mice after primary stimulation with antigen-isologous antibody complexes as compared with antigen alone. J Immunol 107:822–831

Lakey Berg E, Goldstein LA, Jutila MA et al. (1989) Homing receptors and vascular addressins: cell adhesion molecules that direct lymphocyte traffic. Immunol Rev 108:5–18

Levy NS, Malipiero UV, Lebecque SG, Gearhart PJ (1989) Early onset of somatic mutation in immunoglobulin Vh genes during the primary immune response. J Exp Med 169:2007–2019

Linden MD, Fishleder AJ, Katzin WE, Tubbs RR (1988) Absence of B-cell or T-cell clonal expansion in nodular, lymphocyte predominant Hodgkin's disease. Hum Pathol 19:591–594

Liu YJ, Joshud DE, Williams GT, Smith CA, Gordon J, MacLennan ICM (1989) Mechanism of antigen-driven selection in germinal centres. Nature 342:929–931

MacLennan ICM, Gray D (1986) Antigen-driven selection of virgin and memory B cells. Immunol Rev 91:61–85

MacLennan ICM, Gray D, Kumararatne DS, Bazin H (1982) The lymphocytes of splenic marginal zones: a distinct B cell lineage. Immunol Today 3:305–307

Mandel TE, Phipps RP, Abbot A, Tew JG (1980) The follicular dendritic cell: long term antigen retention during immunity. Immunol Rev 53:29–59

Manning MJ (1980) Immunological memory in phylogenetic perspective. In: Manning MJ (ed) Phylogeny of immunological memory. Elsevier/North Holland Biomedical, Amsterdam, pp 311–316

Manning MJ, Turner FRJ (1976) Comparative immunobiology. Blacky, Glasgow

Marlin SD, Springer TA (1987) Purified intercellular adhesion molecule-1 (ICAM-1) is a ligand for lymphocyte function-associated antigen-1 (LFA-1). Cell 51:813–819

Mason DW (1976) The class of surface immunoglobulin on cells carrying IgG memory in rat thoracic duct lymph: the size of the subpopulation mediating IgG memory. J Exp Med 143:1122–1130

Mayer L, Posnett DN, Kunkl HG (1985) Human malignant T cells capable of inducing an immunoglobulin class switch. J Exp Med 161:134–144

Mayrhofer G, Pugh CW, Barclay AN (1983) The distribution, ontogeny and origin in the rat of Ia-positive cells with dendritic morphology and of Ia antigen in epithelia, with special reference to the intestine. Eur J Immunol 13:112–122

McKean D, Huppi K, Bell M, Staudt L, Gerhard W, Weigert M (1984) Generation of antibody diversity in the immune response of BALB/c mice to influenza virus hemagglutinin. Proc Natl Acad Sci USA 81:3180–3184

Meeker TC, Miller RA, Link MP, Bindl J, Warnke R, Levy R (1984) A unique human B lymphocyte antigen defined by a monoclonal antibody. Hybridoma 3:305–320

Melchers F, Andersson J (1984) B cell activation: three steps and their variations. Cell 37:715–720
Menzies DW (1965) The concept of the "centron". Nature 208:163–165
Mietinnen M, Franssila KO, Saxén E (1983) Hodgkin's disease, lymphocytic predominance nodular. Increased risk for subsequent non-Hodgkin's lymphomas. Cancer 51:2292–2300
Mitchell J, Pye J, Holmes MC, Nossal GJV (1972) Antigens in immunity. Antigen localization in congenitally athymic "nude" mice. Aust J Exp Biol Med Sci 50:637
Miyawaki T, Ohzeki S, Ikuta N, Seki H, Taga K, Taniguchi N (1984) Immunohistological localization and immune phenotypes of lymphocytes expressing Tac antigen in human lymphoid tissues. J Immunol 133:2996–3000
Murata H (1959) Comparative studies of the spleen in submammalian vertebrates. II. Minute structure of the spleen, with special reference to the periarterial lymphoid sheath. Bull Yamaguchi Med School 6:83–105
Murray LJ, Swerdlow SH, Habeshaw JA (1984) Distribution of B lymphocyte subsets in normal lymphoid tissue. Clin Exp Immunol 56:399–406
Naiem M, Gerdes J, Abdulaziz Z, Stein H, Mason DY (1983) Production of a monoclonal antibody reactive with human dendritic reticulum cells and its use in the immunohistological analysis of lymphoid tissue. J Clin Pathol 36:167–175
Nettesheim P, Hanna MG (1969) Radiosensitivity of the antigen trapping mechanism and its relation to the suppression of immune response. Adv Exp Med Biol 5:167–175
Nieuwenhuis P (1981) B-cell differentiation in vivo. Immunol Today 2:104–110
Nieuwenhuis P, Ford WL (1976) Comparative migration of B and T lymphocytes in the rat spleen and lymph nodes. Cell Immunol 23:254–267
Nieuwenhuis P, Keuning FJ (1974) Germinal centres and the origin of the B cell system. II. Germinal centres in the rabbit spleen and popliteal lymph nodes. Immunology 26:509–519
Nieuwenhuis P, Lennert K (1980) Histophysiology of normal lymphoid tissue and immune reactions. In: van den Tweel TG, Taylor CR, Bosman FT (eds) Malignant lymphoproliferative diseases. Martinus Nijhoff, The Hague, pp 3–12
Nieuwenhuis P, Opstelten D (1984) Functional anatomy of germinal centres. Am J Anat 170:421–435
Nieuwenhuis P, van Nouhuys CE, Eggens JH, Keuning FJ (1974) Germinal centres and the origin of the B cell system. I. Germinal centres in the rabbit appendix. Immunology 26:497–507
Nossal GJV, Ada GL (1971) Antigens, lymphoid cells and the immune response. Academic, New York
Oberbarnscheidt J, Kölsch E (1978) Direct blockade of antigen-reactive B lymphocytes by immune complexes. An "off" signal for precursors of IgM-producing cells provided by the linkage of antigen- and Fc-receptors. Immunology 35:151–157
Odartchenko N, Lewerenz M, Sordat B, Roos B, Cottier H (1967) Kinetics of cellular death in germinal centers of mouse spleen. In: Cottier H, Odartchenko N, Schindler F, Congdon CC (eds) Germinal centers in immune responses. Springer, Berlin, Heidelberg, New York, pp 212–217
Okumura K, Julius HN, Tsu T, Herzenberg LA, Herzenberg LA (1976) Demonstration that IgG memory is carried by IgG-bearing cells. Eur J Immunol 6:467–472
Opstelten D, Osmond DG (1983) Pre-B cells in mouse bone marrow: immunofluorescence stathmokinetic studies of the proliferation of cytoplasmic μ-chain-bearing cells in normal mice. J Immunol 131:2635–2640
Opstelten D, Stikker R, van der Heijden D, Nieuwenhuis P (1980) Germinal centres and the B cell system. IV. Functional characteristics of rabbit appendix germinal centre (derived) cells. Virchows Arch [B] 34:53–64
Opstelten D, Stikker R, Deenen GJ, Bos L, Nieuwenhuis P (1981) Germinal centers and the B cell system. VI. Migration pattern of germinal center cells of the rabbit appendix. Cell Tissue Res 218:59–73
Opstelten D, Stikker R, Deenen GJ, Nieuwenhuis P (1982) Germinal centers and the B cell system. VII. Complement receptors, antigen receptors, immunoglobulin and alkaline phosphatase in germinal centers of rabbit appendix and popliteal lymph nodes. Cell Tissue Res 224:505–516
Opstelten D, Deenen GJ, Stikker R, Bos L, Nieuwenhuis P (1983) Germinal centers and the B cell system. VIII. Functional characteristics and cell surface markers of germinal center cell subsets differing in density and in sedimentation velocity. Immunobiology 165:1–14

Opstelten D, Deenen GJ, Rozing J, Hunt S (1986) B lymphocyte-associated antigens on terminal deoxynucleotidyl transferase-positive cells and pre-B cells in bone marrow of the rat. J Immunol 137:76–84

Osmond DG, Nossal GJV (1974) Differentiation of lymphocytes in mouse bone marrow. II. Kinetics of maturation and renewal of anti-globulin binding cells studied by double labeling. Cell Immunol 13:132–145

Osmond DG, Melchers F, Paige CJ (1984) Pre-B cells in mouse bone marrow: in vitro maturation of peanut agglutinin binding B lymphocyte precursors separated from bone marrow by fluorescence activated cell sorting. J Immunol 133:86–90

Öst A, Baroni CD, Biberfeld P et al. (1989) Lymphadenopathy in HIV infection histological classification and staging. Acta Pathol Microbiol Immunol Scand [Suppl] 8:7–15

Papamichail M, Gutierrez C, Embling P, Johnson P, Holborow EJ, Pepys MB (1975) Complement dependence of localisation of aggregated IgG in germinal centres. Scand J Immunol 4:343–347

Paradinas F (1985) Primary and secondary immune disorders. In: Stansfeld AG (ed) Lymph node biopsy interpretation. Churchill Livingstone, New York, pp 159–195

Parrott DMV (1967) The integrity of the germinal center: an investigation of the differential localization of labeled cells in lymphoid organs. In: Cottier H, Orartscheko N, Schindler R, Congdon CC (eds) Germinal centres in immune responses. Springer, Berlin Heidelberg New York, pp 168–175

Parwaresch MR, Radzun HJ, Feller AC, Peters KP, Hansmann ML (1983) Peroxidase positive mononuclear leukocytes as possible precursors of human dendritic reticulum cells. J Immunol 131:2719–2725

Pitchappan RM (1980) On the phylogeny of splenic structure and function. Dev Comp Immunol 4:395–416

Pizzolo G, Semenzato G, Chilosi M et al. (1984) Distribution and heterogeneity of cells detected by HNK-1 monoclonal antibody in blood and tissues in normal, reactive and neoplastic conditions. Clin Exp Immunol 57:195–206

Pollard M (1967) Germinal centers in germfree animals. In: Cottier H, Odartchenko N, Schindler R, Congdon CC (eds) Germinal centers in immune responses. Springer, Berlin Heidelberg New York, pp 343–346

Poppema S, Kaiserling E, Lennert K (1979) Nodular paragranuloma and progressively transformed germinal-centers. Virchows Arch [B] 31:211–225

Poppema S, Bahn AK, Reinherz EL, McCluskey RT, Schlossman SF (1981) Distribution of T cell subsets in human lymph nodes. J Exp Med 153:30–41

Poppema S, Visser L, de Leij L (1983) Reactivity of presumed anti-natural killer cell antibody Leu 7 with intrafollicular T lymphocytes. Clin Exp Immunol 54:834–837

Poppema S, Hollema H, Visser L, Vos H (1987) Monoclonal antibodies (MT1, MT2, MB1, MB2, MB3) reactive with leukocyte subsets in paraffin-embedded tissue sections. Am J Pathol 127:418–429

Porwit-Ksiazek A, Ksiazek T, Riberfeld P (1983) Leu 7^+ (HNK-1^+) cells. I. Selective compartmentalization of Leu 7^+ cells with different immunophenotypes in lymphatic tissues and blood. Scand J Immunol 18:485–493

Radoux D, Kinet-Denoël C, Heinen E, Moeremans M, de Mey J, Simar LJ (1985) Retention of immune complexes by Fc receptors on mouse follicular dendritic cells. Scand J Immunol 21:345–353

Raedler A, Raedler E, Arndt R, Thiele HG (1981) Terminal galactosyl residues of cell-surface glycoconjugates exposed on both human and murine immature T- and B- cells. Cell Tissue Res 218:219–226

Rajewsky K, Förster I, Cumano A (1987) Evolutionary and somatic selection of the antibody repertoire in the mouse. Science 238:1088–1094

Ralfkiaer E, Stein H, Ralfkiaer N, Hou-Jensen K, Mason DY (1985) Normal and neoplastic Langerhans cells: phenotypic comparison with other types of macrophages. Adv Exp Med Biol 186:1009–1015

Razzeca KJ, Pillemer E, Weissman IL, Rouse RV (1986) In situ identification of idiotype-positive cells participating in the immune response to phosphorylcholine. Eur J Immunol 16:393–399

Reichert RA, Gallatin WM, Weissman IL, Butcher EC (1983) Germinal center B cells lack homing receptors necessary for normal lymphocyte recirculation. J Exp Med 157:813–827
Rose ML, Malchiodi F (1981) Binding of peanut lectin to thymic cortex and germinal centres of lymphoid tissue. Immunology 42:583–591
Rose ML, Ribbeck MSC, Wallis VJ, Forrester GA, Davies AJS (1980) Peanut lectin binding properties of germinal centres of mouse lymphoid tissue. Nature 28:364–366
Rouse RV, Ledbetter JA, Weissman IL (1982) Mouse lymph node germinal centers contain a selected subset of T cells – the helper phenotype. J Immunol 128:2243–2246
Rouse RV, Reichert RA, Gallatin WM, Weissman IL, Butcher EC (1984) Localization of lymphocyte subpopulations in peripheral lymphoid organs: directed lymphocyte migration and segregation into specific microenvironments. Am J Anat 170:391–405
Rozing J, Brons NHC, van Ewijk W, Benner R (1978) B lymphocyte differentiation in lethally irradiated and reconstituted mice. A histological study using immunofluorescent detection of B lymphocytes. Cell Tissue Res 189:19–30
Schnizlein CT, Kosco MH, Szakal AK, Tew JG (1985) Follicular dendritic cells in suspension: identification, enrichment, and initial characterization indicating immune complex trapping and lack of adherence and phagocytic activity. J Immunol 134:1360–1368
Schriever F, Freedman AS, Freeman G, Messner E, Lee G, Daly J, Nadler LM (1989) Isolated human follicular dendritic cells display a unique phenotype. J Exp Med 169:2043–2058
Schwarting R, Stein H, Wang CY (1985) The monoclonal antibody S-HCL 1 (Leu-14) and S-HCL (Leu-M5) allow the diagnosis of hairy cell leukemia. Blood 65:974–983
Secombes CJ, Manning MJ (1980) Comparative studies on the immune system of fishes and amphibians: antigen localization in the carp *Cyprinus carpio*. J Fish Dis 3:399–412
Seijen HG, Bun JCAM, Wubbena AS, Löhlefink KG (1988) The germinal center precursor cell is surface μ and δ positive. Adv Exp Med Biol 237:233–237
Severson GS, Harrington DS, Johansson SL, McManus BM (1988) Epithelioid germinal-centers in overwhelming childhood infections. Arch Pathol Lab Med 112:917–921
Seymour GJ, Greaves MF, Janossy G (1980) Identification of cells expressing T and p 28,33 (Ia-like) antigens in sections of human lymphoid tissue. Clin Exp Immunol 39:66
Sinclair NRStC, Lees RK, Abrahams S, Chan PL, Fagan G, Stiller CR (1974) Regulation of the immune response. X. Antigen-antibody complex inactivation of cells involved in adoptive transfer. J Immunol 113:1493–1500
Siskind GW, Benacerraf B (1969) Cell selection by antigen in the immune response. Adv Immunol 10:1–50
Sminia T, Janse EM (1982) Distribution of IgM- and IgG-containing cells during the primary immune response in the rat spleen. Cell Tissue Res 224:25–31
Sminia T, Janse EM, Plesch BEC (1983) Ontogeny of Peyer's patches of the rat. Anat Rec 207:309–316
Sordat B, Sordat M, Hess MW, Stoner RD, Cottier H (1970) Specific antibody within lymphoid germinal center cells of mice after primary immunization with horseradish peroxidase: a light and electron microscopic study. J Exp Med 131:77–91
Stansfeld AG (1985) Lymph node biopsy interpretation. Churchill Livingstone, London
Stein H, Bonk A, Tolksdorf G, Lennert K, Rodt H, Gerdes J (1980) Immunohistologic analysis of the organization of normal lymphoid tissue and non-Hodgkin's lymphomas. J Histochem Cytochem 28:746–760
Stein H, Gerdes J, Mason DY (1982) The normal and malignant germinal centre. Clin Haematol 11:531–559
Szakal AK, Holmes KL, Tew JG (1983) Transport of immune complexes from the subcapsular sinus to lymph node follicles on the surface of nonphagocytic cells, including cells with dendritic morphology. J Immunol 131:1714–1727
Szakal AK, Gieringer RL, Kosco MH, Tew JG (1985) Isolated follicular dendritic cells: cytochemical antigen localization, Nomarski, SEM, and TEM morphology. J Immunol 134:1349–1359
Szakal AK, Kosco MH, Tew JG (1988) A novel in vivo follicular dendritic cell dependent iccosome-mediated mechanism for delivery of antigen to antigen-processing cells. J Immunol 140:341–353

Terashima K, Imai Y, Kasajima T, Tsunoda R, Takahashi K, Kojima M (1977) An ultrastructural study on antibody production of the lymph nodes of rats with special reference to the role of germinal centres. Acta Pathol Jpn 27:1–24

Tew JG, Phipps RP, Mandel TE (1980) The maintenance and regulation of the humoral immune response: persisting antigen and the role of follicular antigen-binding dendritic cells as accessory cells. Immunol Rev 53:175–202

Thorbecke GJ (1959) Some histological and functional aspects of lymphoid tissue in germfree animals. I. Morphological studies. Ann NY Acad Sci 78:237–246

Thorbecke GJ, Romano TJ, Lerman SP (1974) Regulatory mechanisms in proliferation and differentiation of lymphoid tissue, with particular reference to germinal centre development. Prog Immunol II, 3:25–34

Thorley-Lawson DA, Schooley RT, Bhan AK, Nadler LM (1982) Epstein-Barr virus super induces a new human B cell differentiation antigen (B-LAST 1) expressed on transformed lymphoblasts. Cell 30:415–425

Timens W, Poppema S (1985) Lymphocyte compartments in human spleen: an immunohistologic study in normal spleens and noninvolved spleens in Hodgkin's disease. Am J Pathol 120:443–452

Timens W, Boes A, Rozenboom-Uiterwyk T, Poppema S (1980) Immuno-architecture of human fetal lymphoid tissues. Virchows Archiv Pathol Anat 413:563–571

Timens W, Visser L, Poppema S (1986) Nodular lymphocyte predominance type of Hodgkin's disease is a germinal center lymphoma. Lab Invest 54:457–461

Timens W, Rozeboom T, Poppema S (1987) Fetal and neonatal development of human spleen: an immunohistological study. Immunology 60:603–609

Timens W, Boes A, Rozenboom-Uiterwyk T, Poppema S (1989) Immaturity of the human splenic marginal zone in infancy. Possible contribution to the deficient infant immune response. J Immunol 143:3200–3206

Tsunoda R, Yaginuma Y, Kojima M (1980) Immunocytochemical studies on the constituent cells of the secondary nodules in human tonsils. Acta Pathol Jpn 30:33–58

van Ewijk W, Rozing J, Brons NHC, Klepper D (1977) Cellular events during the primary immune response in the spleen. A fluorescence-, light- and electronmicroscopic study in germfree mice. Cell Tissue Res 183:471–489

van Rees EP, Döpp EA, Dijkstra CD, Sminia T (1985) The postnatal development of cell populations in the rat popliteal lymph node. An immunohistochemical study. Cell Tissue Res 242:391–398

van Rooijen N (1972) Antigens in the spleen. The non-specificity of the follicles in the process of antigen trapping and the role of antibody. Immunology 22:757–765

van Rooijen N (1980) Immune complex trapping in lymphoid follicles: a discussion on possible functional implications. In: Manning MJ (ed) Phylogeny of immunological memory. Elsevier/North Holland Biomedical, Amsterdam, pp 281–290

van Rooijen N, Claassen E, Eikelenboom P (1986) Is there a single differentiation pathway for all antibody-forming cells in the spleen? Immunol Today 7:193–196

Veerman AJP (1975) The postnatal development of the white pulp in the rat spleen and the onset of immunocompetence against a thymus-independent and a thymus-dependent antigen. Z Immunol Forsch 150:45–59

Veerman AJP, van Ewijk W (1975) White pulp compartments in the spleen of rats and mice. A light and electron microscopy study of lymphoid and non-lymphoid cell types in T- and B-areas. Cell Tissue Res 156:417–441

Velardi A, Mingari MC, Moretta L, Grossi CE (1988) Functional analysis of cloned germinal center $CD4^+$ cells with natural killer cell-related features; divergence from typical T helper cells. J Immunol 137:2808–2813

Villena A, Zapata A, Rivera-Pomar JM, Barrutia MG, Fonfria J (1983) Structure of the non-lymphoid cells during the postnatal development of the rat lymph nodes. Cell Tissue Res 229:219–232

Weinberg WC, Howard JC, Iannaccone PM (1984) Histological demonstration of mosaicism in a series of chimeric rats produced between congenic strains. Science 227:524–527

Weinberg DS, Ault KA, Gurley M, Pinkus GS (1986) The human lymph node germinal center cell: characterization and isolation by using two-color flow cytometry. J Immunol 137:1486–1497
Weissman IL, Gutman GA, Friedberg SH, Jerabek L (1976) Lymphoid tissue architecture. III. Germinal centers, T cells, and thymus-dependent vs. thymus-independent antigens. Adv Exp Med Biol 66:229–237
Westerga J, Timens W (1989) Immunohistological analysis of human fetal lymph nodes. Scand J Immunol 29:103–112
White RG, Henderson DC, Eslami MB, Nielsen KH (1975) Localization of a protein antigen in the chicken spleen: effects of various manipulative procedures on the morphogenesis of the germinal centre. Immunology 28:1–21
Zaitoun AM (1980) Cell population kinetics of the germinal centers of lymph nodes of Balb/c mice. J Anat 130:131–137

T Lymphocytes in Non-neoplastic Lymph Nodes

J.J. van den Oord, F. Facchetti, J. Delabie, and C. de Wolf-Peeters

1 Introduction

Over the past 10 years, advances in diverse areas of basic research and technology have elucidated the functions of T lymphocytes. These include helper activity on B and T cells, release of various cytokines that act on nonlymphoid cells, e.g., macrophages, dendritic cells, and endothelial cells, cytolytic effector activity directed towards nonself or altered-self target cells, and suppressor activity on both B and T lymphocytes (Reinherz and Schlossman 1980).

Demonstration of surface receptors capable of binding the Fc portion of either IgM or IgG and studies with monoclonal antibodies to unique cell surface glycoproteins on T cells disclosed that helper/inducer and suppressor/cytotoxic T cells reside in phenotypically distinct T-cell subpopulations; the former display the $CD4^+$ phenotype and bear receptors for the Fc portion of IgM, whereas the latter express the CD8 antigen and bear receptors for the Fc portion of IgG (Moretta et al. 1984). Recent experiments, however, indicate that the correlation between phenotype and function is not as strict as was formerly believed. Single cloned T cells may display simultaneous cytolytic and helper activity and cytotoxic T cells directed to a variety of viruses may express the $CD4^+$ helper/inducer immunophenotype (Meuer et al. 1983a); conversely, $CD8^+$ T cells have been found to display functions comparable to those of helper T cells (Schwartz 1986). Since antigen recognition by T cells requires simultaneous display of products encoded by the major histocompatibility complex (MHC), it is now generally believed that the CD4 and CD8 antigens indicate the class of MHC antigens with which a particular T-cell subset will interact in an immune response, rather than the precise function of that T-cell subset (Romain and Schlossman 1984).

Early reports by GUTMAN and WEISSMAN (1972) showed that the paracortex corresponds to the lymph node compartment in which T lymphocytes home. The paracortex is localized in the cortical region beneath the lymphoid follicles. It extends down to the corticomedullary boundary; its upper margins are not well defined and may even reach as far as the subcapsular sinus (LENNERT et al. 1978). The paracortex of the human lymph node is rich in high endothelial venules, several types of reticulum cell, including interdigitating reticulum cells, and lymphocytes. These lymphocytes are small cells that have an irregular or more rounded nucleus with coarse, condensed chromatin and scant cytoplasm. Occasionally, blastic forms, i.e., T immunoblasts, are observed; these cells have large round or irregular nuclei with one or more nucleoli, and moderately abundant cytoplasm. Although electron-microscopic criteria specific for T cells have been reported (POLLIACK et al. 1973; WATANABE et al. 1974), it is generally believed that T lymphocytes cannot reliably be distinguished from B lymphocytes on the basis of pure morphology.

The identification of paracortical lymphocytes as thymus-derived cells has evolved from enzyme- and immunohistochemical studies (MÜLLER-HERMELINK et al. 1974; STEIN et al. 1980). In the early 1970s, several authors succeeded in demonstrating T cells in situ applying the E-rosette assay to cryostat sections (SILVEIRA et al. 1972; TONDER et al. 1974). When the cytochemical profile of peripheral T lymphocytes was unraveled, enzyme-histochemical techniques were introduced to study the composition of the paracortex (MÜLLER-HERMELINK et al. 1974; PANGALIS et al. 1978; CHILOSI et al. 1981). Nonspecific acid α-naphthyl acetate esterase positive lymphocytes were found in largest numbers in the lumen of high endothelial venules (MÜLLER et al. 1975; KNOWLES and HOLEK 1978); diaminopeptidase IV positive cells, considered to represent T lymphocytes with receptors for the Fc portion of IgM, were found diffusely throughout the paracortex as well as in blood vessels and sinuses (FELLER 1982). In situ studies with a variety of *lectins* have shown that T lymphocytes react with most lectins in a cap-like staining pattern; only wheat germ agglutinin, concanavalin A, and *Ricinus communis* A show a membranous staining of T lymphocytes in formalin-fixed, paraffin-embedded tissue (HSU and REE 1983).

The definite localization of T-cell subsets in lymphoid tissues has only recently become possible and has awaited the production of a large variety of *monoclonal antibodies* directed to T cells and their subsets. Application of these monoclonal antibodies to snap-frozen lymphoid tissue, together with the refinement of single and double immunohistochemical labeling techniques, has allowed a precise localization of the various T-cell subsets in normal and reactive lymphoid tissues and has permitted a better understanding of the overall lymph node architecture and its changes during an immune response (MASON et al. 1981, 1982; VAN DER VALK and MEIJER 1987).

2 Distribution of T Cells and T-Cell Subsets in the Unstimulated Lymph Node

In situ immunohistochemical studies have confirmed that T lymphocytes are located mainly in the paracortex of the lymph node. Studies on the distribution of T-cell subsets have revealed a predominance (POPPEMA et al. 1981) of $CD4^+$ helper/inducer T cells, ranging from 60% (JANOSSY et al. 1981; HSU et al. 1983) up to 80% of all paracortical lymphocytes (JANOSSY et al. 1980; VAN DER VALK et al. 1984). A minority of paracortical T cells display the $CD8^+$ suppressor/cytotoxic T cell phenotype; however, considerable variations in the relative percentages of both subsets appear to exist (DELSOL et al. 1984). In contrast to peripheral blood, a small but significant number of paracortical T cells express the interleukin-2 (IL-2) receptor, a feature that may reflect continuous antigenic stimulation due to contact with the environment (MIYAWAKI et al. 1984; TAKACS et al. 1985; SHEIBANI et al. 1987; STRAUCHEN and BREAKSTONE 1987).

Separate nests of aggregates of immunoreactive T cells can be found in the paracortex upon staining for the various polypeptides of the CD45 or leukocyte common antigen family (JANOSSY et al. 1989). Whether these clusters of T cells respond to the same antigen, or whether their clustering is caused by the sharing of certain adhesive properties, remains to be investigated.

A minority of the $CD8^+$ T cells in the paracortex have been found to display the β chain of S-100 protein (TAKAHASHI et al. 1985). By virtue of their suppressive capabilities, these cells may play a regulatory role in the immune response (FERRARI et al. 1988).

Scattered T cells are also found in B-lymphoid follicles and in the lymph node medulla. In the medullary cords, the majority of T cells express the helper/inducer phenotype, as do the lymphocytes present in the afferent lymph (LUKOMSKA et al. 1980; OLSZEWSKI et al. 1982). The follicle center localization of T cells was detected in 1972 in murine lymph nodes by GUTMAN and WEISSMAN, who used an immunofluorescent technique. Similar results were obtained in human lymphoid tissue (HOFFMANN-FEZER et al. 1976; LAMELIN et al. 1978; HOFFMANN-FEZER et al. 1981; SEYMOUR et al. 1981). T cells represent between 10% and 40% of all cells that populate the follicle center (DVORETSKY et al. 1982; ROUSE et al. 1982; HSU et al. 1983). Their number varies considerably and is thought to reflect the functional stage of follicle center development (SI and WHITESIDE 1983; SWERDLOW and MURRAY 1984). Intrafollicular T cells belong almost exclusively to the $CD4^+$ helper/inducer T-cell subset and form a crescentic rim of immunoreactive cells at the border between the follicle center and lymphocytic corona; variable numbers of $CD4^+$ T cells are found scattered throughout the follicle center as well (LAMELIN et al. 1978; JANOSSY et al. 1980; WARNKE and LEVY 1980; POPPEMA et al. 1981; ROUSE et al. 1982; DVORETSKY et al. 1982; HSU et al. 1983). The majority of the $CD4^+$ intrafollicular cells react with the monoclonal antibody Leu-7 (HNK-1), directed against natural killer cells (BANERJEE and THIBERT 1983; MORI et al. 1983; POPPEMA et al. 1983; RITCHIE et al. 1983; SI and WHITESIDE 1983; PIZZOLO et al. 1984; SWERDLOW and MURRAY 1984) but differ markedly from the recirculating Leu-7$^+$ natural killer cells (VON GAUDECKER 1984). In contrast to extrafollicular T cells, those in the follicle center lack the antigen recognized by the monoclonal antibody Leu-8 (KANSAS et al. 1985). Finally, intrafollicular T cells have been found to display diaminopeptidase IV (MENTHEIN et al. 1984) but no discernible nonspecific esterase activity (KNOWLES and HOLEK 1978; FELLER 1982).

T cells recognize antigen in association with MHC products by a receptor consisting of α/β heterodimers associated with the CD3 complex. Using monoclonal antibodies to nonpolymorphic determinants on the T-cell receptor β chain, almost all CD3$^+$ T cells in the paracortex and lymphoid follicles were found to express the β chain (PICKER et al. 1987). Recently, a subpopulation of T cells was described that lacks CD4 and CD8 antigens, and whose antigen receptor consists of a γ/δ heterodimer associated with the CD3 complex (BRENNER et al. 1987; BANK et al. 1986). The latter T cells represent only between 1% and 5% of cells of the paracortex and are virtually absent from B-lymphoid follicles (PICKER et al. 1988).

3 Distribution of T Cells and T-Cell Subsets in the Lymph Node During an Immune Response

In both the primary and the secondary immune response (FORD 1975), T lymphocytes are recruited from the recirculating pool of cells, enter the lymph node parenchyma via high endothelial venules, and follow a labyrinthic route through the paracortex towards the efferent lymphatic vessels (PARROTT and DE SOUSA 1971). In the paracortex, these T cells encounter the antigen at the surface of antigen-presenting cells. The exact identity of this accessory cell is unknown. Based on the close contacts between interdigitating reticulum cells and T lymphocytes, it has been postulated that interdigitating reticulum cells create a microenvironment necessary for the homing and subsequent proliferation of recirculating T lymphocytes (VELDMAN 1970; VEERMAN and VAN EWIJK 1975; VELDMAN and KEUNING 1978; VELDMAN et al. 1978). The strong expression of HLADR antigens at their surface and the finding of finger-like protrusions of lymphocytes into interdigitating reticulum cells (LEENE 1971) have led to the hypothesis that these cells play a crucial role in the presentation of antigens to helper/inducer T lymphocytes (SILBERBERG-SINAKIN et al. 1976). This hypothesis has been supported by the finding of a selective accumulation of CD4$^+$ lymphocytes around paracortical interdigitating reticulum cells (JANOSSY et al. 1980, 1981); however, neither antigens nor antigen-antibody complexes have been demonstrated thus far at the surface of interdigitating reticulum cells. More recently, B lymphocytes, loaded with antigen bound to their surface immunoglobulins, have been claimed to serve as the principal antigen-presenting cell in the lymph node (JANEWAY et al. 1987; RON and SPRENT 1987). Since antigen presentation by B cells depends on their size and activation status (KRIEGER et al. 1985), medium-sized marginal zone B cells may act as antigen-presenting cells for T cells. Marginal zone B cells are located at a place where they are among the first to come into contact with foreign antigens that enter the lymph node (VAN DEN OORD et al. 1986a). They are equipped with a variety of receptors such as C3b receptors (VAN DER VALK et al. 1984), receptors for the Fc portion of IgG (JAFFE et al. 1975), surface immunoglobulins, and HLADR antigens (VAN DEN OORD et al. 1985e); moreover, marginal zone B cells are in an activated stage, and have been found to bind various antigenic particles and immune complexes (NOSSAL et al. 1966; MITCHELL and ABBOT 1971; BROWN et al. 1973; VAN ROOIJEN 1973; VEERMAN and VAN ROOIJEN 1975). All these features render marginal zone B cells in the spleen and lymph node excellent candidates to serve as antigen-presenting cells for T lymphocytes.

Upon antigenic stimulation, the human paracortex gains a "mottled appearance" by virtue of the appearance of large numbers of scattered interdigitating reticulum cells and acquires a nodular configuration, thereby resembling the T area described in several animal species in normal (KELLY 1975; BÉLISLE and SAINTE-MARIE 1981a–c) and pathological conditions (MYKING 1974; DAVIES et al. 1969; VELDMAN and KEUNING 1978). Nodular transformation of the human paracortex was studied in detail by REE and FANGER (1975) in reactive lymph nodes. These so-called T nodules showed a characteristic "starry sky" appearance and were composed of variable numbers of small lymphocytes, high endothelial venules, and histiocytic elements. On the basis of their localization and cellular composition, T nodules were considered to represent a stage of local immune reaction (REE and FANGER 1975). Using antibodies directed against interdigitating reticulum cells and T-cell subsets, we analyzed the morphological and immunohistochemical characteristics of the successive developmental stages of these T nodules (VAN DEN OORD et al. 1985c).

Primary T nodules, predominantly situated near the subcapsular sinus, appeared to originate from small clusters of veiled cells that had entered the lymph node via the afferent lymph and had settled in the interfollicular or paracortical area (Fig. 1). Upon recruitment of helper/inducer T cells in these clusters, T-cell proliferation takes place and results in a gradual expansion of these clusters with peripheral distribution of interdigitating reticulum cells and high endothelial venules, thus giving rise to a primary T nodule. Its cellular composition, i.e., an almost pure population of $CD4^+$ helper/inducer T cells admixed with $HLADR^+$ interdigitating reticulum cells (Fig. 1), strongly resembles the dendritic cell–T cell clusters observed in vitro during the early phases of the immune response (INABA et al. 1984). Similar T-cell aggregates occur in cutaneous delayed-type hypersensitivity reactions (PLATT et al. 1983) and in the synovium of patients with severe, active rheumatoid arthritis (MALONE et al. 1984). These primary T nodules likely represent the morphological expression of the early phase of the cellular immune response in which antigen-specific helper/inducer T lymphocytes are recruited and proliferate in response to signals delivered by antigen-presenting cells. Under the inductive influences of T cells and interdigitating reticulum cells, high endothelial

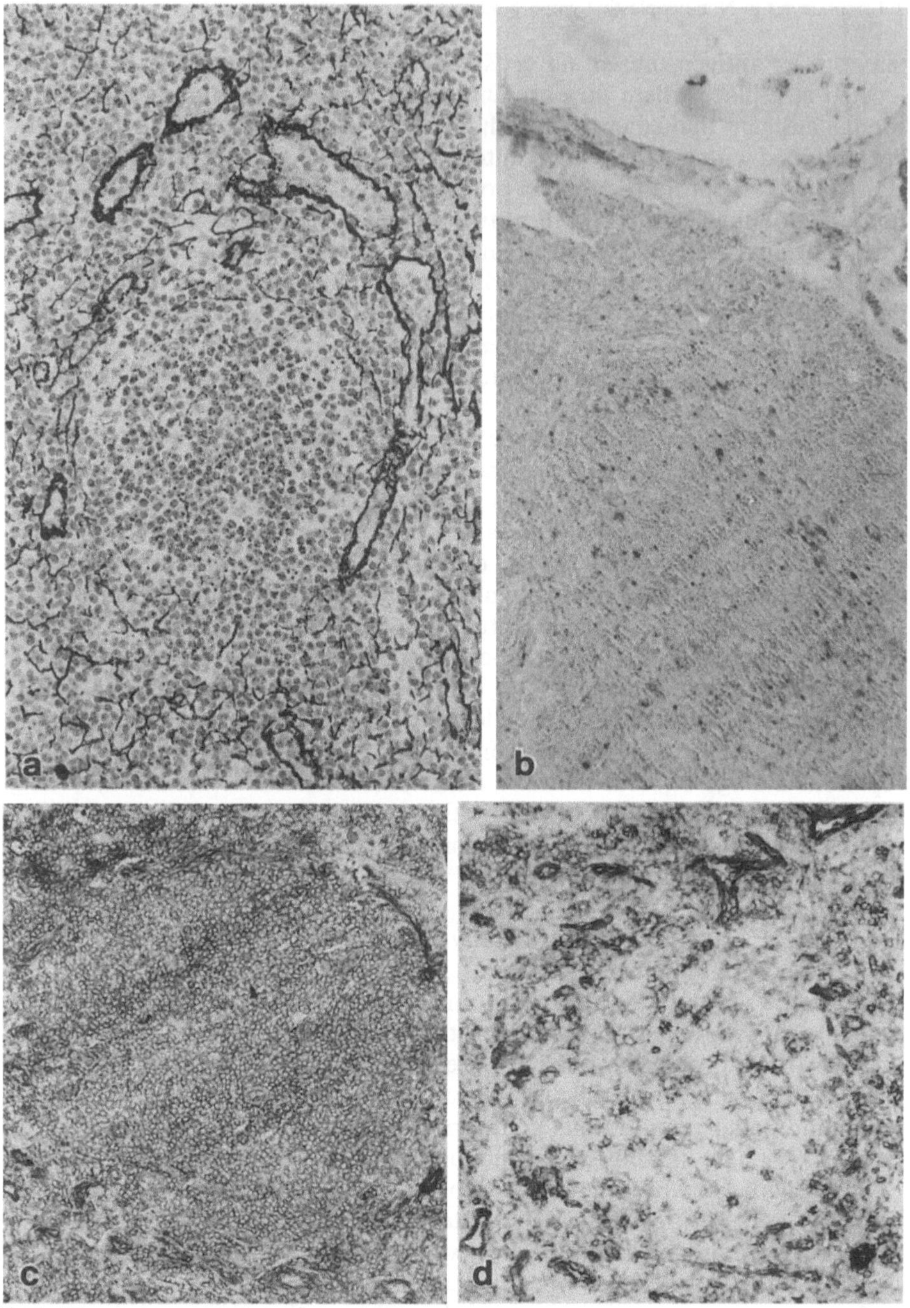

Fig. 1. Morphology and histochemistry of a primary T nodule in fixed (**a** and **b**) and frozen (**c** and **d**) sections of a lymph node with nonspecific reactive lymphadenitis. **a** High endothelial venules and **b** S-100β$^+$ interdigitating reticulum cells are situated preferentially at the periphery of the nodule. Combined enzyme-immunohistochemical staining for alkaline phosphatase and CD4 (**c**) and DC8 (**d**) reveals numerous helper/inducer T cells (**c**) but few CD8$^+$ suppressor-cytotoxic T cells (**d**) within the nodule, delineated by alkaline phosphatase positive venules. **a** reticulin stain; **b** anti-S-100β antiserum, PAP method; **c** combined enzyme-immunohistochemistry for alkaline phosphatase and OKT4/Leu-3a; **d** combined enzyme-immunohistochemistry for alkaline phosphatase and OKT8. All figures ×90

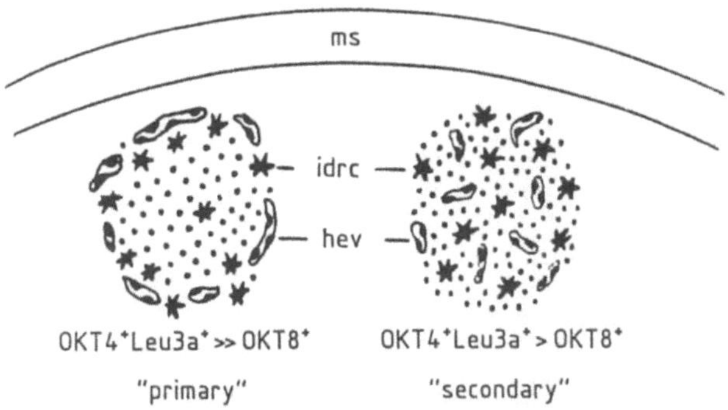

Fig. 2. Schematic illustration of primary and secondary T nodules. *idrc*, interdigitating reticulum cells; *hev*, high endothelial venules; *ms*, marginal (subcapsular) sinus

venules proliferate and grow into the nodules, thus providing a further supply of T cells. On immunohistochemistry, the T cells in these nodules are considered to be in an activated state since they react very strongly with anti-CD4 monoclonal antibodies, and since at least some of them express HLADR antigens (VAN DEN OORD et al. 1985c). In vitro experiments have indeed shown that, once T cells are appropriately activated, a number of interrelated events occur, i.e., a three- to fourfold increased expression of CD4 antigens (MEUER et al. 1983b), the appearance of variable amounts of HLADR antigens (REINHERZ et al. 1979), and the acquisition of receptors for IL-2 on cells which are largely located in the paracortical area (TAKACS et al. 1985). Proliferation of activated $CD4^+$ helper/inducer T cells then results in the generation of $CD8^+$ antigen-specific suppressor/cytotoxic T cells, and a consequent decrease in the CD4–CD8 ratio in the T nodule (Fig. 2). Such a nodule corresponds to what we term a *secondary T nodule* (Fig. 3), which likely represents the later stage of the cellular immune response (VAN DEN OORD et al. 1985c).

Using combined enzyme-immunohistochemical techniques, a striking topographical relationship was observed between secondary paracortical T nodules on the one hand, and adjacent B-lymphoid follicles on the other, resulting in distinctive nodular structures which we term *composite nodules* (VAN DEN OORD et al. 1986b). In its most characteristic form, the composite nodule is an ovoid structure, composed of two separate domains (Fig. 4). The upper part is a classical B domain and corresponds to a B-lymphoid follicle; the lower part is a T domain with the light microscopic, enzyme- and immunohistochemical features of a secondary T nodule. B cells that have been recruited in the follicle center, where they undergo a series of morphological and phenotypical transformations, subsequently leave the follicle, transform into immunoblasts under the influence of helper T cells, and finally appear as Ig-secreting plasma cells in the medullary cords (LENNERT et al. 1978; LUKES and COLLINS 1975). The T domain of the composite nodule seems well equipped to serve as the place where antigen-stimulated B cells become segregated when they have left the deep or dark part of the follicle center through the thinned lymphocytic

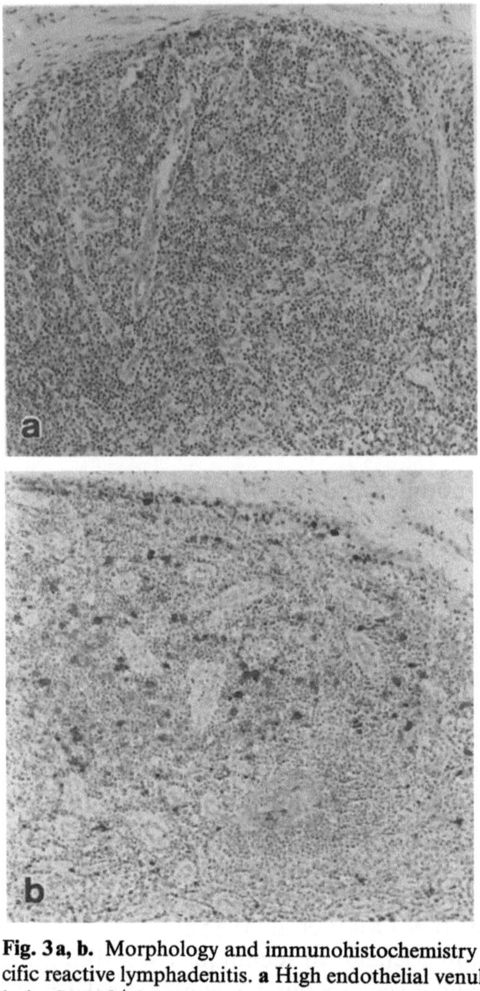

Fig. 3 a, b. Morphology and immunohistochemistry of a secondary T nodule in a case of nonspecific reactive lymphadenitis. **a** High endothelial venules are present throughout the nodule. **b** Similarly, S-100β$^+$ interdigitating reticulum cells are distributed scattered throughout the secondary T nodule. **a** hematoxylin and eosin; **b** anti-S-100β antiserum, PAP method. Both figures ×90

▶

Fig. 4 a–d. Morphology and histochemistry of a composite nodule. **a** The T domain of the composite nodule shows the features of a secondary T nodule and contains many scattered S-100β$^+$ interdigitating reticulum cells. **b** Combined enzyme-immunohistochemical staining for pan-T marker CD5 and alkaline phosphatase reveals numerous immunoreactive cells in the T domain of the composite nodule, which is delineated by high endothelial venules. Analysis of T cell subsets shows numerous helper/inducer T cells (**c**) but few suppressor/cytotoxic T cells (**d**). **a** PAP method, anti-S-100β antiserum; **b** combined enzyme-immunohistochemistry for Leu-1 and alkaline phosphatase; **c, d** three-step indirect immunoperoxidase method for OKT4/Leu-3a and OKT8 respectively. All figures ×90

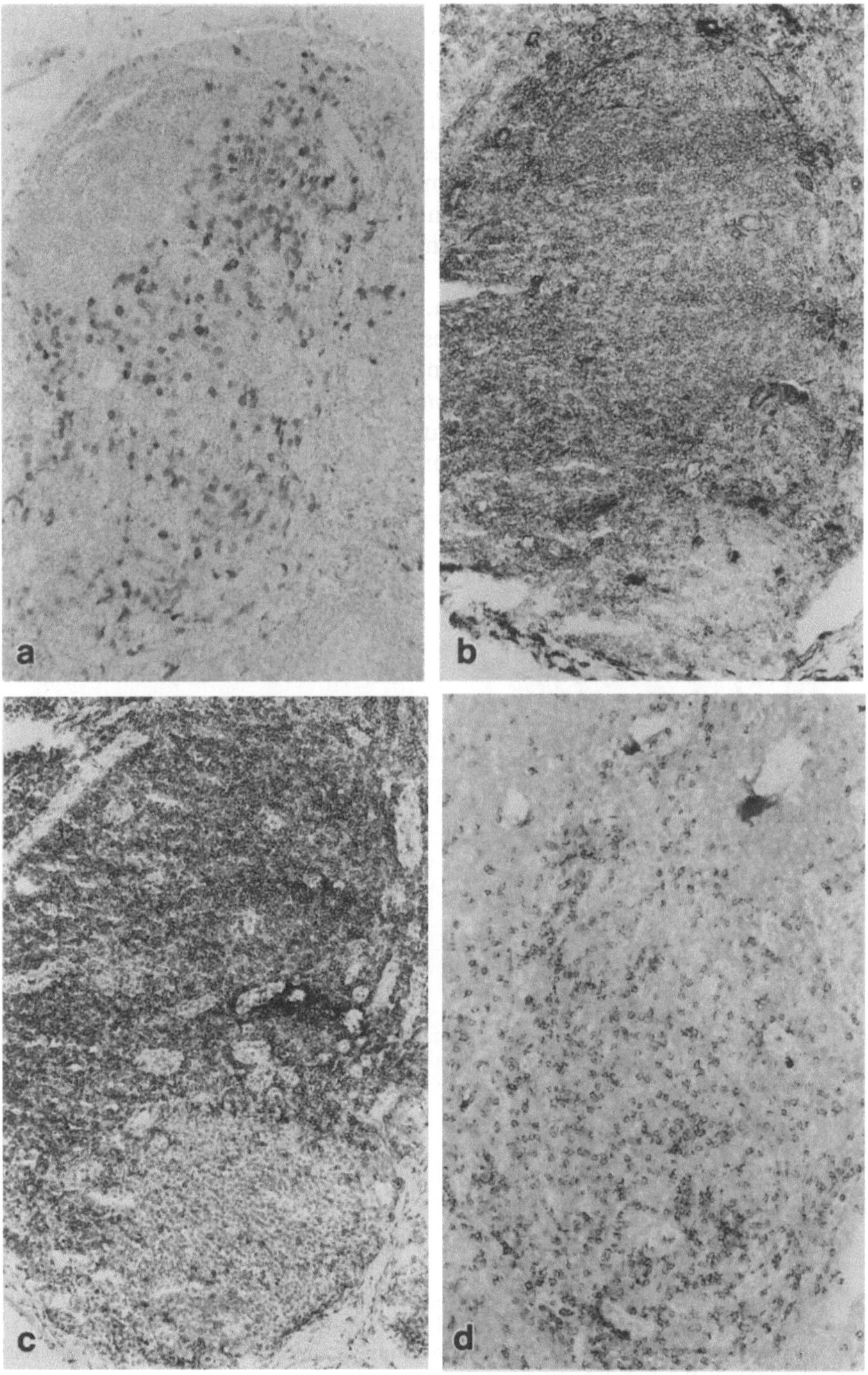
a
b
c
d

mantle at its lower pole, and where these B cells interact with immunoregulatory T cells (Fig. 5). This is supported by studies in experimental animals that suggest that B cell–T cell interactions take place in the area immediately adjacent to lymphoid follicles (Nieuwenhuis and Ford 1976). Due to its sharp demarcation from the surrounding tissues by high endothelial venules, sinuses, and fibroblastic reticulum cells, the T domain of the composite nodule possesses the features of a distinct compartment. Various mitogenic factors released by activated T cells will be operative only within the limits of this compartment.

By virtue of its cellular composition, the composite nodule is a dynamic, transient anatomical structure that represents the morphological expression of an immune response at a given moment. Therefore, composite nodules are *continuously changing and remodeling structures,* the histological aspect and cellular composition of either domain fluctuating with the type of challenging antigen and course of the immune response (Fig. 6). A simultaneous develop-

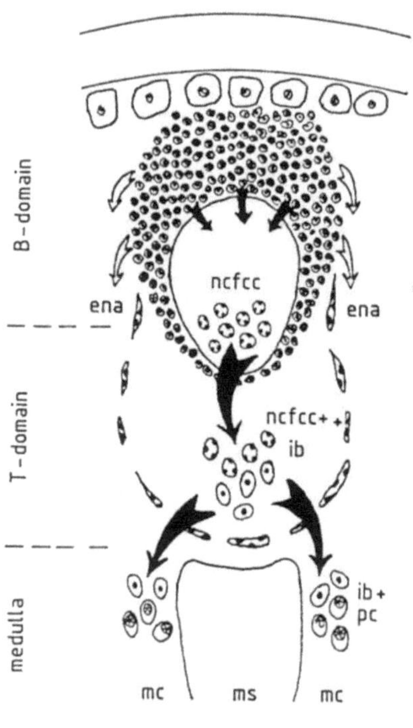

Fig. 5. Schematic illustration of the composite nodule as the site of T cell–B cell interactions. Antigen-stimulated follicle center cells segregate in the T domain of the composite nodule (*large arrow*), where they interact with activated T cells and transform into immunoblasts and plasma cells which accumulate in the medullary cords; nonstimulated B cells traverse the lymph node via the extranodular area (*open arrows*). *ncfcc,* noncleaved follicle center cells; *ib,* immunoblasts; *pc,* plasma cells; *mc,* medullary cords; *ms,* medullary sinus; *ena,* extranodular area

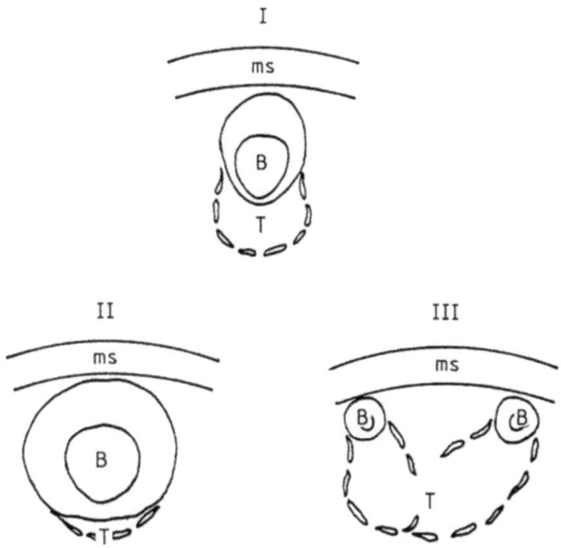

Fig. 6. Schematic illustration of the fluctuating nature of the composite nodule in nonspecific reactive lymphadenitis (*I*), follicular hyperplasia (*II*), and T-zone hyperplasia (*III*). *ms*, marginal or subcapsular sinus; *B*, B domain; *T*, T domain of the composite nodule

ment of both the B and the T domain results in the formation of typical composite nodules which are seen mainly in nonspecific reactive lymphadenitis. In follicular hyperplasia, the T domain of the composite nodule is reduced to a narrow crescent, and the hyperplastic lymphoid follicle constitutes the major part of the composite nodule. In T-zone hyperplasia, T domains of adjacent composite nodules fuse together and give rise to a large, semicircular structure containing one or more small lymphoid follicles in its periphery (VAN DEN OORD et al. 1986b).

Certain reaction patterns in the lymph node are characterized by a peculiar aspect of composite nodules, such as the nodular structures that occur in dermatopathic lymphadenitis. In this reactive lymphadenitis in response to a chronic itching skin disease, very large nodules occur that are composed of predominantly $CD4^+$ T lymphocytes and small numbers of $CD8^+$ T cells which show a weak and random positivity for IL-2 receptors (Fig. 7; VAN DEN OORD et al. 1984a; BURKE et al. 1986; WEISS et al. 1985, 1986). These nodules, which we term *tertiary T-nodules* (VAN DEN OORD et al. 1985c), contain massive amounts of $CD1^+S\text{-}100\beta^+$ dendritic cells (HERRERA 1987; GOULD et al. 1988). Similar dendritic cells also appear in the subcapsular afferent sinus, and correspond ultrastructurally to Langerhans cells, interdigitating reticulum cells, and intermediate forms between these two cell types (VAN DEN OORD et al. 1984 a). The large size of the tertiary T nodules may be indicative of a continuous influx of Langerhans cells; the persistence of the CD1 antigen on a large

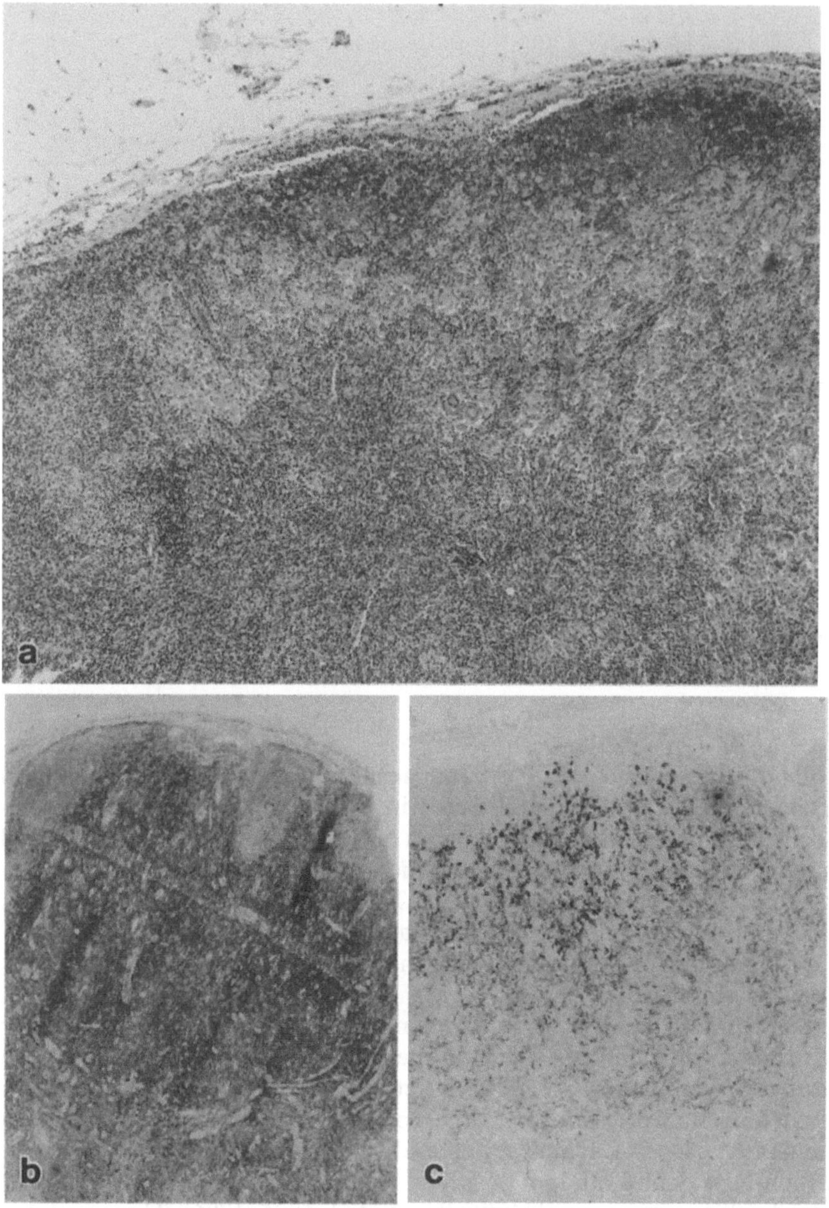

Fig. 7 a–c. Morphology and histochemistry of a tertiary T nodule. **a** On routine staining, lymphocyte-rich and reticulum cell-rich parts can be recognized in the nodule. **b** The lymphocytes belong mainly to the helper/inducer subset; note several unstained B-lymphoid follicles in the periphery of the nodule. **c** The reticulum cells display variable reactivity for the CD1 antigen. **a** hematoxylin and eosin; **b, c** three-step indirect immunoperoxidase method for OKT4/Leu-3a and OKT6 respectively. **a** ×215; **b, c** ×90

proportion of these accessory cells might reflect their defective maturation into classical interdigitating reticulum cells. Together with the poor development of high endothelial venules in these nodules, tertiary T nodules may represent a less optimal microenvironment for T-cell responses to occur, and hence may result in a chronic lymphadenopathy (VAN DEN OORD 1985).

A second type of aberrant composite nodule is known as *progressively transformed follicle centers*. These are large lymphocytic nodules that may occur in a variety of lymph node conditions in which excessive hyperplasia of B-lymphoid follicles takes place (LENNERT and MÜLLER-HERMELINK 1975). In contrast to well-organized secondary lymphoid follicles, progressively transformed follicle centers consist of small round lymphocytes admixed with small clusters of follicle center cells and dendritic reticulum cells (LENNERT and MÜLLER-HERMELINK 1975). On immunohistochemistry, these follicles contain most elements of the composite nodule, i.e., dendritic and interdigitating reticulum cells, small B lymphocytes, follicle center cells, and large numbers of $CD4^+$ helper/inducer T cells, some of which express the Leu-7 marker (VAN DEN OORD et al. 1985d). All these elements are distributed in a disordered, not yet organized fashion. The dendritic reticulum cells show a poorly cohesive arrangement and do not reveal an elaborated meshwork of IgM; tingible body macrophages are absent and terminally differentiated B cells are lacking. All these features suggest that progressively transformed follicle centers represent an early, transient stage in the development of a composite nodule (VAN DEN OORD 1985).

The very presence of a single nodular structure, unifying both cortical and paracortical lymph node parenchyma, necessitates a new concept of compartmentalization of the reactive lymph node (Fig. 8). Instead of the classical division of the lymph node parenchyma along an axis parallel to the lymph node capsule into an outer, cortical region and a deep, paracortical region, a compartmentalization of the reactive lymph node along axes perpendicular to the lymph node capsule, i.e., parallel to the traffic of antigens, has to be considered (VAN DEN OORD 1985). The latter division results in the recognition of an extranodular compartment (FACCHETTI et al. 1989b), which is situated outside composite nodules and which corresponds to the lymph node pulp (LENNERT et al. 1978). It consists of a mixture of T and B lymphocytes, macrophages, and plasma cells which surround high endothelial venules and lymph sinuses.

This extranodular compartment of the lymph node plays an important role in the migration of cells and antigens. Antigens enter the lymph node along the lymphatic route, either as soluble antigens, as antigen-antibody complexes, or as antigens bound to the surface of antigen-presenting veiled cells (BALFOUR et al. 1984). Lymphatics also represent the site of entry for macrophages, dendritic cells, and a minority of lymphocytes (HALL 1985), whereas high endothelial venules are actively involved in the entrance of lymphocytes from the blood into the lymphoid parenchyma. Following migration across the high endothelium, B and T lymphocytes segregate and home into the cortex and paracortex respectively (NIEUWENHUIS and FORD 1976).

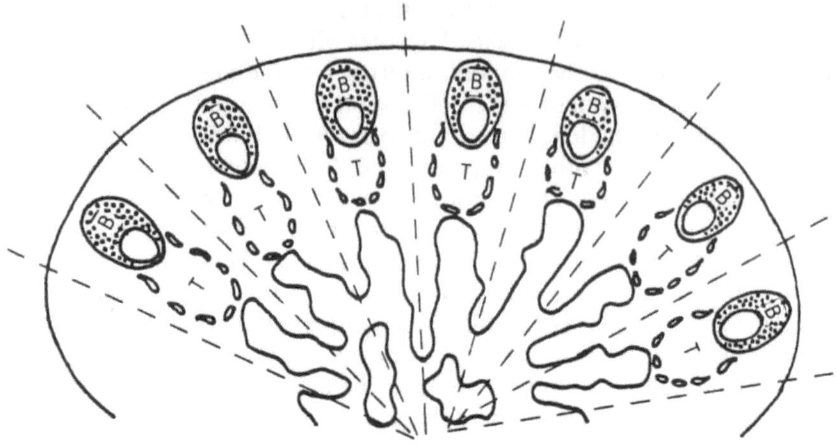

Fig. 8. Schematic illustration of the division of the reactive lymph node along axes perpendicular to the lymph node capsule, resulting in the delineation of structural and functional units (composite nodules), each consisting of a B and a T domain

Finally, the extranodular compartment selectively contains a subset of dendritic cells reactive with the monoclonal antibody Mac 387 (DELABIE et al. 1989) as well as plasmacytoid monocytes (so-called plasmacytoid T cells) (FACCHETTI et al. 1989b). The latter cells were formerly designated "lymphoblasts" because of their cytological characteristics. They are rounded lymphoid cells with uniform pale, oval or round nuclei containing a small nucleolus and abundant, weakly basophilic cytoplasm (Fig. 9a; LENNERT and REMMELE 1958). On electron microscopy, these cells demonstrate abundant profiles of rough endoplasmic reticulum and a prominent Golgi apparatus, suggesting a secretory function (MÜLLER-HERMELINK et al. 1973); for this reason, they were considered to represent a special type of plasma cell, and were renamed "T-associated plasma cells" (LENNERT et al. 1975). Immunohistochemical studies failed to show Ig secretion but disclosed the surface phenotype $CD4^{+}HLADR^{+}$, and hence the cells were renamed "plasmacytoid T cells," thought to be involved in the production and secretion of lymphokines (LENNERT et al. 1984; FELLER et al. 1983; MÜLLER-HERMELINK et al. 1983). Using monoclonal antibodies reactive in paraffin-embedded tissue, FACCHETTI

▶

Fig. 9. **a** A plasmacytoid monocyte cluster in a case of non-specific reactive lymphadenitis, showing medium-sized, rounded cells with pale nuclei and abundant cytoplasm, near several high endothelial venules. **b, c** Involvement of plasmacytoid monocytes in granulomas occurring in the extranodular compartment. Large numbers of plasmacytoid monocytes in close association with multinucleated giant cells and epithelioid histiocytes appear upon staining with **b** LN2 and **c** KP1. **a** hematoxylin and eosin, ×215; **b, c** three-step indirect immunoperoxidase method for LN2 and KP1 respectively, both ×90

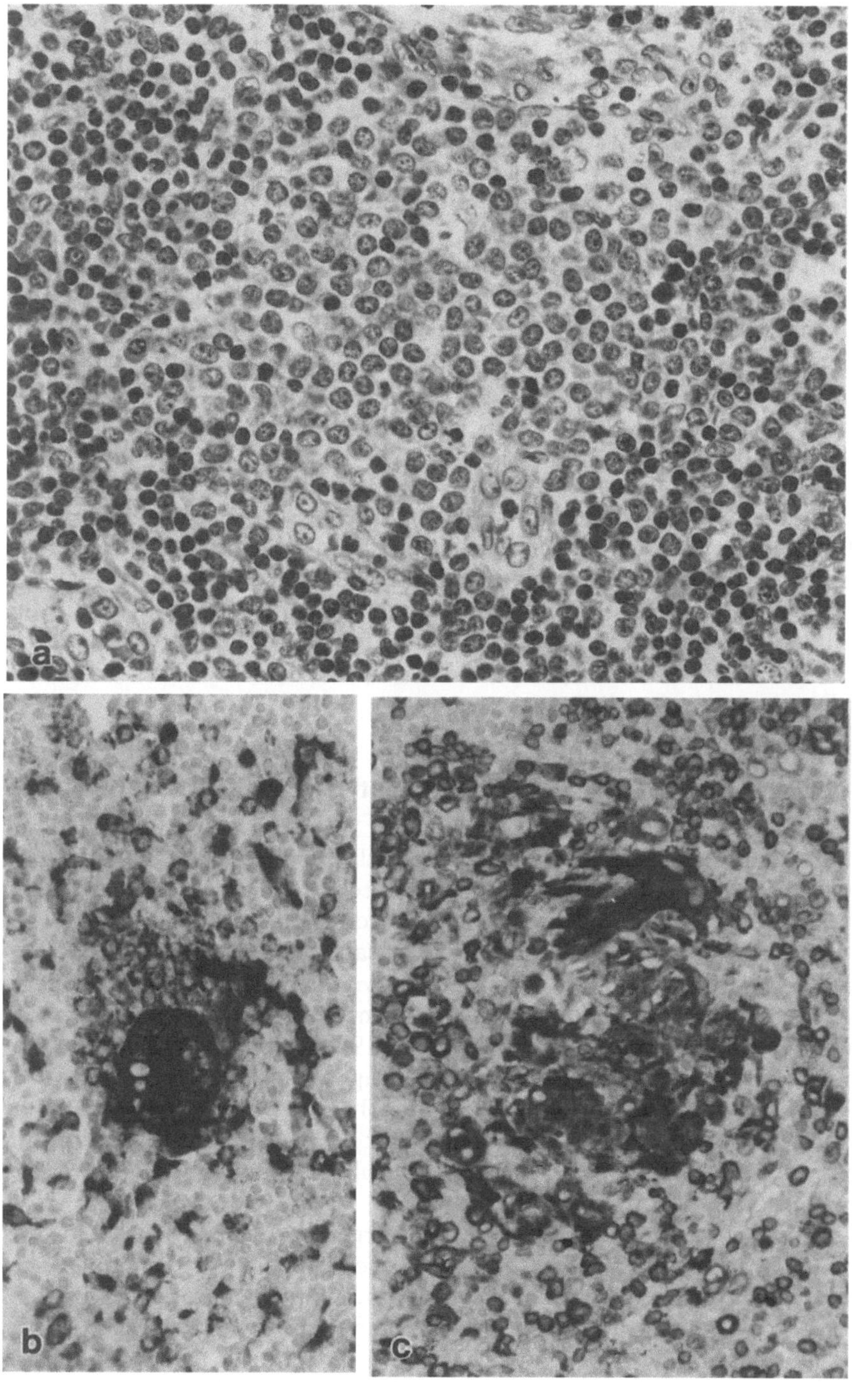
a
b
c

et al. (1987) showed that plasmacytoid T cells are not as rare as formerly believed. They can be found in the majority of reactive lymph nodes either as singular cells or in small aggregates, as well as in a variety of extranodal lymphoid tissues. They therefore belong to the normal constituents of the lymph node, and represent one of the normal components of the lymphoid tissue in general as well (Facchetti et al. 1988 a).

Using a large battery of monoclonal antibodies, the phenotype of plasmacytoid T cells was compared with that of other cell populations of the lymph node. In addition to the CD4 antigen, plasmacytoid T cells were found to express several myelomonocytic and purely monocytic markers, but to lack purely myeloid as well as B- and T-markers, including the β and δ chains of the T-cell antigen receptor. For this reason, it was concluded that plasmacytoid T cells belong to the family of monocyte-derived cells, and they received the name plasmacytoid monocytes (Facchetti et al. 1988 b). Since plasmacytoid monocytes express the $OKM5^{+}OKM1^{-}HLADR^{+}$ immunophenotype, which is also found on a small subset of peripheral blood monocytes involved in the autologous mixed lymphocyte reaction (Shen et al. 1983), they might exert inductive influences on immigrating T cells in the extranodular compartment. By virtue of their strategic position in the near proximity of high endothelial venules, plasmacytoid T cells might play an important role in the recruitment of lymphocytes into the lymph node parenchyma (Facchetti 1989).

4 Distribution of T Cells in Various Reactive Lymphadenopathies

During the immune response, the extranodular compartment of the lymph node represents the site where IgM- and IgG-secreting plasma cells mature and migrate towards the medullary cords. A reactive condition that largely involves the extranodular compartment is so-called *polymorphous pulp hyperplasia* (Lennert et al. 1978). This reactive lymph node pattern is regularly found in viral infections, in enlarged lymph nodes that emerge one or more weeks after smallpox vaccination (Hartsock 1968), and in the lymphadenopathy provoked by intake of anticonvulsant drugs (Saltzstein and Ackerman 1959). Although this condition primarily involves a diffuse hyperplasia of the extranodular compartment, the T-dependent areas may additionally be involved to a variable degree, whereas follicular hyperplasia usually is not prominent (Lennert et al. 1978).

On histology, a mixture of small and large transformed lymphoid cells dysplaying variable sizes and cytoplasmic basophilia are found. Initially considered to represent a sequela of a cellular immune reaction (Lennert et al. 1978), polymorphous pulp hyperplasia is now believed to represent a later stage of a humoral immune response (Morris et al. 1983). On immunohistochemistry, some of the large transformed lymphoid cells represent T immunoblasts and some contain cytoplasmic IgG, IgM, or IgA (Stein et al.

1980). This polyclonal B-cell proliferation is accompanied by increased numbers of CD4$^+$ helper/inducer T cells which may coexpress the OKT10 marker, normally found on activated T and B cells (Audouin et al. 1985; Morgan-Capner et al. 1986; Krueger et al. 1987; Frizzera 1987).

A reactive lymph node condition with similar histological features has recently been described in patients with autoimmune or immunecomplex diseases, under the name "autoimmune disease associated lymphadenopathy" (Koo et al. 1984). It has to be noted that a completely different reactive pattern is seen in the lymphadenopathy in rheumatoid arthritis; in this condition, the B-lymphoid follicles show a hyperplastic appearance but contain only small numbers of T cells on immunohistochemistry (Willkens et al. 1980).

Lymphadenopathies in the *acquired immunodeficiency syndrome* (AIDS) reflect the severe immunological defects caused by the immunodeficiency virus (Said 1988). This retrovirus uses the CD4 molecule as a receptor to enter cells (Dalgleish et al. 1984), resulting in an absolute reduction in CD4$^+$ cells and a reversal of the CD4–CD8 ratio. Since the CD4 molecule is expressed not only by helper/inducer T cells but also by monocytes, macrophages, dendritic cells, Langerhans cells, and glial cells, the human immunodeficiency virus affects a pleiade of cells, a feature that significantly contributes to the defects in immunological response occurring in AIDS patients. The histological features of the involved lymph nodes range from florid follicular hyperplasia to profound lymphoid depletion (Guarda et al. 1983; Ioachim et al. 1983; Brynes et al. 1983; Amberson et al. 1984; Biberfeld et al. 1987). The follicular hyperplasia is characterized by irregular lymphoid follicles which may lose their follicle mantles, and which may show hemorrhage and follicle lysis due to piecemeal infiltration by lymphocytes (Wood et al. 1985; Parravicini et al. 1986). The latter lymphocytes have previously been considered to represent mantle zone B lymphocytes, but have now definitely been characterized as CD8$^+$ cytotoxic/suppressor T cells, accompanied by accessory cells (Baroni et al. 1985).

In the paracortex, large collections of interdigitating reticulum cells, reminiscent of dermatopathic lymphadenitis, may be found. The extranodular compartment contains a polymorphic mixture of lymphocytes, immunoblasts, plasma cells, eosinophils, and histiocytes as well as large aggregates of monocytoid B lymphocytes (Said 1988). The very presence of the latter B cells may elucidate the polyclonal B-cell activation in AIDS patients that results in elevated levels of serum immunoglobulins and circulating immune complexes (van den Oord et al. 1985 b). On immunohistochemistry, an absolute decrease in the number of CD4$^+$ helper/inducer T cells is evident within all lymph node compartments and parallels the changes in the peripheral blood (Said et al. 1984); on the other hand, increased numbers of CD8$^+$ T cells are found. This increase occurs predominantly in the T-suppressor subset (Wood et al. 1986) and is accompanied by elevated numbers of HLADR$^+$ activated T cells and decreased numbers of IL-2 receptor positive cells (Said 1988).

The introduction of monoclonal antibodies has clarified several aspects of the immunopathology of granulomatous lymphadenitis. *Hypersensitivity-type granulomas*, such as those that occur in tuberculous and sarcoidal lymphadenitis, contain a variety of cells, i.e., epithelioid histiocytes, multinucleated giant cells, fibroblasts, plasma cells, and lymphocytes. The epithelioid histiocytes, but not the giant cells, are in an activated state since they contain large amounts of IL-1 related molecules (CHILOSI et al. 1988). The majority of lymphocytes within the granuloma belong to the $CD4^+$ helper/inducer subset (Fig. 10; VAN DEN OORD et al. 1984b); these T cells are in an activated state by virtue of their HLADR antigen and IL-2 receptor expression (MODLIN et al. 1984; SEMENZATO et al. 1984). They probably secrete mediators that attract monocytes to the site of injury and that modulate granuloma formation (HUNNINGHAKE et al. 1980). The numerically minor $CD8^+$ suppressor/cytotoxic subset (Fig. 10; SEMENZATO et al. 1982; MODLIN et al. 1983; VAN DEN OORD et al. 1984b) is located at the edge of the granuloma as a single row of cells. This ring-like distribution has been associated with the possible role of these cells in the restriction and localization of the immunopathological process (MODLIN et al. 1983; NARAYANAN et al. 1983). Around the granuloma, variable numbers of proliferating and activated $CD4^+$ T cells are present; these cells create an environment rich in diffusing lymphokines, which in turn may activate macrophages and modulate granuloma formation (CHILOSI et al. 1988).

In *suppurative granulomatous lymphadenitis*, a shift in the predominating T-cell subset takes place during the successive phases of the immune response (VAN DEN OORD et al. 1985a). In the early stage of the disease, the intragranulomatous T cells belong mainly to the $CD4^+$ subset. Upon activation by antigen-presenting epithelioid histiocytes and multinucleated giant cells, $CD8^+$ suppressor/cytotoxic T cells are generated and progressively replace the $CD4^+$ subset during the later stages of the disease. The cytotoxic activity and/or the suppression of intragranulomatous immune reactions by the $CD8^+$ subset results in the necrosis characteristically found in these granulomas. The apparent lack of a perigranulomatous rim of $CD8^+$ T cells permits $CD4^+$ T cells to assist in the local maturation of surrounding B cells, resulting in large numbers of plasma cells around these granulomas (VAN DEN OORD et al. 1985a). This feature resembles the hypersensitivity-type granulomas observed in immunodeficient patients, in which $CD4^+$ T cells are reduced in number and $CD8^+$ T cells are found throughout the granuloma but never form a perigranulomatous rim (SHEN et al. 1988).

The exact origin of epithelioid histiocytes, as well as the differentiation pathways from precursors into fully mature epithelioid cells, is still debated (SUTTON and WEISS 1966; TURK et al. 1978). Moreover, more than one cell might serve as a precursor of epithelioid histiocytes, and the very type of precursor might well be determined by the site where the granuloma forms. VEERMAN (1974) found ultrastructural and functional evidence that epithelioid histiocytes originate from interdigitating reticulum cells that are arrested in their locomotion and phagocytic capacities by migration inhibition factor, produced by nearby activated T lymphocytes (VEERMAN 1974). This view is supported by recent immunohistochemical studies demonstrating that sarcoid

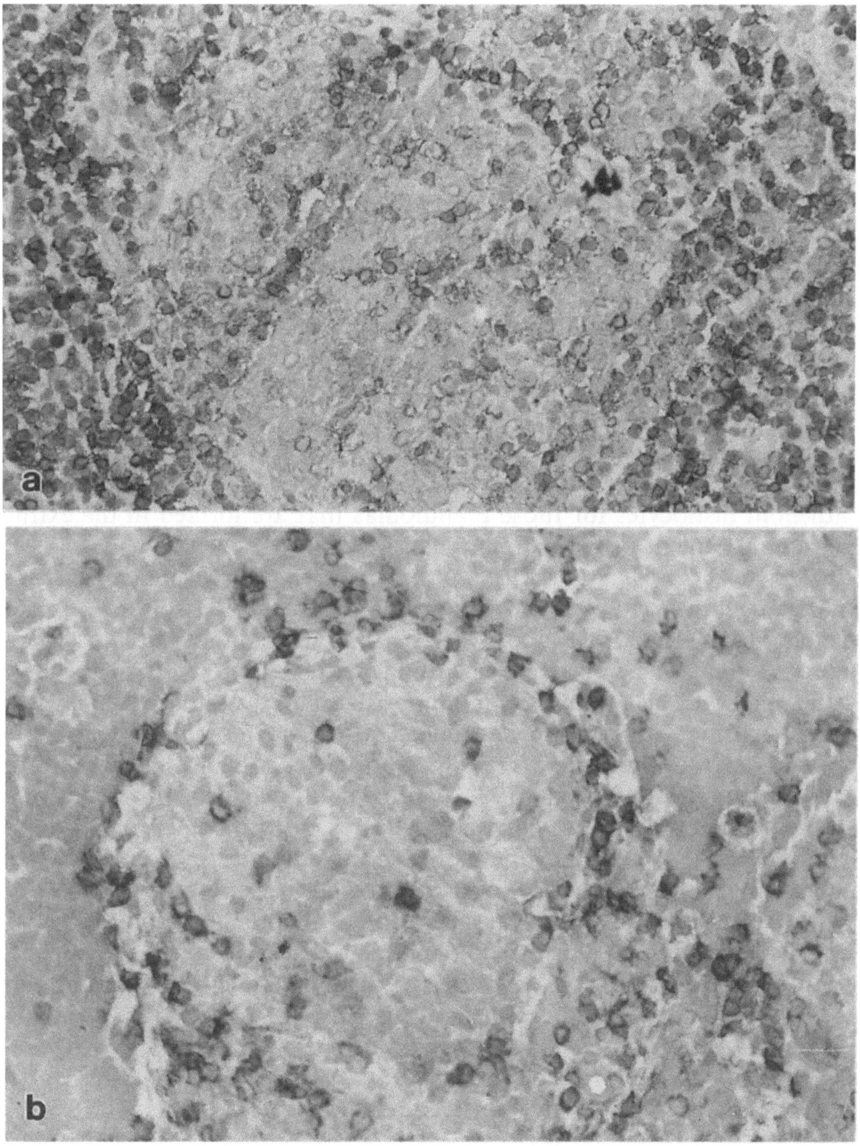

Fig. 10 a, b. T-cell subsets in hypersensitivity-type granulomas. **a** Many $CD4^+$ helper/inducer T cells are found throughout the granuloma and are also present in the surrounding lymphocytic cuff. **b** $CD8^+$ suppressor/cytotoxic T cells are distributed in a ring-like manner around the granuloma. Three-step indirect immunoperoxidase method for **a** OKT4/Leu-3a and **b** OKT8; both figures ×215

(MISHRA et al. 1983) and leprosy granulomas (POULTER et al. 1984) are surrounded by a rim of interdigitating reticulum cells. Moreover, epithelioid histiocytes share the membranous ATP-ase expression with interdigitating reticulum cells (MCKERROW et al. 1985). As such, some hypersensitivity-type granulomas actually represent transformed T domains of the composite nodule (Fig. 11; VAN DEN OORD 1986); the fibrosis in and around granulomas may result from fibroblastic reticulum cells, which are a component of the composite nodule and which are stimulated by soluble factors produced by activated T lymphocytes within the granuloma (ROMAIN and SCHLOSSMAN 1984); the confluence of singular granulomas may reflect the tendency of expanding T domains to fuse together. On the other hand, granulomas accompanied by numerous plasmacytoid monocytes were found to be situated outside the composite nodule, i.e., in the *extranodular compartment* (Fig. 9b, c). In addition to their topographical relationships within these lymph nodes, epithelioid histiocytes and plasmacytoid monocytes share several monocyte-related antigens. For this reason, plasmacytoid monocytes may well represent a precursor of epithelioid histiocytes for those granulomas that are formed in the extranodular compartment of the lymph node (FACCHETTI et al. 1989a).

Histiocytic necrotizing or Kikuchi's lymphadenitis is a self-limiting disease that affects mainly young women who usually present with isolated cervical lymphadenopathy (DORFMAN and BERRY 1988). On histology, circumscribed paracortical areas of necrosis are surrounded by collections of histiocytes, dendritic cells, variable numbers of immunoblasts and lymphocytes, and large clusters of plasmacytoid monocytes, many of which show nuclear pyknosis and death. Polymorphonuclear granulocytes and epithelioid histiocytes are notably absent (PILERI et al. 1982). On immunohistochemistry, strong HLADR expression is observed on the histiocytes, dendritic cells, and plasmacytoid monocytes, whereas the immunoblasts and admixed small lymphocytes belong mainly to the $CD8^+$ suppressor/cytotoxic T-cell subset (RIVANO et al. 1987). These features suggest a local generation of $CD8^+$ T cells and a cytotoxic T-cell response towards plasmacytoid monocytes. This results in their death, in variably sized areas of tissue necrosis, and in an impaired transformation of plasmacytoid monocytes into epithelioid histiocytes. Histiocytic necrotizing lymphadenitis consequently represents an *"abortive" granulomatous lymphadenitis* (FACCHETTI et al. 1989c), similar to what occurs in lepromatous leprosy (MODLIN et al. 1983; VAN VOORHIS et al. 1982).

▶

Fig. 11. a A small epithelioid granuloma is situated in close apposition to a lymphoid follicle, suggesting a process of granulomatous transformation of the T domain of the composite nodule. **b, c** On immunohistochemistry for a pan-B marker (**b**) or C3b receptors (**c**), the adjacent B domain is well preserved (**b**) or reduced to a narrow crescent (**c**). **d** Several epithelioid granulomas have fused to form a large tubercle; at the edge of the lesion, collections of dendritic reticulum cells reflect the remaining B domains of the granulomatous transformed composite nodules. **a,** hematoxylin and eosin, × 90; **b, c** three-step indirect immunoperoxidase method for Leu-1 and To5 respectively, both × 90; **d** three-step indirect immunoperoxidase for To5, × 40

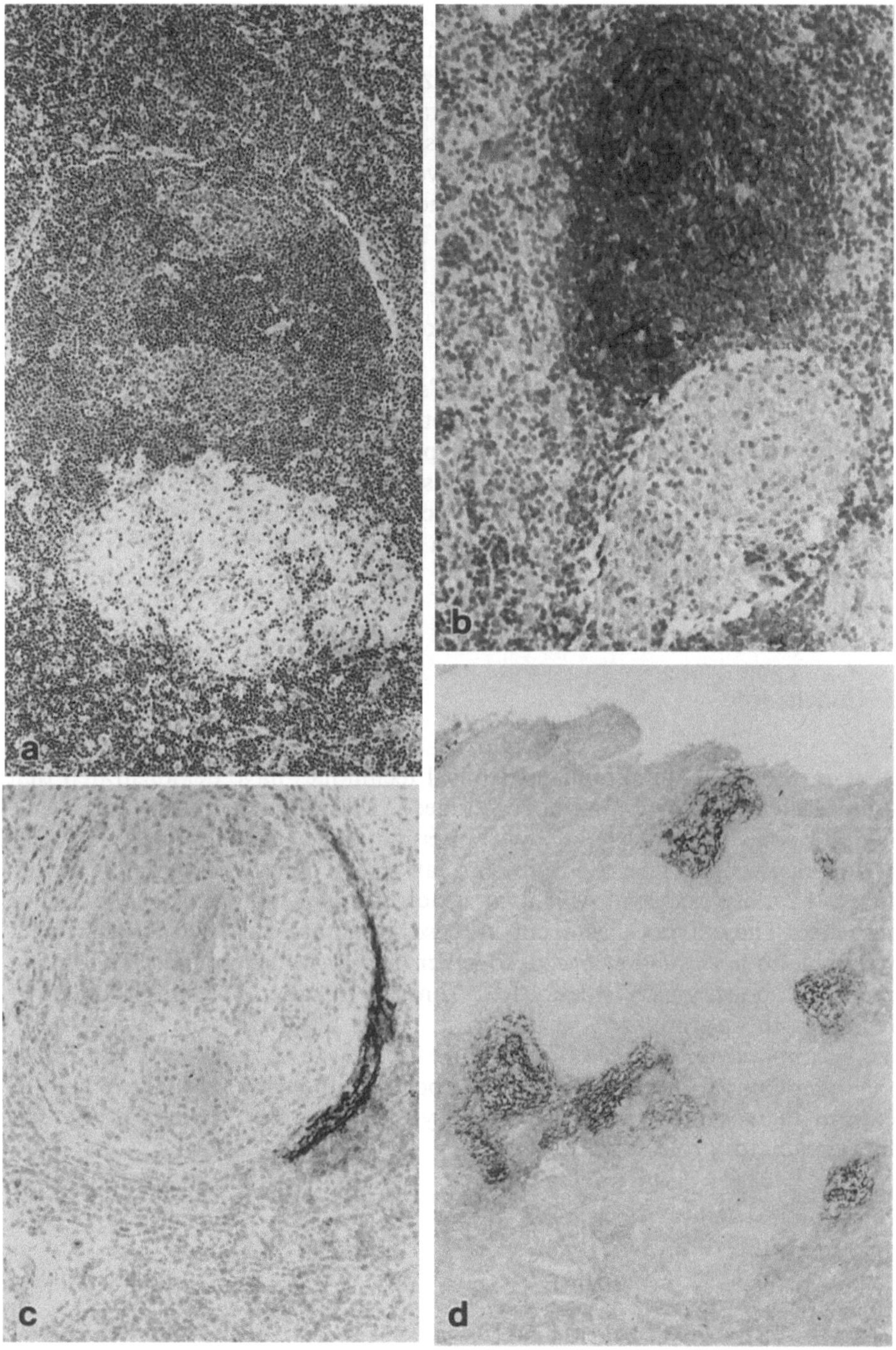
a
b
c
d

Angiofollicular lymph node hyperplasia or *Castleman's disease* occurs as a localized or multicentric disease, and can be separated into different types on histological and clinical grounds (Frizzera 1988). In the hyaline-vascular type, the involved lymph nodes are characterized by large lymphoid follicles with burnt-out, hyalinized follicle centers. They are composed mainly of dendritic reticulum cells and small blood vessels, and they are surrounded by concentric layers of lymphocytes. Enzyme- and immunohistochemical studies have demonstrated that helper/inducer T cells and Leu-7^+ cells are almost completely lacking in these regressively transformed follicle centers and are replaced by $CD8^+$ suppressor/cytotoxic T cells (Jones et al. 1984; van den Oord et al. 1984c). The onion skin-like mantle, however, contains many $CD4^+$ helper/inducer T cells among the mantle B lymphocytes.

The plasma cell variant of Castleman's disease, which is much less frequent and which may be associated with a variety of constitutional symptoms, shows hyperplastic follicle centers and a dense plasma cell infiltrate in the remaining lymph node parenchyma. On immunohistochemistry, T-cell subsets are present in normal proportions. Normal T-cell numbers are similarly found in follicle centers and interfollicular areas in the multicentric form of Castleman's disease (Frizzera 1988).

5 Conclusion

New investigative immunohistochemical techniques have demonstrated that the paracortex of the lymph node is indeed rich in T cells. In this area of the lymph node, T cells together with interdigitating reticulum cells and high endothelial venules give rise to the formation of T nodules or organoid structures, the morphology of which varies according to the stage of the immune response. These T nodules occur in close topographical association with B-lymphoid follicles of the cortex. Together they form the composite nodule of the lymph node, which is delineated from the extranodular compartment by high endothelial venules.

T lymphocytes occur not only in the T nodule and paracortex but also in the other compartments of the lymph node, i.e., the lymphoid follicle and the extranodular compartment, where they similarly play an important, immunoregulatory role.

References

Amberson JB, Di Carlo EF, Metroka CE, Koizumi JH, Mouradian JA (1984) Diagnostic pathology in the acquired immunodeficiency syndrome. Arch Pathol Lab Med 109:345–351

Angermeier PA, Hartman AL, Swerdlow SH (1987) T-cells in follicular hyperplasia and follicular center-cell lymphomas: an immunoultrastructural study of the T-cell receptor-associated CD3 antigen. J Histochem Cytochem 35:1433–1438

Audouin J, Le Tourneau A, Aubert J-P, Diebold J (1985) Herpes simplex virus lymphadenitis mimicking tumoral relapse in a patient with Hodgkin's disease in remission. Virchows Arch [A] 408:313–321

Balfour BM, Drexhage HA, Kamperdijk EWA, Hoefsmit ECM (1984) Antigen-presenting cells, including Langerhans cells, veiled cells and interdigitating cells. In: Porter R, Whelan J (eds) Microenvironments in haemopoietic and lymphoid differentiation (Ciba Found Symp). Pitman, London, pp 281–298

Banerjee D, Thibert RF (1983) Natural killer-like cells found in B-cell compartments of human lymphoid tissues. Nature 204:270–272

Bank I, DePinho RA, Brenner MB, Cassimeris J, Alt FW, Chess L (1986) A functional T3 molecule associated with a novel heterodimer on the surface of immature human thymocytes. Nature 322:179–181

Baroni CD, Pezzella F, Stoppaciaro A et al. (1985) Systemic lymphadenopathy (LAS) in intravenous drug abusers. Histology, immunohistochemistry and electron microscopy: pathogenic correlations. Histopathology 9:1275–1293

Bélisle C, Sainte-Marie G (1981 a) Tridimensional study of the deep cortex of the rat lymph node. I. Topography of the deep cortex. Anat Rec 199:45–59

Bélisle C, Sainte-Marie G (1981 b) Tridimensional study of the deep cortex of the rat lymph node. II. Relation of deep cortex units to afferent lymphatic vessels. Anat Rec 199:61–72

Bélisle C, Sainte-Marie G (1981 c) Tridimensional study of the deep cortex of the rat lymph node. III. Morphology of the deep cortex units. Anat Rec 199:213–226

Biberfeld P, Ost A, Porwit A et al. (1987) Histopathology and immunohistology of HTLV-III/LAV related lymphadenopathy and AIDS. Acta Pathol Microbiol Immunol Scand [A] 95:47–65

Brenner MB, McLean J, Scheft H, Warnke RA, Jones N, Strominger JL (1987) Characterization and expression of the human α-β T cell receptor by using a framework monoclonal antibody. J Immunol 138:1502–1509

Brown JC, Harris G, Papamichail M, Slijvic VS, Holborow E (1973) The localization of aggregated human γ-globulin in the spleens of normal mice. Immunology 24:955–968

Brynes RK, Chan WC, Spira TJ et al. (1983) Value of lymph node biopsy in unexplained lymphadenopathy in homosexual men. JAMA 250:1313–1317

Burke JS, Sheibani K, Rappaport H (1986) Dermatopathic lymphadenopathy. An immunophenotypic comparison of cases associated and unassociated with mycosis fungoides. Am J Pathol 123:256–263

Chilosi M, Pizzolo G, Menestrina F, Ianucci AM, Bonetti F, Fiore-Donati L (1981) Enzyme histochemistry on normal and pathologic paraffin-embedded lymphoid tissues. Am J Clin Pathol 76:729–736

Chilosi M, Menestrina F, Capelli P et al. (1988) Immunohistochemical analysis of sarcoid granulomas. Evaluation of Ki67$^+$ and interleukin-1$^+$ cells. Am J Pathol 131:191–198

Dalgleish AG, Beverley PCL, Clapham PR, Crawford DH, Greaves MF, Weiss RA (1984) The CD4 (T4) antigen is an essential component of the receptor for the AIDS retrovirus. Nature 312:763–767

Davies AJS, Carter RL, Leuchars E, Wallis V (1969) The morphology of immune reactions in normal, thymectomized and reconstituted mice. II. The response to oxalozone. Immunology 17:111–126

Delabie J, de Wolf-Peeters C, van den Oord JJ, Desmet VJ (1990) Differential expression of the calcium-binding proteins MRP8 and MRP14 in granulomatous conditions: an immunohistochemical study. Clin exp Immunol, in press

Delsol G, Al Saati T, Caveriviere P, Voigt JJ, Ancelin E, Rigal-Huguet F (1984) Etude en immunoperoxydase du tissu lymphoide normal et pathologique. Interêt des anticorps monoclonaux. Ann Pathol 4:165–183

Dorfman RD, Berry GJ (1988) Kikuchi's histiocytic necrotizing lymphadenitis: an analysis of 108 cases with emphasis on differential diagnosis. Semin Diagn Pathol 5:329–345

Dvoretsky P, Wood GS, Levy R, Warnke RA (1982) T-lymphocyte subsets in follicular lymphomas compared with those in non-neoplastic lymph nodes and tonsils. Hum Pathol 13:618–625

Facchetti F (1989) The plasmacytoid monocyte (the so-called plasmacytoid T cell): an enigmatic cell of the human lymph node. PhD Thesis, Catholic University of Leuven, ACCO, Leuven

Facchetti F, de Wolf-Peeters C, van den Oord JJ, Desmet VJ (1987) Immunohistochemical visualization of plasmacytoid T cells in paraffin sections. Hum Pathol 18:61

Facchetti F, de Wolf-Peeters C, van den Oord JJ, de Vos R, Desmet VJ (1988 a) Plasmacytoid T cells: A cell population normally present in the reactive lymph node. An immunohistochemical and electronmicroscopic study. Hum Pathol 19:1085–1092

Facchetti F, de Wolf-Peeters C, Mason DY, Pulford K, van den Oord JJ, Desmet VJ (1988 b) Plasmacytoid T cells. Immunohistochemical evidence for their monocyte/macrophage origin. Am J Pathol 133:15–21

Facchetti F, de Wolf-Peeters C, de Vos R, van den Oord JJ, Pulford KAF, Desmet VJ (1989 a) Plasmacytoid monocytes (so-called plasmacytoid T-cells) in granulomatous lymphadenitis. Hum Pathol 20:588–593

Facchetti F, de Wolf-Peeters C, van den Oord JJ, Meijer CJLM, Pals ST, Desmet VJ (1989 b) Anti-high endothelial venule monoclonal antibody HECA-452 recognizes plasmacytoid T cells and delineates an "extranodular" compartment in the reactive lymph node. Immunol Lett 20:277–282

Facchetti F, de Wolf-Peeters C, van den Oord JJ, de Vos R, Desmet VJ (1989 c) Plasmacytoid monocytes (so-called plasmacytoid T cells) in Kikuchi's lymphadenitis. An immunohistochemical study. Am J Clin Pathol 92:42–50

Feller AC (1982) Cytochemical reactivity of T-μ lymphocytes in human lymphatic tissue for dipeptidylaminopeptidase IV. Histochem J 14:889–895

Feller AC, Lennert K, Stein H, Bruhn HD, Wuthe HH (1983) Immunohistology and aetiology of histiocytic necrotizing lymphadenitis. Report of three instructive cases. Histopathology 7:825–839

Ferrari C, Sansoni P, Rowden G, Manara GC, Torresani C, de Panfilis G (1988) One half of the $CD11b^+$ human peripheral blood T lymphocytes coexpresses the S-100 protein. Clin Exp Immunol 72:357–361

Fiore-Donati L (1982) Dipeptidyl (amino)peptidase IV (DAP-IV) histochemistry on normal and pathologic lymphoid tissues. Am J Clin Pathol 77:714–719

Ford WL (1975) Lymphocyte migration and immune responses. Prog Allergy 19:1–59

Frizzera G (1987) The clinico-pathological expressions of Epstein-Barr virus infection in lymphoid tissues. Virchows Arch [B] 53:1–12

Frizzera G (1988) Castleman's disease and related disorders. Semin Diagn Pathol 5:346–364

Gould E, Porto R, Albores-Saavedra J, Ibe MJ (1988) Dermatopathic lymphadenitis. The spectrum and significance of its morphologic features. Arch Pathol Lab Med 112:1145–1150

Guarda LA, Butler JJ, Mansell P, Hersh ME, Reuben J, Nervell GR (1983) Lymphadenopathy in homosexual men: morbid anatomy with clinical and immunologic correlations. Am J Clin Pathol 79:559–568

Gutman GA, Weisman IL (1972) Lymphoid tissue architecture. Experimental analysis of the origin and distribution of T-cells and B-cells. Immunology 23:465–479

Hall JG (1985) The functional anatomy of lymph nodes. In: Stansfeld AG (ed) Lymph node biopsy interpretation. Churchill Livingstone, Edinburgh, pp 1–25

Hartsock RJ (1968) Postvaccinial lymphadenitis – hyperplasia of lymphoid tissue that simulates malignant lymphomas. Cancer 21:632–649

Herrera GA (1987) Light microscopic, S-100 immunostaining, and ultrastructural analysis of dermatopathic lymphadenopathy, with and without associated mycosis fungoides. Am J Clin Pathol 87:187–195

Hoffmann-Fezer G, Rodt H, Eulitz M, Thierfelder S (1976) Immunohistochemical identification of T- and B-lymphocytes delineated by the unlabeled antibody enzyme method. I. Anatomical distribution of theta-positive and Ig-positive cells in lymphoid organs of mice. J Immunol Methods 13:261–270

Hoffmann-Fezer G, Lohrs U, Rodt HV, Thierfelder S (1981) Immunohistochemical identification of T- and B-lymphocytes delineated by the unlabelled antibody enzyme method. Cell Tissue Res 216:361–375

Hsu S-M, Jaffe ES (1985) Phenotypic expression of T lymphocytes in thymus and peripheral lymphoid tissues. Am J Pathol 121:69–78

Hsu S-M, Ree HJ (1983) Histochemical studies on lectin binding in reactive lymphoid tissue. J Histochem Cytochem 31:538–546

Hsu S-M, Cossman J, Jaffe ES (1983) Lymphocyte subsets in normal human lymphoid tissues. Am J Clin Pathol 80:21–30

Hunninghake GW, Gadek JE, Young RC et al. (1980) Maintenance of granuloma formation in pulmonary sarcoidosis by T lymphocytes within the lung. N Engl J Med 302:594–598

Inaba K, Witmer MD, Steinman RM (1984) Clustering of dendritic cells, helper T lymphocytes, and histocompatible B cells during primary antibody responses in vitro. J Exp Med 160:858–876

Ioachim HL, Lerner CW, Tapper ML (1983) The lymphoid lesions associated with the acquired immunodeficiency syndrome. Am J Surg Pathol 7:543–553

Jaffe ES, Shevach EM, Sussman EH, Frank M, Green I, Berard CW (1975) Membrane receptor sites for the identification of lymphoreticular cells in benign and malignant conditions. Br J Cancer 31 (Suppl II):107–120

Janeway CA Jr, Ron J, Katz ME (1987) The B cell is the initiating antigen-presenting cell in peripheral lymph nodes. J Immunol 138:1051–1055

Janossy G, Tidman N, Selby WS, Thomas JA, Granger S, Kung PC, Goldstein G (1980) Human T lymphocytes of inducer and suppressor type occupy different microenvironments. Nature 287:81–84

Janossy G, Thomas JA, Pizzolo G (1981) The analysis of lymphoid populations in normal and malignant tissues by immunofluorescence technique. J Cancer Res Clin Oncol 101:1–11

Janossy G, Bofill M, Rowe D, Muir J, Beverley PCL (1989) The tissue distribution of T lymphocytes expressing different CD45 polypeptides. Immunology 66:517–525

Jones EL, Crocker J, Gregory J, Guibarra M, Curran RC (1984) Angiofollicular lymph node hyperplasia (Castleman's disease): an immunohistochemical and enzymehistochemical study of the hyaline-vascular form of lesion. J Pathol 144:131–147

Kansas GS, Wood GS, Fishwild DM, Engleman EG (1985) Functional characterization of human T lymphocyte subsets distinguished by monoclonal anti-Leu-8. J Immunol 134:2995–3002

Kelly RH (1975) Functional anatomy of lymph nodes. I. The paracortical cords. Int Arch Allergy Appl Immunol 48:836–849

Knowles DM, Holek S (1978) Tissue localization of T-lymphocytes by the histochemical demonstration of acid α-naphthyl acetate esterase. Lab Invest 39:70–76

Koo CH, Nathwani BN, Winberg CD, Hill LR, Rappaport H (1984) Atypical lymphoplasmacytic and immunoblastic proliferation in lymph nodes of patients with autoimmune disease (autoimmune disease-associated lymphadenopathy). Medicine 63:274–290

Krieger JI, Grammaer SF, Grey HM, Chesnut RW (1985) Antigen presentation by splenic B cells: resting B cells are ineffective, whereas activated B cells are effective accessory cells for T cell responses. J Immunol 135:2937–2945

Krueger GRF, Papadakis T, Schaefer H-J (1987) Persistent active Epstein-Barr virus infection and atypical lymphoproliferation. Report of two cases. Am J Surg Pathol 11:972–981

Lamelin J-P, Thomasset N, Andre C, Brochier J, Revillard JP (1978) Study of human T and B lymphocytes with heterologous antisera. III. Immunofluorescence studies on tonsil sections. Immunology 35:463–469

Leene W (1971) Origin and fate of lymphoid cells in the developing palatine tonsil of the rabbit. A possible mechanism of homing of lymphoid cells. Z Zellforsch 116:502–522

Lennert K (1961) Lymphknoten. Diagnostik in Schnitt und Ausstrich. Cytologie und Lymphadenitis. Handb Spez Pathol Anat Histol, vol 1, part 3a. Springer, Berlin Heidelberg New York

Lennert K, Müller-Hermelink HK (1975) Lymphozyten und ihre Funktionsformen – Morphologie, Organisation und immunologische Bedeutung. Verh Anat Ges 69:19–62

Lennert K, Remmele W (1958) Karyometrische Untersuchungen an Lymphknotenzellen des Menschen. I. Germinoblasten, Lymphoblasten und Lymphozyten. Acta Haematol (Basel) 19:99–113

Lennert K, Kaiserling E, Müller-Hermelink HK (1975) T-associated plasma cells. Lancet I:1031–1032

Lennert K, Mohri N, Stein H, Kaiserling E, Müller-Hermelink HK (1978) Malignant lymphomas other than Hodgkin's disease. Springer, Berlin Heidelberg New York

Lennert K, Stein H, Müller-Hermelink HK, Vollenweider R (1984) T cells with plasmacytoid features. In: Bernard A, Boumsell L, Dausset J, Milstein C, Schlossman SF (eds) Leucocyte typing. Human leucocyte differentiation antigens detected by monoclonal antibodies. Springer, Berlin Heidelberg New York, p 711

Lukes RJ, Collins RD (1975) New approaches to the classification of lymphomata. Br J Cancer 31:1–28

Lukomska B, Olszewski L, Engeset A (1980) Immunologic characteristics of human peripheral lymph cell populations. Lymphology 13:186–191

Malone DG, Wahl SM, Tsokos M, Cattell H, Decker JL, Wilder RL (1984) Immune functions in severe, active rheumatoid arthritis: a relationship between peripheral blood mononuclear cell proliferation to soluble antigens and synovial tissue immunohistologic characteristics. J Clin Invest 74:1173–1185

Marrack P, Kappler J (1987) The T cell receptor. Science 238:1073–1077

Mason DY, Stein H, Naiem N, Abdulaziz Z (1981) Immunohistological analysis of human lymphoid tissue by double immunoenzymatic labelling. J Cancer Res Clin Oncol 101:13–22

Mason DY, Naiem M, Abdulaziz Z, Nash JRG, Gatter KC, Stein H (1982) Immunohistochemical labelling of cryostat sections with monoclonal antibody. In: McMichael AJ, Fabre JW (eds) Monoclonal antibodies in clinical medicine. Academic, London, pp 632–635

McKerrow JH, Jeong KH, Beckstead JH (1985) Enzyme histological comparison of *Biomphalaria glabrata* amebocytes with human granuloma macrophages. J Leukocyte Biol 37:341–347

Menthein R, Heymann E, Scholz W, Feller AC, Flad H-D (1984) Dipeptidyl peptidase IV as a new surface marker for a subpopulation of human T-lymphocytes. Cell Immunol 89:11–19

Meuer SC, Hodgdon JC, Cooper DA, Hussey RE, Fitzgerald KA, Schlossman SF, Reinherz EL (1983a) Human cytotoxic T cell clones directed at autologous virus transformed targets: further evidence for linkage of genetic restriction to T4 and T8 surface glycoproteins. J Immunol 131:186–190

Meuer SC, Acuto O, Hussey RE, Hodgdon JC, Fitzgerald KA, Schlossman SF, Reinherz EL (1983b) Evidence for the T3-associated 90K heterodimer as the T-cell antigen receptor. Nature 303:808–810

Mishra BB, Poulter LW, Janossy G, Geraint James D (1983) The distribution of lymphoid and macrophage like cell subsets of sarcoid and Kveim granulomata: possible mechanism of negative PPD reaction in sarcoidosis. Clin exp Immunol 54:705–715

Mitchell J, Abbot A (1971) Antigens in immunity: XVI. A light and electron microscope study of antigen localization in the rat spleen. Immunology 21:207–224

Miyawaki T, Ohzeki S, Ikuta N, Seki H, Taga K, Taniguchi N (1984) Immunohistologic localization and immune phenotypes of lymphocytes expressing Tac antigen in human lymphoid tissues. J Immunol 133:2996–3000

Modlin RL, Hofman FM, Meyer PR et al. (1983) in situ demonstration of T lymphocyte subsets in granulomatous inflammation: leprosy, rhinoscleroma and sarcoidosis. Clin Exp Immunol 51:430

Modlin RL, Hofman FM, Horwits DA, Husmann LA, Gillis S, Taylor CR, Rea TH (1984) In situ identification of cells in human leprosy granulomas with monoclonal antibodies to interleukin-2 and its receptor. J Immunol 132:3085–3090

Moretta A, Pantaleo G, Maggi E, Mingari MC (1984) Recent advances in the phenotypic and functional analysis of human T lymphocytes. Semin Hematol 21:257–269

Morgan-Capner P, Morris JA, McIllmurray MB, Thomas JA, Crawford DH, Azim T (1986) Immunohistological studies of lymphoproliferative lesions in a fatal case of Epstein-Barr virus infection. J Clin Pathol 39:1317–1322

Mori S, Mohri N, Morita H, Yamaguchi K, Shimamine T (1983) The distribution of cells expressing a natural killer cell marker (HNK-1) in normal human lymphoid organs and malignant lymphomas. Virchows Arch [B] 43:253–263

Morris MB, Mason DY, Stein H, Lennert K (1983) An immunohistological study of reactive lymphoid tissue. Histopathology 7:809–823

Müller J, Brun del Re G, Buerki H, Keller H-U, Hess MWX, Cottier H (1975) Nonspecific acid esterase activity: a criterion for differentiation of T and B lymphocytes in mouse lymph nodes. Eur J Immunol 5:270–274

Müller-Hermelink HK, Kaiserling E, Lennert K (1973) Pseudofollikulaere Nester von Plasmazellen (eines besonderen Typs?) in der paracorticalen Pulpa menschlicher Lymphknoten. Virchows Arch [B] 14:47–56

Müller-Hermelink HK, Heusermann U, Stutte HJ (1974) Enzyme histochemical observations on

the localization and structure of the T-cell and B-cell regions in the human spleen. Cell Tissue Res 154:167–179
Müller-Hermelink HK, Steinman G, Stein H, Lennert K (1983) Malignant lymphoma of plasmacytoid T-cells. Morphologic and immunologic studies characterizing a special type of T-cell. Am J Surg Pathol 7:849–862
Myking AO (1974) Histologic changes in mouse lymph nodes and skin following repeated skin painting with oxalozone. Acta Pathol Microbiol Scand [A] 82:249–254
Narayanan RB, Bhutani LK, Sharma AK et al. (1983) T cell subsets in leprosy lesions: in situ characterization using monoclonal antibodies. Clin Exp Immunol 51:421
Nieuwenhuis P, Ford WL (1976) Comparative migration of B- and T-lymphocytes in the rat spleen and lymph nodes. Cell Immunol 23:254–267
Nossal GJV, Austin CM, Pye J, Mitchell J (1966) Antigens in immunity: XII. Antigen trapping in the spleen. Int Arch Allergy 29:368–383
Olszewski WL, Grzelak I, Engeset A (1982) Cells in lymph draining normal human skin – monoclonal antibody analysis. Lymphology 15:168–173
Pangalis GAZ, Weldman SR, Rappaport H (1978) Cytochemical findings in human nonneoplastic blood and tonsillar B and T lymphocytes. Am J Clin Pathol 69:314–318
Parravicini CL, Vago L, Costanzi GC et al. (1986) Follicle lysis in lymph nodes from homosexual men. Blood 68:595–596
Parrott DMV, de Sousa MAB (1971) Thymus-dependent and thymus-independent populations: origin, migratory patterns and life span. Clin Exp Immunol 8:663–684
Picker JL, Brenner MB, Weiss LM, Smith SD, Warnke RA (1987) Discordant expression of CD3 and T-cell receptor β-chain antigens in T-lineage lymphomas. Am J Pathol 129:434–440
Picker LJ, Brenner MB, Michie S, Warnke RA (1988) Expression of T cell receptor delta chains in benign and malignant T lineage lymphoproliferations. Am J Pathol 132:401–405
Pileri S, Kikuchi M, Dagmar H, Lennert K (1982) Histiocytic necrotizing lymphadenitis without granulocytic infiltration. Virchows Arch [A] 395:257–271
Pineiro Maccira JM, Fukuyama K, Epstein WL, Rowden G (1984) Immunohistochemical demonstration of S-100 protein antigen-containing cells in beryllium-induced, zirconium-induced and sarcoidosis granulomas. Am J Clin Pathol 81:563–568
Pizzolo G, Semenzato G, Chilosi M et al. (1984) Distribution and heterogeneity of cells detected by HNK-1 monoclonal antibody in blood and tissues in normal, reactive and neoplastic conditions. Clin Exp Immunol 57:195–206
Platt JL, Grant BW, Eddy AA, Michael AF (1983) Immune cell populations in cutaneous delayed-type hypersensitivity. J Exp Med 158:1227–1242
Polliack A, Lampen N, Clarkson BD, de Harven E, Bentwich Z, Siegal FP, Kunkel HG (1973) Identification of human B and T lymphocytes by scanning electron microscopy. J Exp Med 138:607–624
Poppema S, Bhan AK, Reinherz EL, McCluskey RT, Schlossman SF (1981) Distribution of T cell subsets in human lymph nodes. J Exp Med 153:30–41
Poppema S, Visser L, de Ley L (1983) Reactivity of presumed antinatural killer cell antibody Leu 7 with intrafollicular T lymphocytes. Clin Exp Immunol 54:834–837
Poulter LW, Collings LI, Tung KS, Waters MFR (1984) Parasitism of antigen presenting cells in hyperbacillary leprosy. Clin Exp Immunol 55:611–617
Ree H, Fanger H (1975) Paracortical alteration in lymphadenopathic and tumor-draining lymph nodes: histologic study. Hum Pathol 6:363–372
Reinherz EL, Schlossman SF (1980) The differentiation and function of human T lymphocytes: a review. Cell 19:821–827
Reinherz EL, Kung PC, Pesando JM (1979) Ia determinants on human T-cell subsets defined by monoclonal antibody: activation stimuli required for expression. J Exp Med 150:1472–1482
Ritchie AWS, James K, Micklem HS (1983) The distribution and possible significance of cells identified in human lymphoid tissue by the monoclonal antibody HNK-1. Clin Exp Immunol 51:439–447
Rivano MT, Falini B, Stein H et al. (1987) Histiocytic necrotizing lymphadenitis without granulocytic infiltration (Kikuchi's lymphadenitis). Morphological and immunohistochemical study of eight cases. Histopathology 11:1013–1027

Romain PL, Schlossman SF (1984) Human T lymphocyte subsets. Functional heterogeneity and surface recognition structures. J Clin Invest 74:1559–1565

Ron Y, Sprent J (1987) T cell priming in vivo: a major role for B cells in presenting antigen to T cells in lymph nodes. J Immunol 138:2848–2856

Rouse RV, Ledbetter JA, Weisman IL (1982) Mouse lymph node germinal centers contain a selected subset of T cells – the helper phenotype. J Immunol 128:2243–2246

Said JW (1988) AIDS-related lymphadenopathies. Semin Diagn Pathol 5:365–375

Said JW, Sintaku IP, Teitelbaum A, Chien K, Sassoon AF (1984) Distribution of T-cell phenotypic subsets and surface immunoglobulin-bearing lymphocytes in lymph nodes from male homosexuals with persistent generalized lymphadenopathy. An immunohistochemical and ultrastructural study. Hum Pathol 15:785–790

Saltzstein SL, Ackerman LV (1959) Lymphadenopathy induced by anticonvulsant drugs and mimicking clinically and pathologically malignant lymphoma. Cancer 12:164–182

Schwartz RH (1986) The role of gene products of the major histocompatibility complex in T cell activation and cellular interactions. In: Paul WE (ed) Fundamental immunology. Raven, New York, pp 379–438

Semenzato G, Pezzuto A, Chilosi M, Pizzolo G (1982) T lymphocyte redistribution in the lymph nodes of sarcoidosis patients. N Engl J Med 306:48–49

Semenzato G, Agostini C, Frentin L et al. (1984) Evidence of cells bearing interleukin-2 receptor at sites of disease activity in sarcoid patients. Clin Exp Immunol 57:331–337

Seymour GJ, Greaves MJ, Janossy G (1981) Identification of cells expressing Tac and p28,33 (Ia-like) antigens in sections of human lymphoid tissue. Clin Exp Immunol 36:66–75

Sheibani K, Winberg CD, van de Velde S, Blayney DW, Rappaport H (1987) Distribution of lymphocytes with interleukin-2 receptors (TAC antigens) in reactive lymphoproliferative processes, Hodgkin's disease, and non-Hodgkin's lymphomas. An immunohistologic study of 300 cases. Am J Pathol 127:27–37

Shen HH, Talle MA, Goldstein G, Chess L (1983) Functional subsets of human monocytes defined by monoclonal antibodies: a distinct subset of monocytes contains the cells capable of inducing the autologous mixed lymphocyte culture. J Immunol 130:698–705

Shen J-Y, Barnes PF, Rea TH, Meyer PR (1988) Immunohistology of tuberculous adenitis in symptomatic HIV infection. Clin Exp Immunol 72:186–189

Si L, Whiteside TL (1983) Tissue distribution of human NK cells studied with anti-Leu7 monoclonal antibody. J Immunol 130:2149–2155

Si L, Roscoe G, Whiteside TL (1983) Selective distribution and quantitation of T-lymphocyte subsets in germinal centers of human tonsils. Arch Pathol Lab Med 107:228–231

Silberberg-Sinakin I, Thorbecke GJ, Baer RL, Rosenthal SA, Berezowski V (1976) Antigen-bearing Langerhans cells in skin, dermal lymphatics and in lymph nodes. Cell Immunol 25:137–151

Silveira PA, Mendes NF, Tolnai MEA (1972) Tissue localization of two populations of human lymphocytes distinguished by membrane receptors. J Immunol 108:1456–1460

Stein H, Bonk A, Tolksdorf G, Lennert K, Rodt H, Gerdes J (1980) Immunohistologic analysis of the organization of normal lymphoid tissue and non-Hodgkin's lymphomas. J Histochem Cytochem 28:746–760

Strauchen JA, Breakstone BA (1987) IL-2 receptor expression in human lymphoid lesions. Immunohistochemical study of 166 cases. Am J Pathol 126:506–512

Sutton JS, Weiss L (1966) Transformation of monocytes in tissue culture into macrophages, epithelioid cells and multinucleated giant cells. J Cell Biol 28:303–332

Swerdlow SH, Murray LJ (1984) Natural killer (Leu 7^+) cells in reactive lymphoid tissues and malignant lymphomas. Am J Clin Pathol 81:459–463

Takacs L, Osawa H, Toro I, Diamantstein T (1985) Immunohistochemical localization of cells reacting with monoclonal antibodies directed against the interleukin-2 receptor of murine, rat and human origin. Clin Exp Immunol 59:37–44

Takahashi K, Isobe T, Ohtsuki Y, Sonobe H, Yamaguchi H, Akagi T (1985) S-100 protein positive human T-lymphocytes. Am J Clin Pathol 83:69–72

Tonder O, Morse PA Jr, Humphrey LJ (1974) Similarities of Fc receptors in human malignant tissue and normal lymphoid tissue. J Immunol 113:1162–1167

Turk JL, Badenoch-Jones P, Parker D (1978) Ultrastructural observation on epithelioid cell granulomas induced by zirconium in the guinea-pig. J Pathol 124:45–49
van den Oord JJ (1985) The immune response in the human lymph node. A morphological, enzyme- and immunohistochemical study. PhD Thesis, Catholic University of Leuven, Leuven, Belgium. ACCO, Leuven
van den Oord JJ, de Wolf-Peeters C, de Vos R, Desmet VJ (1984a) The paracortical area in dermatopathic lymphadenitis and other reactive conditions of the lymph node. Virchows Arch [B] 45:289–299
van den Oord JJ, de Wolf-Peeters C, Facchetti F, Desmet VJ (1984b) Cellular composition of hypersensitivity-type granulomas. Immunohistochemical analysis of tuberculous and sarcoidal lymphadenitis. Hum Pathol 15:559–565
van den Oord JJ, de Wolf-Peeters C, Tricot G, Desmet VJ (1984c) Distribution of lymphocyte subsets in a case of angiofollicular lymph node hyperplasia. Am J Clin Pathol 82:491–495
van den Oord JJ, de Wolf-Peeters C, Desmet VJ (1985a) Cellular composition of suppurative granulomas. An immunohistochemical study of suppurative granulomatous lymphadenitis. Hum Pathol 16:1009–1014
van den Oord JJ, de Wolf-Peeters C, Desmet VJ (1985b) Immature sinus histiocytes in the lymphadenopathic stage of AIDS: relationship to polyclonal B-cell activation? J Pathol 145:63–64
van den Oord JJ, de Wolf-Peeters C, Desmet VJ, Takahashi K, Ohtsuki Y, Akagi T (1985c) Nodular alteration of the paracortical area. An in situ immunohistochemical analysis of primary, secondary, and tertiary T-nodules. Am J Pathol 120:55–66
van den Oord JJ, de Wolf-Peeters C, Desmet VJ (1985d) Immunohistochemical analysis of progressively transformed follicular centers. Am J Clin Pathol 83:560–564
van den Oord JJ, de Wolf-Peeters C, de Vos R, Desmet VJ (1985e) Immature sinus histiocytosis. Light- and electronmicroscopic features, immunologic phenotype, and relationship with marginal zone lymphocytes. Am J Pathol 118:266–277
van den Oord JJ, de Wolf-Peeters C, Desmet VJ (1986a) The marginal zone in the human reactive lymph node. Am J Clin Pathol 86:475–479
van den Oord JJ, de Wolf-Peeters C, Desmet VJ (1986b) The composite nodule. A structural and functional unit of the reactive lymph node. Am J Pathol 122:83–91
van der Valk P, Meijer CJLM (1987) The histology of reactive lymph nodes. Am J Surg Pathol 11:866–882
van der Valk P, van der Loo EM, Jansen J, Daha MR, Meyer CJLM (1984) Analysis of lymphoid and dendritic cells in human lymph node, tonsil and spleen. A study using monoclonal and heterologous antibodies. Virchows Arch [B] 45:169–185
van Rooijen N (1973) Mechanism of follicular antigen trapping: migration of antigen-antibody complexes from marginal zone towards follicle centres. Immunology 25:847–852
van Voorhis WC, Kaplan G, Nunes Sarno-E (1982) The cutaneous infiltrates of leprosy: cellular characteristics and the predominant T-cell phenotypes. N Engl J Med 307:1593–1597
Veerman AJP (1974) On the interdigitating cells in the thymus dependent area of the rat spleen: a relationship between the mononuclear phagocyte system and T-lymphocytes. Cell Tissue Res 148:247–257
Veerman AJP, van Ewijk W (1975) White pulp compartments in the spleen of rats and mice. A light and electron microscopic study of lymphoid and non-lymphoid cell types in T- and B-areas. Cell Tissue Res 156:417–441
Veerman AJP, van Rooijen N (1975) Lymphocyte capping and lymphocyte migration as associated events in the in vivo antigen trapping process: an electron-microscopic autoradiographic study in the spleen of mice. Cell Tissue Res 161:211–217
Veldman JE (1970) Histophysiology and electron microscopy of the immune response. Doctoral Thesis, State University of Groningen, Groningen, The Netherlands
Veldman JE, Keuning FJ (1978) Histophysiology of cellular immunity reactions in B-cell deprived rabbits. An X-irradiation model for delineation of an "isolated T-cell system". Virchows Arch [B] 28:203–216

Veldman JE, Molenaar I, Keuning FJ (1978) Electron microscopy of cellular immunity reactions in B-cell deprived rabbits. Thymus-derived antigen-reactive cells, their micro-environment and progeny in the lymph node. Virchows Arch [B] 28:217–228

von Gaudecker B, Pfingsten U, Müller-Hermelink H-K (1984) Localization and characterization of T-cell subpopulations and natural killer cells ($HNK1^+$ cells) in the human tonsilla palatina. An ultrastructural-immunocytochemical study. Cell Tissue Res 238:135–143

Warnke R, Levy R (1980) Detection of T and B cell antigens with hybridoma monoclonal antibodies: a biotin-avidin-horseradish peroxidase method. J Histochem Cytochem 28:771–776

Watanabe Y, Tamaoki N, Habu S, Tashiro Y, Akatsuka S, Enomoto Y (1974) Fine structural study on human T- and B-lymphocytes. Acta Haematol Jpn 37:655–666

Weiss LM, Wood GS, Warnke RA (1985) Immunophenotypic differences between dermatopathic lymphadenopathy and lymph node involvement in mycosis fungoides. Am J Pathol 120:179–185

Weiss LM, Beckstead JH, Warnke RA, Wood GS (1986) Leu-6-expressing cells in lymph nodes: dendritic cells phenotypically similar to interdigitating reticulum cells. Hum Pathol 17:179–184

Willkens RF, Roth GF, Husby G, Williams RC (1980) Immunocytological studies of lymph nodes in rheumatoid arthritis and malignant lymphoma. Ann Rheum Dis 39:147–151

Wood GS, Garcia C, Dorfman RF et al. (1985) The immunohistochemistry of follicle lysis in lymph node biopsies from homosexual men. Blood 66:1092–1097

Wood GS, Burns BF, Dorfman RF et al. (1986) In situ quantitation of lymph node helper, suppressor, and cytotoxic T cell subsets in AIDS. Blood 67:596–603

The Plasmacytoid T Cell or Plasmacytoid Monocyte – A Sessile Lymphoid Cell with Unique Immunophenotype and Unknown Function, Still Awaiting Lineage Affiliation

B. Brado and P. Möller

1 Introduction

Plasmacytoid T cells (PTCs) were first described in 1958, as clusters of cells with the light-microscopic appearance of "lymphoblasts" (Lennert and Remmele 1958). The electron-microscopic features conformed to the criteria for secretory cells, which were then thought to represent a special type of plasma cell (Müller-Hermelink et al. 1973). These plasma cell-like cells have been identified in T zones of human lymphoid tissue, in reactive (Feller et al. 1983; Vollenweider and Lennert 1983) and in neoplastic (Beiske et al. 1986; Müller-Hermelink et al. 1983; Prasthofer et al. 1985) conditions. In accordance with the topographical relation between these plasmacytoid cells and T regions of lymph nodes, they were designated "T-associated plasma cells" (Lennert et al. 1975). Because of immunohistological features indicative of a T-cell nature (Feller et al. 1983), they were subsequently renamed "plasmacytoid T cells." A recent study, however, has suggested a myelomonocytic origin of this cell type (Horny et al. 1987); this view is not generally accepted (Harris and Bahn 1987; Papadimitriou et al. 1983), but it has led to the alternative designation "plasmacytoid monocyte" (Facchetti et al. 1989).

In order to obtain further information about the origin and functional equipment of this cell type, we comprehensively studied its immunophenotype. Using a broad panel of clustered monoclonal antibodies (mAbs) against T-cell, B-cell, and myelo/monocyte-restricted and -associated differentiation and activation antigens (McMichael et al. 1987; Knapp et al. 1989), we examined three cases of lymphadenitis with nests of PTCs considerably enlarged and increased in number.

2 Materials and Methods

Three specimens containing a considerable number of large nests of PTCs were selected from our stock of fresh-frozen lymph nodes affected by various types of lymphadenitis. These lymph nodes were removed from three middle-aged women, all presenting with mild axillary and inguinal lymphadenopathy in the absence of other clinical symptoms. Red and white cell counts were within the normal range, and human immunodeficiency virus 1 titers and antistreptolysin-O tests were negative.

The lymph nodes were snap-frozen in liquid nitrogen and stored at −70 °C until sectioning. Serial frozen sections (4–6 μm) were cut, extensively air dried, acetone fixed (10 min at room temperature), and immediately immunostained.

The mAbs used in this study are listed in Table 1. Some were gifts of Drs. L. GRAF, Seattle, WA (ISCR3); A. ZIEGLER, Tübingen, FRG (Tü22); W. KNAPP, Vienna, Austria (VIC-Y1); B. DÖRKEN and G. MOLDENHAUER, Heidelberg, FRG (HD37, HD28); J.H. LEDBETTER, Seattle (G28-8, G28-5); and P.A. TETTEROO, Amsterdam (CLB-Gran/B Ly). Others were obtained commercially from Becton Dickinson, Mountain View, CA (B7/21, anti-Leu-M1, anti-Leu-M4, anti-Leu-M5, anti-Leu-7/HNK-1, anti-Leu-11 b), from Ortho Diagnostics, Raritan, NJ (OKT1, OKT3, OKT4, OKT6, OKT8, OKT9, OKT10, OKT11, OKT16, OKT17), from Behring-Werke, Frankfurt, FRG (Ki-M2, Ki-M5, Ki-M6, Ki-M7, Ki-M8, Vim-2, Vim-C6, BMA031), from Dianova GmbH, Hamburg, FRG (B1.49.9, B1.19.2, J3D3, GO22, 2E-1, BEAR-1, BEAR-2), from Coulter Immunology, FL (My7, PCA-1), and from Dakopatts, Glostrup, Denmark (Ki-1, Ki-67). A polyclonal biotinylated sheep antibody to mouse immunoglobulin (Ig) (reactive with all mouse isotopes) and a streptavidin-biotinylated peroxidase complex (from Amersham Buchler, High Wycombe, UK) served as the detection system for the monoclonal primary antibodies.

After rehydration with phosphate buffered saline (PBS), the frozen sections were incubated for 1 h with culture supernatants or purified mAbs at appropriate dilutions. Incubation times of tissue for the second-step and third-step reagents were 30 min. In order to avoid cross-reactions, the second antibody was used in the presence of 5% pooled human IgG. All incubation steps were performed in a humid chamber at room temperature and were rinsed with PBS. The binding of antibody was visualized by 10 min incubation with 0.4 mg/ml 3-amino-9-ethylcarbazole (Sigma, St. Louis, MO), 5% dimethylformamide (Sigma), and 0.0015% H_2O_2 in 0.1 M acetate buffer, pH 5.2. The sections were counterstained with Harris' hematoxylin and mounted with glycerol gelatine.

Intrinsic positive controls for the immunoreactivity of HLA-D associated invariant chain (Ii) and class II mAbs were interstitial dendritic cells, endothelial cells, and macrophages, indicating by their staining the reliability of the reaction and thus excluding false-negative results. Negative controls were acquired by omitting the primary antibody. Endogenous peroxidase activity of

Table 1. Immunophenotype of PTCs

Antigen[a]	Clone(s)	Result[b]
T cell restricted antigens		
CD2	9.6	(+)
CD3	OKT3, Leu-4	–
TCR/CD3	BMA031	–
T cell associated		
CD1	OKT6	–
CD4	OKT4	+
CD5	OKT1	–
CD6	OKT17	–
CD7	OKT16	–
CD8	OKT8	–
CD16	GO22	–
CD57	Leu-7	–
B cell specific		
CD19	HD37	–
CD20	B1	–
CD22	HD39	–
B cell associated		
CD24	CLB-Gran/B Ly	–
CD37	HD28	–
CD39	G28-8	–
CD40	G28-5	–
PCA-1	PCA-1	–
Nonlineage antigens (LFA-1 family)		
CD11b	OKM1	–
CD11b	BEAR-1	–
CD11b	Ki-M5	–
CD11c	S-HCL-3	+
Granulocyte/monocyte/macrophage		
CD13	My7	–
CD14	BEAR-2	–
CD15	MMA; Vim-C6	–
CDw65	Vim-2	–
CD68	Ki-M6; Ki-M7	+
Group 11D	Ki-M8	–
88KDa	OKM5	+
	Ki-M5	–
Activation and proliferation antigens		
CD30	Ki-1	–
	Ki-67	–
CD25	Tac; B1.49.9	–
CD71	OKT9	–
CD38	OKT10	–
CD26	B1.19.2	+
MHC antigens		
HLA-ABC	W6/32	+
Ii	VIC-Y1	+
HLA-DR	ISCR3	+
HLA-DP	B7/21	(+)
HLA-DQ	Tü22	–
Miscellaneous antigens		
CD35	J3D3	–
CDw32	2E-1	–

[a] 4th Workshop antigen designation (KNAPP et al. 1989)
[b] +, positive on the plasmacytoid T-cell population; (+), weakly positive on the plasmacytoid T-cell population; –, negative on the plasmacytoid T-cell population

sparse granulocytes was not blocked in order to ensure optimal antigenicity and because it was easily distinguishable from specific immunostaining.

3 Results

The foci mainly consisting of PTCs were chiefly located in the interfollicular areas, in the T zone of the lymph nodes, and frequently in the vicinity of epithelioid venules (Fig. 1). These nests contained a small number of tingible

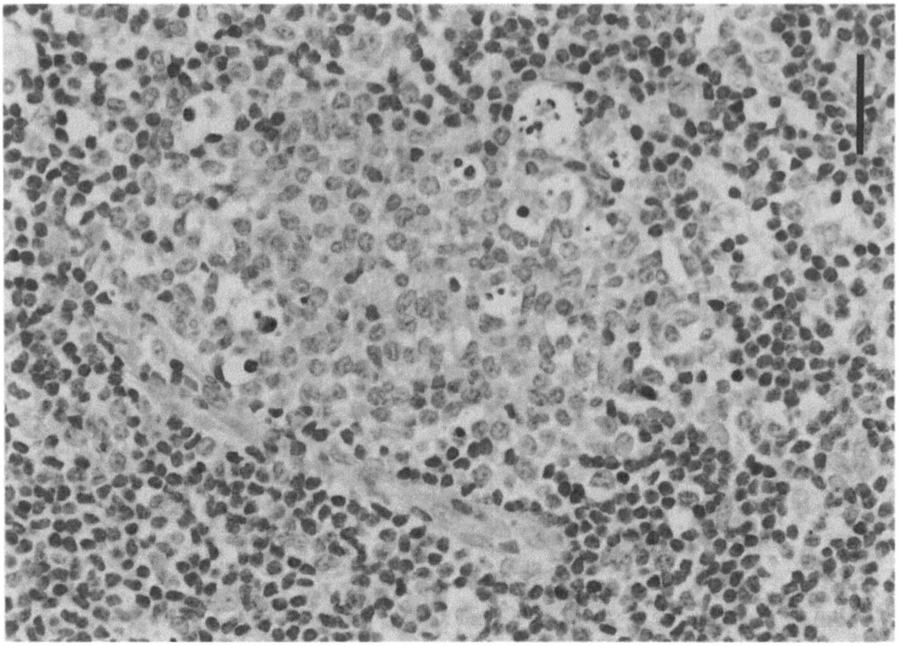

Fig. 1. Giemsa-stained paraffin section of a lymph node with one of numerous foci of PTCs. The nests of pale medium-sized lymphoid cells with leptochrome nuclei are often situation in the vicinity of postcapillary epithelioid venules and regularly contain (some) tingible body macrophages. Mitoses are absent in these foci. Nuclei are stained with hematoxylin. *Bar* = 50 µm

body macrophages and very few "true" plasma cells; some of them displayed a very small number of granulocytes. The PTCs were about 1.5 times larger than peripheral T lymphocytes and had a rather broad rim of faintly eosinophilic cytoplasm, oval nuclei with small dots of chromatin, and a prominent but minute nucleolus. There were small numbers of single cell necroses but no mitotic figures whatsoever.

The immunohistological results are summarized in Table 1. PTCs expressed the T-cell antigen (CD4) in amounts comparable to those of small T helper cells (Fig. 4c). The sheep erythrocyte receptor CD2 was detectable, but only at a very low density (Fig. 2). CD1, CD3, CD5, CD6, CD7, CD8, and CD57 antigens expressed on the common T cells around the PTC nests could not be identified in/on PTCs (Fig. 4b, d). The following B-cell antibodies were shown not to react with the PTCs: HD37, B1, HD39, CLB-Gran/B Ly, HD28, G28-8, G28-5, and PCA-1 (Fig. 4a).

Out of the large panel of mAbs recognizing granulocytes, monocytes, and macrophages, the PTCs were strongly stained by CD68 (Ki-M6 and Ki-M7) (Fig. 4g, h). Furthermore, PTCs expressed the CD11c antigen (Fig. 4e) and reacted with the mAb OKM5 (Fig. 4f), which recognizes a 88-kD antigen. The pan-myelomonocytic antigens CD13, CD14, and M2 were not detectable. The

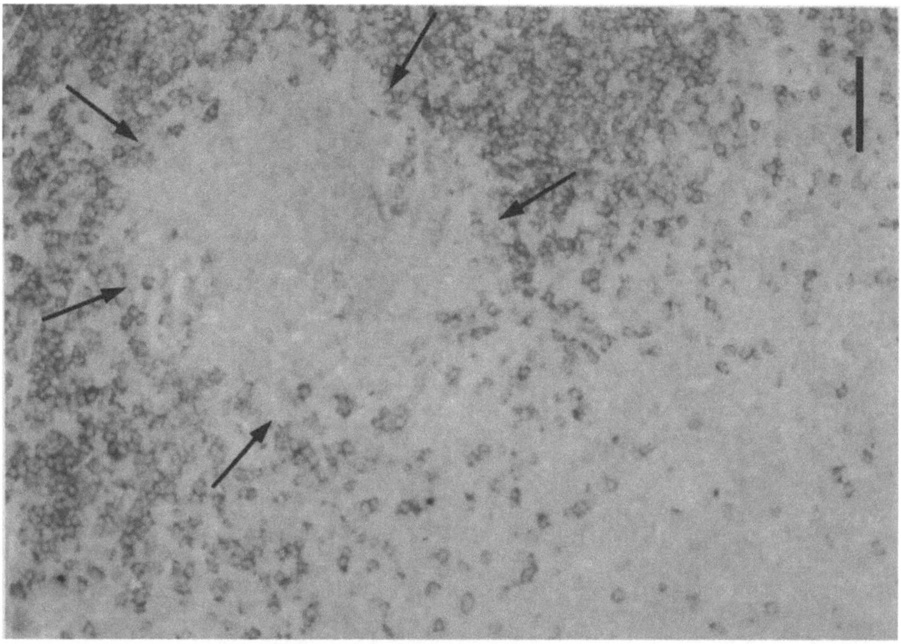

Fig. 2. Indirect immunoperoxidase reaction on a frozen section of a lymph node. mAb OKT11, being specific for the CD2 antigen, reveals high antigenic density in small T lymphocytes, lack of CD2 in B lymphocytes, and a very low antigenic distribution on PTCs (*arrows*). Nuclei are stained with hematoxylin. *Bar* = 50 μm

Ki-M2, Ki-M5, and Ki-M8 binding antigens, however, as well as the CD15 and CD11 b antigens, were likewise lacking in/on PTCs. CD26, a "late" T-cell activation antigen, was present on PTCs in all three cases examined. In addition to a strong HLA-ABC positivity, there was a differential expression of major histocompatibility complex (MHC) class II antigens and Ii in the following order of antigenic density: Ii > HLA-DR > HLA-DP, while HLA-DQ antigens were not detectable (Fig. 3). The transferrin receptor, the interleukin-2 receptor, i.e., CD71 and CD25, and the CD38 antigen, along with the CD30 antigen and the nuclear proliferation antigen recognized by the mAb Ki-67, could not be detected in/on PTCs. This pattern of antigen expression was found in each individual PTC in every area examined.

4 Discussion

Our results extend the present knowledge of PTCs in that they show that PTCs, being a cell type with well-defined morphology, express a small set of T-cell antigens and antigens so far ascribed to the myelomonocytic lineage (cf.

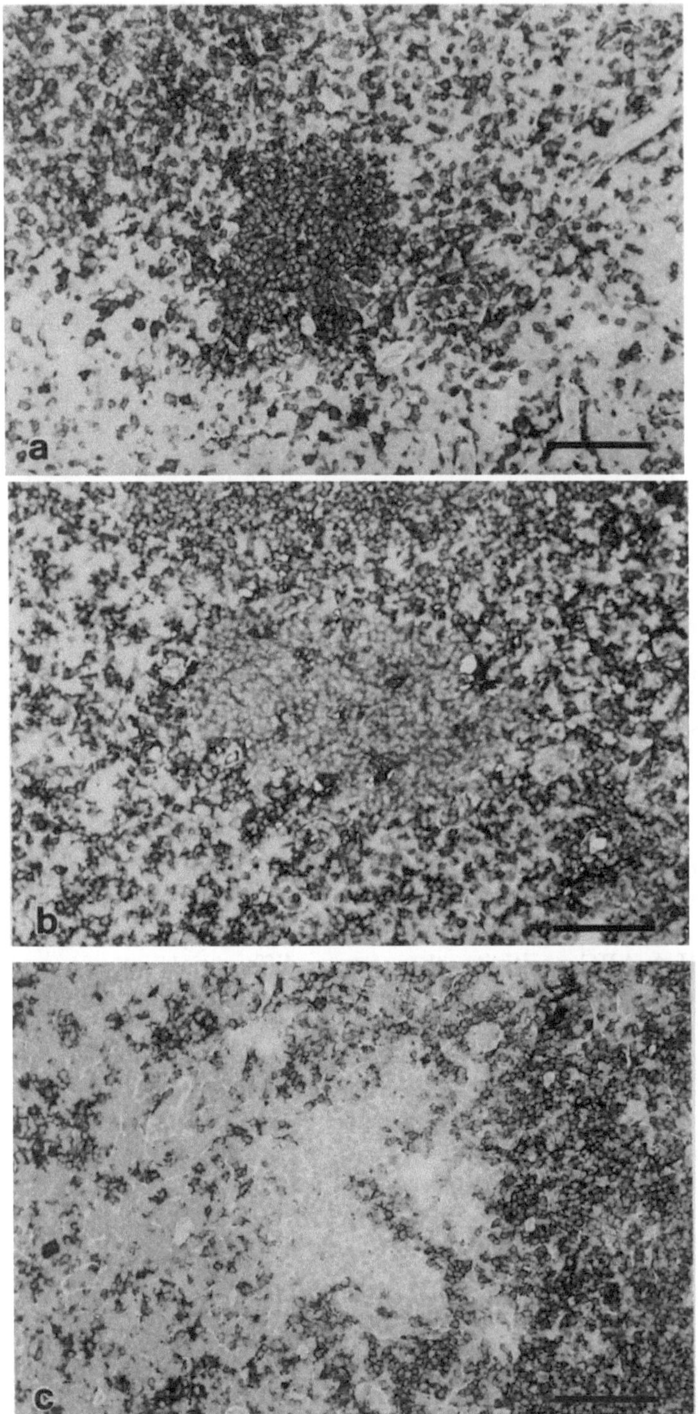
a
b
c

Table 1). Although the obtained immunoprofile as a whole is unique and thus represents a clear-cut immunophenotypic definition of PTCs, it is yet not unambiguous in terms of lineage affiliation.

We confirm the expression of the CD4 antigen on PTCs. CD4 is a 62-kD membrane glycoprotein, which characterizes T helper lymphocytes. CD4 antigen bearing T lymphocytes are liable to recognize class II molecules as part of their specificity. The CD4 molecule does not participate in antigen recognition; it might interact with the constant regions of the respective MHC molecules and increase cell-to-cell interactions between the T cell and its target cell (Dembic et al. 1987; Sleckman et al. 1987). CD4 could be detected on monocytes (Wood et al. 1983), histiocytes, Langerhans cells, and glial cells (Sattentau and Weiss 1988, Spickett and Dalgleish 1988). Therefore, the expression of the CD4 antigen on PTCs is only a feeble argument for a T-cell origin of PTCs.

The CD2 molecule was expressed in low density by PTCs. CD2 (50 kD) is the receptor by which the T lymphocytes form rosettes with sheep red blood cells (Howard et al. 1981). The role of CD2 in T-cell function is not clear. Recent studies suggest that it might play a role in the alternative pathway of T-cell activation distinct from that mediated through the T-cell antigen receptor heterodimer (TCR) (Martin et al. 1983; Meuer et al. 1984). Neither in normal PTCs nor in tumor-like proliferations of PTCs or alleged "PTC" lymphomas could the sheep erythrocyte receptor be found by the immunohistological methods applied (Feller et al. 1983; Beiske et al. 1986; Müller-Hermelink et al. 1983; Prasthofer et al. 1985; Harris and Bhan 1987). In contrast, we could demonstrate in all three cases a very weak but definite staining of PTCs with CD2 (OKT11). This discrepancy we attribute to the sensitivity of the detection systems used. Although CD2 was found to be expressed in some cases of acute myeloid leukemia (i.e., on malignant cells), there is no evidence that this antigen is not T cell specific within the leukocyte cell population. Therefore, the presence of the sheep erythrocyte receptor on non-neoplastic PTCs favors its T-cell origin.

Plasmacytoid T cells were found to be TCR/CD3$^-$, CD5$^-$, CD6$^-$. It has been shown that phorbolesters and synthetic diacylglycerols inducing T-cell activation cause a rapid down-regulation of the TCR and the CD3 antigen together with the acquisition of an unresponsive state to interaction with specific antigen (Ando et al. 1985; Cantrell et al. 1985; Crumpton et al. 1987). It is therefore conceivable that the lack of the TCR/CD3 molecule complex on PTCs is due to a special functional state in which T cells can be

◀ **Fig. 3a–c.** Immunostained serial frozen sections of a lymph node. **a** mAb VIC-Y1 detecting Ii reveals high antigenic density in B lymphocytes, in the majority of histiocytic and dendritic cells, and in PTCs. **b** mAb ISCR3, being specific for HLA-DR antigens, discloses large amounts of antigen in B lymphocytes and histiocytes, and a lower antigenic density on PTCs. The rest of the T-cell population does not express detectable HLA-DR antigens. **c** mAb Tü22, being specific for HLA-DQ antigens, reveals an antigenic distribution comparable to that of HLA-DR except for PTCs that are completely unreactive. Nuclei are stained with hematoxylin. *Bar* = 100 μm

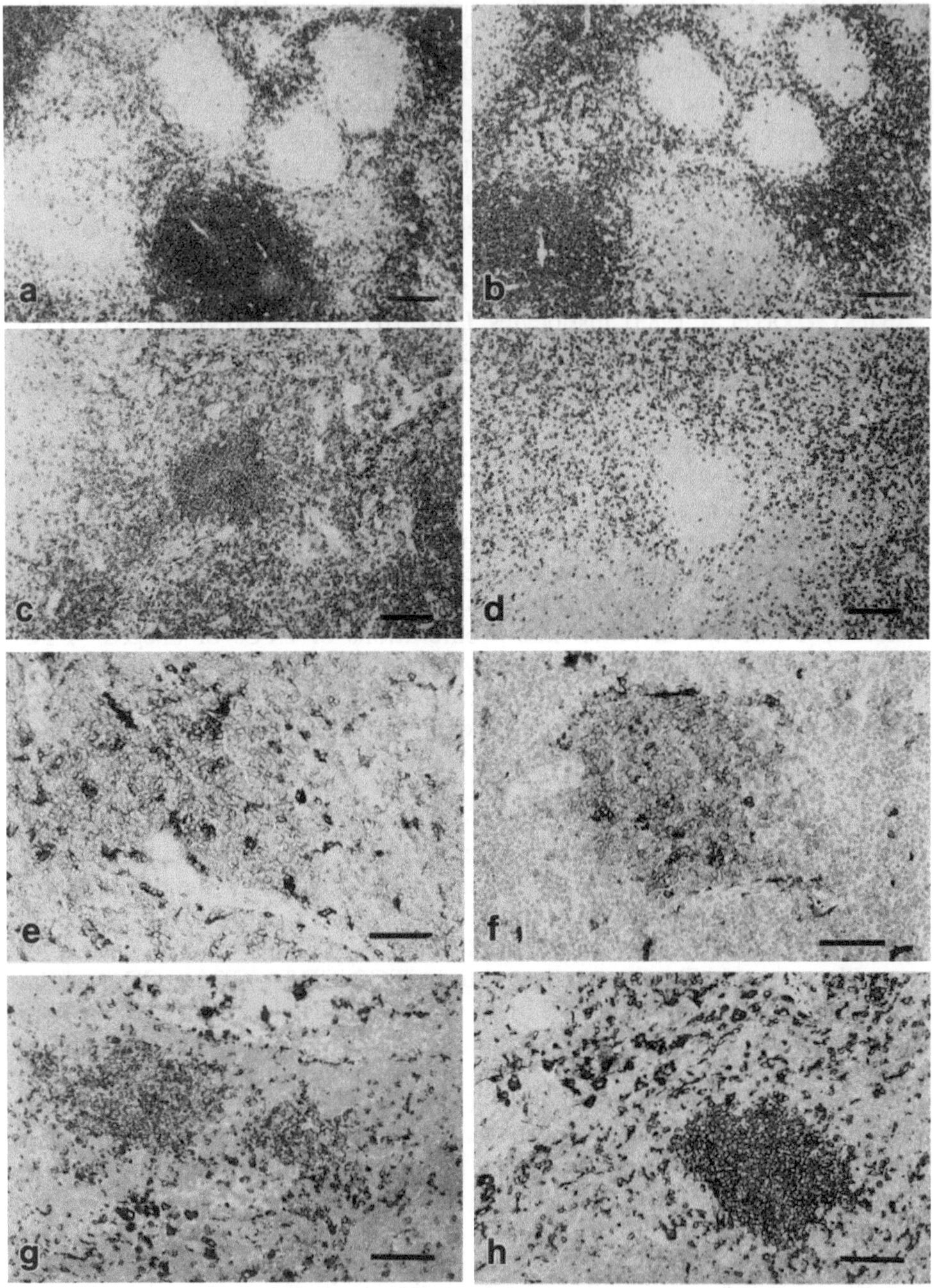
a
b
c
d
e
f
g
h

found after activation or persistent antigen contact. This loss of TCR/CD3 at a functional end-stage would then have its parallel in B-cell maturation characterized by a complete abrogation of "pan-B" antigens (e.g., CD19, CD20, CD22) at the plasma cell stage (NADLER 1986).

The CD6 antigen (49 kD) is present on the majority of resting normal peripheral T cells, but is expressed only on a subset of $CD4^+$ lymphocytes after activation. THOMAS et al. (1982) ascribed a radiosensitive helper function to activated peripheral T lymphocytes with the phenotype $CD4^+CD6^-$. PTCs lacking the CD6 antigen, while expressing the CD4 antigen on the cell surface membrane, show the same phenotype as this functionally mature subset of activated peripheral T lymphocytes.

It is in line with these arguments that PTCs did not express well-known granulocyte/monocyte/macrophage-associated antigens such as CD13, CD14, and CD15. However, PTCs did react with CD68 (Ki-M6) and CD68 (Ki-M7), which are directed against intracytoplasmically localized antigens not yet characterized. CD68 mAbs were reported to have high specificity for the myelomonocytic cell lineage (KREIPE et al. 1987; PARWARESCH et al. 1986) whereas they did not recognize dendritic reticulum cells of lymphoid follicles and interdigitating reticulum cells of lymphoid T zones. Meanwhile, it has been shown that CD68 (Ki-M7) also labels granulocytes and platelets (HOGG and MORTON 1987). FRANKLIN et al. (1987) found a positive reaction with these CD68 antibodies with a bronchial carcinoid. We detected a positive reaction of both antibodies with so-called monocytoid B cells (synonym: sinusoidal B cells) and also with a subset of B-cell lymphomas (unpublished data). Thus, in contrast to HORNY et al. (1987), we hold that the binding of CD68 mAbs does not at all favor a myelomonocytic origin of PTCs. We disagree, as well, with the conclusions drawn by FACCHETTI et al. (1988), who described positive staining of PTCs with the mAbs MT1 and LN2. These two mAbs do not stain only monocytes and macrophages, but also T cells, erythrocyte precursors, and B cells (WEST et al. 1986; POPPEMA et al. 1987). During the last Workshop on Leukocyte Differentiation Antigens (KNAPP et al. 1989), the mAb LN2 was shown to recognize the MHC class II associated invariant chain (Ii) and now belong to the cluster CD74. Thus, it has become evident that LN2 binding does not at all favor a monocyte derivation of the target cell.

◀ **Fig. 4a–h.** Indirect immunoperoxidase on serial frozen sections of a lymph node with numerous PTC nests. **a** mAb HD39 reveals high amounts of the CD22 antigen on a B-cell follicle; the three PTC foci depicted, however, are completely unreactive. **b** mAb OKT1 shows CD5 antigen in the T-cell areas, while the B-cell follicle and the PTC foci depicted lack this antigen. **c** mAb OKT4 clearly demonstrates CD4 antigen in/on PTCs and in/on small T lymphocytes around the PTC nest. **d** mAb OKT8 reveals lack of CD8 antigen in PTCs, but displays a positive CD8 expression on small T lymphocytes around the PTC nest. **e** mAb Leu-M5, recognizing the CD11c antigen, moderately stains PTC foci. **f** mAb OKM5, recognizing a polypeptide of 88 kD, reveals positively stained PTC foci. **g** mAb Ki-M6 (CD68) clearly stains PTC foci and tissue macrophages. **h** mAb Ki-M7 (CD68) reveals a staining pattern comparable to that of Ki-M6. Nuclei are stained with hematoxylin. *Bars* = 150 μm on **a–d** and 100 μm on **e–h**

Plasmacytoid T cells expressed high amounts of CD11 c antigen. The C3bi receptor (CD11 b, 165,96 kD) and the (CD11 c) p150,95 antigen are structurally related glycoproteins that function in cell-to-cell adhesion reactions of myeloid and lymphoid cells (Anderson et al. 1986; Springer et al. 1986). Each of these two glycoproteins, as well as the third member, the LFA-1 antigen (CD11 a, 177,95 kD), is an α,β heterodimer in which one of three different α subunits is associated with a common β subunit (Sanchez-Madrid et al. 1983). The α chains, which have a discrete and different tissue distribution, can be distinguished by mAbs. CD11 c is present on neutrophils, monocytes, and macrophages (Springer and Anderson 1986), in low amounts on populations enriched with large granular lymphocytes (Lanier et al. 1985), and on the hairy cells of hairy cell leukemia (Schwarting et al. 1985). Phorbol ester stimulation of chronic B lymphocytic leukemia cells causes strong expression of CD11 c (Caligaris-Cappio et al. 1985). Although p150,95 is not expressed on peripheral T lymphocytes, it is clearly expressed on cytotoxic lymphocyte clones (Miller et al. 1986). The present results show that p150,95 can be expressed on certain types of activated or transformed B and T lymphocytes. The function of this molecule has not been elucidated. Solubilized p150,95 has been shown to bind C3b receptor (C3bi) (Cantrell et al. 1985). These findings predict that inducing p150,95 expression on activated B and T lymphocytes may result in acquisition of complement receptors by these cells. Thus, PTC precursors could perhaps be able to migrate into the lymph nodes and become sessile PTCs.

Plasmacytoid T cells were clearly stained by the mAb OKM5. The OKM5 binding surface antigen, a polypeptide of 88 kD (Talle et al. 1985), is expressed on the majority of large adherent peripheral blood monocytes, on thrombocytes (Talle et al. 1985), and on most endothelial cells, especially the capillary venular and arteriolar endothelium in lymph nodes and tonsils (Knowels et al. 1984). The function of this lineage-unspecific antigen is still obscure. Thus, the expression of the 88-kD polypeptide on PTCs at present illuminates neither the origin nor the function of PTCs.

Plasmacytoid T cells were CD26 antigen positive. CD26 is a 240-kD protein found on a subset of activated T lymphocytes (Cotner et al. 1981) after DNA synthesis and is accordingly classified as a "late" activation antigen (Cotner et al. 1983). Given this and the finding that PTCs lack the proliferation-associated unknown antigen recognized by Ki-67, it follows that PTCs are in a postproliferative, late stage of activation, which, at least for T cells, is accompanied by HLA-DR expression (Cotner et al. 1983).

In line with this argument, we proved that PTCs differentially express HLA class II (HLA-DR, -DP, -DQ) antigens. Feller et al. (1983) characterized PTCs as HLA-DR antigen negative. Harris and Bhan (1987), however, found a weak HLA-DR antigen expression in PTCs by applying a commercial HLA-DR antibody not further characterized. Horny et al. (1987) took the reactivity of PTCs with the mAbs Tü35, Tü39, and Leu-10 for a global HLA-DR, -DP, -DQ antigen expression in these cells. However, since Tü35 and Tü39 fail to discriminate between HLA-DR and HLA-DP determinants (Pawelec et al.

1982) and Tü39 is reported also to bind to class II-like molecules other than HLA-DR, -DQ, and -DP (WERNET et al. 1987), these antibodies do not represent class II sublocus-specific reagents. Using well-characterized class II sublocus-specific mAbs (Table 1), we could demonstrate a differential expression of HLA class II antigens on PTCs, according to the following scheme: HLA-DR$^+$, HLA-DQ$^+$, HLA-DP$^-$.

Data on functional properties of PTCs are scarce. Here we must mention that tumor-like proliferations of PTCs or alleged "PTC" lymphomas have repeatedly been reported to be associated with a myeloproliferative disorder mimicking acute myelomonocytic leukemia (BEISKE et al. 1986, 1987; PRASTHOFER et al. 1985; PAPADIMITRIOU et al. 1983). These authors concluded from this observation that the hyperplastic PTC pool might have secreted a myeloproliferative factor. BEISKE et al. (1986), who kept neoplastic PTCs in short-term culture, failed to detect granulocyte/monocyte-progenitor colony stimulating factor (GM-CSF) or interleukins-1 and -2. Recently, a novel human T-cell product, presently called interleukin-3, has been characterized as a potent stimulator of colonies composed of erythroid as well as myeloid progenitors (YANG et al. 1986). In our three cases the white cell counts were at the upper extremity of the normal range, and the differential cell counts were inconspicuous (data not shown).

In summary, the immunoprofile of the PTC is suggestive of a terminally differentiated, activated tissue T lymphocyte having abrogated the TCR/CD3 complex, which is nonmobile and is most likely to exert a secretory function.

5 Summary

Clusters of cells with a plasmacytoid appearance have been identified in T zones of human lymphoid tissue. These cells were shown to express the CD4 antigen in the absence of B-cell antigens. Thus, they were named "plasmacytoid T cells" (PTCs). Recent studies, however, have suggested a myelomonocytic origin of this cell type, which led to the designation "plasmacytoid monocytes." In order to obtain a comprehensive immunophenotype of this cell, we used frozen serial sections of lymph nodes, an indirect immunoperoxidase technique, and a broad panel of well-defined monoclonal antibodies (mAbs). On PTCs, the antigenic density was high for CD4 and CD26 antigens and low for CD2; they furthermore reacted with the mAb OKM5 recognizing an undefined antigen associated with the myelomonocytic lineage and expressed the monocyte-associated antigen CD68. PTCs expressed HLA-A,B,C, HLA-DR, and the HLA-D associated invariant chain (Ii) while HLA-DP antigens were expressed only in low amounts and HLA-DQ antigens were lacking entirely. PTCs further expressed the adhesion molecule CD11 c. The absence of detectable transferrin receptor and the proliferation antigen defined by Ki-67 indicated that PTCs were nonproliferating. Other well-defined antigens confined to the T-, B-, and myelomonocyte lineages could not be detected in the target cell population. For us, antigenic equipment is still suggestive of a sessile, terminally differentiated T cell likely to exert a secretory function as yet unknown.

Acknowledgement. This work was supported by the Tumorzentrum Heidelberg/Mannheim and the state of Baden-Württemberg (AIDS-Forschung).

References

Anderson DC, Miller LJ, Schmalstieg FC, Rothlein R, Springer TA (1986) Contributions of the Mac-1 glycoprotein family to adherence-dependent granulocyte functions: structure-function assessments employing subunit-specific monoclonal antibodies. J Immunol 137:15–27

Ando I, Hariri G, Wallace D, Beverley P (1985) Tumor promoter phorbol-esters induce unresponsiveness to antigen and expression of interleukin 2 receptor on T cells. Eur J Immunol 15:196–199

Beiske K, Langholm R, Godal T, Marton PF (1986) T-zone lymphoma with predominance of 'plasmacytoid T-cells' associated with myelomonocytic leukaemia – a distinct clinicopathological entity. J Pathol 150:247–255

Beiske K, Munthke-Kaas A, Davies CDL, Marton PF, Godal T (1987) Single cell studies on the immunological marker profile of plasmacytoid T-zone cells. Lab Invest 56:381–393

Caligaris-Cappio F, Pizzolo G, Chilosi M et al. (1985) Phorbol ester induces abnormal chronic lymphocytic leukemia cells to express features of hairy cell leukemia. Blood 66:1035–1042

Cantrell DA, Davies AA, Crumpton MJ (1985) Activators of protein kinase C down-regulate and phosphorylate the T3/T-cell antigen receptor complex of human T lymphocytes. Proc Natl Acad Sci USA 82:8158–8162

Cotner T, Hemler M, Strominger JL (1981) Human T cell proteins recognized by rabbit heteroantisera and monoclonal antibodies. Int J Immunopharmacol 3:255–268

Cotner T, Williams JM, Christenson L, Shapiro HM, Strom TB, Strominger J (1983) Simultaneous flow cytometric analysis of human T cell activation antigen expression and DNA content. J Exp Med 157:461–472

Crumpton MJ, Cantrell DA, Davies AA, Verbi W (1987) The effect and role of protein kinase C activation in the stimulation of human T-lymphocytes. In: McMichael AJ et al. (eds) Leucocyte typing III, white cell differentiation antigens. Oxford University Press, Oxford, pp 918–923

Dembic Z, Haas W, Zamoyska R, Parnes J, Steinmetz M (1987) Transfection of the CD8 gene enhances T-cell recognition. Nature 326:510–515

Facchetti F, De Wolf-Peeters C, van den Oord J, De Vos R, Desmet VJ (1988) Plasmacytoid T cells: a cell population normally present in the reactive lymph node. Hum Pathol 19:1085–1092

Facchetti F, De Wolf-Peters C, van den Oord J, De Vos R, Desmet VJ (1989) Plasmacytoid monocytes (so-called plasmacytoid T-cells) in Kikuchi's lymphadenitis. An immunohistologic study. Am J Clin Pathol 92:42–50

Feller AC, Lennert K, Stein H, Bruhn H-D, Wuthe H-H (1983) Immunohistology and aetiology of histiocytic necrotizing lymphadenitis. Report of three instructive cases. Histopathology 7:825–839

Franklin WA, Bogen S, Hartley JP et al. (1987) Reaction patterns of workshop myeloid antibodies with peripheral blood leucocytes, leukaemic cells, normal solid tissues, and neuroendocrine neoplasms. In: McMichael AJ et al. (eds) Leucocyte typing III, white cell differentiation antigens. Oxford University Press, Oxford, pp 672–678

Harris NL, Bhan AK (1987) "Plasmacytoid T cells" in Castleman's disease. Immunohistologic phenotype. Am J Surg Pathol 11:109–113

Hogg N, Horton MA (1987) Myeloid antigens: new and previously defined clusters. In: McMichael AJ et al. (eds) Leucocyte typing III, white cell differentiation antigens. Oxford University Press, Oxford, pp 576–602

Horny H-P, Feller AC, Horst HA, Lennert K (1987) Immunocytology of plasmacytoid T cells: marker analysis indicates a unique phenotype of this enigmatic cells. Hum Pathol 18:28–32

Howard FD, Ledbetter JA, Wong J, Bieber CP, Stinson EB, Herzenberg LA (1981) A human T lymphocyte differentiation marker defined by monoclonal antibodies that block E rosette formation. J Immunol 126:2117–2122

Knapp W et al. (1989) Leukocyte typing IV. Oxford University Press, Oxford

Knowels DM, Tolidjian B, Marboe C, D'Agati V, Grimes M, Chess L (1984) Monoclonal anti-human monocyte antibodies OKM1 and OKM5 possess distinctive tissue distributions including differential reactivity with vascular endothelium. J Immunol 132:2170–2173

Kreipe H, Radzun HJ, Parwaresch MR, Haislip A, Hansmann M-L (1987) Ki-M7 monoclonal antibody specific for myelomonocytic cell lineage and macrophages in human. J Histochem Cytochem 35:1117–1126

Lanier LL, Arnaout MA, Schwarting R, Warner NL, Ross GD (1985) p150/95, third member of the LFA-1/CR3 polypeptide family identified by anti-Leu-M5 monoclonal antibody. Eur J Immunol 15:713–720

Lennert K, Remmele W (1958) Karyometrische Untersuchungen an Lymphknotenzellen des Menschen. I. Mitteilung, Germinoblasten, Lymphoblasten und Lymphozyten. Acta Haematol (Basel) 19:99–108

Lennert K, Kaiserling E, Müller-Hermelink HK (1975) T-associated plasma cells. Lancet I:1031–1032

Malhotra V, Hogg N, Sim RB (1986) Ligand binding by the p150,95 antigen of U937 monocytic cells: properties in common with complement receptor type 3 (CR3). Eur J Immunol 16:1117–1123

Martin PJ, Longton G, Ledbetter JA, Newman W, Braun MP, Beatty PG, Hansen JA (1983) Identification and functional characterization of two distinct epitopes on the human T cell surface protein Tp50. J Immunol 131:180–185

McMichael AJ et al. (eds) (1987) Leucocyte typing III, white cell differentiation antigens. Oxford University Press, Oxford

Meuer SC, Hussey RE, Fabbi M et al. (1984) An alternative pathway of the T-cell activation: a functional role for the 50 kD T11 sheep erythrocyte receptor protein. Cell 36:897–906

Miller LJ, Schwarting R, Springer TA (1986) Regulated expression of the Mac-1, LFA-1, p150,95 glycoprotein family during leukocyte differentiation. J Immunol 137:2891–2900

Müller-Hermelink HK, Kaiserling E, Lennert K (1973) Pseudofollikuläre Nester von Plasmazellen (eines besonderen Typs?) in der paracorticalen Pulpa menschlicher Lymphozyten. Virchows Arch [B] (Cell Pathol) 14:47–56

Müller-Hermelink HK, Stein H, Steinmann G, Lennert K (1983) Malignant lymphoma of plasmacytoid T-cells. Morphologic and immunologic studies characterizing a special type of T-cell. Am J Surg Pathol 7:849–862

Nadler LM (1986) B cell/leukemia panel workshop: Summary and comments. In: Reinherz EL et al. (eds) Leukocyte typing II. Springer, Berlin Heidelberg New York

Papadimitriou CS, Stephanaki-Nikou SN, Malamou-Mitsi VD (1983) Comparative immunostaining of T-associated plasma cells and other lymph node cells in paraffin sections. Virchows Arch [B] (Cell Pathol) 43:31–36

Parwaresch MR, Radzun HJ, Kreipe H, Hansmann M-L, Barth J (1986) Monocyte/macrophage-reactive monoclonal antibody Ki-M6 recognizes an intracytoplasmatic antigen. Am J Pathol 125:141–151

Pawelec GP, Shaw S, Ziegler A, Müller C, Wernet P (1982) Differential inhibition of HLA-D- or SB-directed secondary lymphoproliferative responses with monoclonal antibodies detecting human Ia-like antigens. J Immunol 129:1070–1075

Poppema S, Hollema S, Visser L (1987) Monoclonal antibodies (MT1, MT2 MB1, MB2, MB3) reactive with leukocyte subsets in paraffin-embedded tissue sections. Am J Pathol 127:418–429

Prasthofer EF, Grizzle WE, Prchal JT, Grossi CE (1985) Plasmacytoid T-cell lymphoma associated with chronic myeloproliferative disorder. Am J Surg Pathol 9:380–387

Sanchez-Madrid F, Nagy J, Robbins E, Simon P, Springer TA (1983) A human leukocyte differentiation antigen family with distinct α subunits and a common β subunit: the lymphocyte-function associated antigen (LFA-1), the C3bi complement receptor (OKM1/Mac-1), and the p150,95 molecule. J Exp Med 158:1785–1803

Sattentau QJ, Weiss RA (1988) The CD4 antigen physiological ligand and HIV receptor. Cell 52:631–633

Schwarting R, Stein H, Wang CY (1985) The monoclonal antibodies αS-HCL 1 (αLeu-14) and αS-HCL3 (αLeu-M5) allow the diagnosis of hairy cell leukemia. Blood 65:974–983

Sleckman BP, Peterson A, Jones WK, Foran JA, Greenstein JL, Seed B, Burakoff SJ (1987) Expression and function of CD4 in a murine T-cell hybridoma. Nature 328:351–353

Spickett GP, Dalgleish AG (1988) Cellular immunology of HIV-infection. Clin Exp Immunol 71:1–7

Springer TA, Anderson DC (1986) The importance of the Mac-1, gLFA-1 glycoprotein family in monocyte and granulocyte adherence, chemotaxis and migration into inflammatory sites: insights from an experiment of nature. Ciba Found Symp 118:102–126

Springer TA, Miller LJ, Anderson DC (1986), p150,95, the third member of the Mac-1, LFA-1 human leukocyte adhesion glycoprotein family. J Immunol 136:240–245

Talle MA, Rao PE, Makowski M, Boselli C, Allegar N, Goldstein G (1985) Null cell identification and characterization with OKT16: an anti-p40 monoclonal antibody. Blood 66:1124–1132

Thomas Y, Rogozinski L, Irigoyen OH, Shen HH, Talle MA, Goldstein G, Chess L (1982) Functional analysis of human T cell subsets defined by monoclonal antibodies. V. Suppressor cells within the activated OKT4$^+$ population belong to a distinct subset. J Immunol 128:1386–1390

Vollenweider R, Lennert K (1983) Plasmacytoid T-cell clusters in non-specific lymphadenitis. Virchows Arch [B] 44:1–14

Wernet P, Fernandez N, Schneider EM, Festenstein H, Pawelec G (1987) HLA-<DY>-determinants, possibly associated with novel class II molecules, stimulate autoreactive CD4$^+$ T cells with suppressive activity. Immunobiology 175:360

West KP, Warford A, Fray L (1986) The demonstration of B-cell, T-cell and myeloid antigens in paraffin sections. J Pathol 150:89–101

Wood GS, Warner NL, Warnke RA (1983) Anti-Leu-3/T4 antibodies react with cells of monocyte/macrophage and Langerhans lineage. J Immunol 131:212–216

Yang YC, Ciarletta AB, Temple PA et al. (1986) Human IL-3 (Multi-CSF): identification by expression cloning of a novel hematopoietic growth factor related to murine IL-3. Cell 47:3–10

Accessory Cells in Normal Human and Rodent Lymph Nodes: Morphology, Phenotype, and Functional Implications

H.-H. WACKER, H.J. RADZUN, and M.R. PARWARESCH

1 Introduction and Terminology

The recent progress in our understanding of the significance of accessory cell function and of the actual cells underlying this important process preparatory to immune reaction has been closely associated with the ill-defined terms "dendritic cells" and "reticulum cells." This is probably the reason why dendritic or reticulum cells are generally regarded as the only accessory cells. In fact there is convincing evidence that not only dendritic or reticulum cells, with their mononuclear precursors, but also nondendritic cells such as B lymphocytes, epithelial cells of the thymus gland, virus-infected cells, and some endothelial cells are capable of functioning as accessory cells, presenting certain antigens to T or B lymphocytes (Table 1).

The terms "dendritic cells" and "reticulum cells" have been applied to cells with an arachnoid morphology and long, stretched dendrites. In the past there was considerable controversy as to the nature of these cells, until it became possible to separate them from collagen-synthesizing fibroblasts, myofibroblasts, stroma cells, phagocytosing macrophages and histiocytes, and endothelial cells. The observations made by FREI et al. (1965), UNANUE and ASKONAS (1968), and OPPENHEIM et al. (1968) were successfully extended by STEINMAN and COHN (1973), who discovered the precise functional relevance for the immune response of a distinct cell population designated "lymphoid dendritic cells." The term "dendritic cells" has become a synonym for terms like "reticulum cells" and "reticular cells," which are increasingly being dismissed. In

Table 1. Main accessory cells proposed to be involved in various types of immune response. Accessory cells other than those of secondary cell-mediated immunity have or develop a dendritic (arachnoid, reticular) morphology. Cell types marked by an asterisk have not been specifically detailed in this review

Primary cell-mediated immunity
Lymphoid dendritic cells (Steinman's cells)
Indeterminate cells*
Langerhans cells*
Veiled cells
Interdigitating dendritic (reticulum) cells (IDCs)
Secondary cell-mediated immunity
B lymphocytes*
Others, thymus epithelia, virus-infected cells*
Primary humoral immunity
Unknown possibly a macrophage-related cell
Sinus-lining cells of lymph nodes
Secondary humoral immunity
Follicular dendritic (reticulum) cells (FDCs)

contrast, the terms "accessory cells" (ACs) and "antigen trapping and presenting cells" are generally used in a broader sense, as generic terms covering dendritic and nondendritic immune ACs.

More specific reference will be made to this issue later in this chapter. Here, however, it appears important to give a brief description of the properties specific to dendritic ACs to rule out possible confusion. Dendritic ACs:

1. Have a typical reticular or dendritic morphology
2. Have a constant and highly characteristic tissue distribution pattern
3. Are positive to or can easily express major histocompatibility (MHC) glycoproteins, complement, and FC receptors
4. Are nonphagocytosing, antigen trapping, processing, and presenting cells
5. Produce and secrete the cell-stimulatory factors interleukin-1 and -6

Considering the above-mentioned properties it is evident that ACs constitute a well-defined group of cells with regard to morphology and function. This again underlines the need for observation of the recommendations made by the Reticuloendothelial Society Committee on Nomenclature (TEW et al. 1982). Terms like "dendritic cells" and "reticulum cells" should be restricted to antigen trapping, processing, and presenting immunostimulatory cells.

Before discussing dendritic ACs in detail, reference will be made to the functional aspects and to the finer mechanisms involved in antigen processing and presentation.

2 Function of Accessory Cells in the Immune System

Our present knowledge on the biological significance of accessory cell function is based on numerous experimental observations:

1. There is a quantitative as well as a qualitative critical requirement for adherent cells in spleen cell and blood cell suspensions or blood cells exposed to antigen to undergo blast transformation or mitogenesis, or to produce lymphokines or specific antibodies. Depletion of adherent cells, among which ACs are to be expected, reduces or even blocks lymphocyte reaction. In a similar manner, metabolic inhibitors cause a blockade of lymphocyte response (FREI et al. 1965; UNANUE and ASKONAS 1968).
2. Adherent cells exposed to soluble antigens retain their immunogenicity even after vigorous washings, indicating that at least a significant part of the applied antigen is protected against catabolic degradation (UNANUE and ASKONAS 1968).
3. Humoral immunity is readily inducible against tertiary structures of unaltered molecules presented by adherent cells, whereas cellular immunity requires prior denaturation resolving sequential immunogenic determinants of the antigen-designated antigen processing (GELL and BENACERRAF 1959; ISHIZAKA et al. 1974; SCHIRRMACHER and WIGZELL 1974).
4. In vitro antigen exposure of adherent cells primes the immune reaction only in an MHC-restricted manner (ROSENTHAL and SHEVACH 1973).

The experiments performed by OPPENHEIM et al. (1968) and ROSENTHAL and SHEVACH (1973) provided impressive evidence of the functional implications of ACs, which were referred to as "macrophages" or "adherent cells" in these studies. It was brilliantly shown that the depletion of "adherent cells" from human lymphocyte suspensions exposed to streptolysin-O, vaccinia vaccine, or purified protein derivative of tuberculin prevented the typical antigen-derived blast transformation. Similar results were presented by WALDRON et al. (1973) from observations on inbred rodent strains. Animal experiments also confirmed the immunobiological importance of an AC population. Peritoneal exudate cells exposed to antigen failed to activate lymphocytes following a passage through a glass column. Antigen-pulsed macrophages, however, could restore the immune reaction. Additional work showed that antigen presentation was not specific in an immunological sense. Adherent cells from tolerant animals proved to be as effective. The ACs were described as a nondividing low density cell population. The specific density of ACs appeared to be below the values of other mononuclear blood cells. Density gradients ranging from 1.045 to 1.065 g/ml are apparently appropriate for providing a good separation of ACs, as compared with a usual density of 1.077 g/ml for the separation of other mononuclear cells (BOYUM 1968).

Accessory cells are believed to bind antigens, and specifically soluble proteins, transported to the lymph nodes and spleen by the afferent lymph stream or blood. Such molecules represent the original antigen to which the individual has been exposed. Antigens may also derive from the catabolic degradation or phagocytic digestion of particulate matter by macrophages. Such soluble proteins are bound to the surface membrane of ACs and are highly concentrated within the lymphoid organs. This is generally referred to as "antigen trapping." The exact mechanism by which the primary binding of unprocessed antigen to the surface membrane of ACs is established still remains obscure, though some authors have speculated that Fc receptors account for the nonspecific antigen binding. This has become one of the most fascinating unsolved enigmas in the field.

Extensive research work has shown that T and B lymphocytes react differently in response to one and the same antigen. During a primary humoral immune response, recirculating B-lymphocyte clones bearing specifically rearranged surface immunoglobulins are retained and stimulated within the lymphatic tissue. The specificity of such B lymphocytes is directed against exposed immunogenic domains of more or less unaltered antigenic structures attached to the surface membrane of ACs. In the case of B lymphocytes the antigen seems to become an immunogen as soon as surface fixation has been effected by the ACs. The specific immunoglobulins on the surface of virgin B lymphocytes recognize epitopes of the unaltered tertiary structure of the antigen (Ishizaka et al. 1974; Schirrmacher and Wigzell 1974; Benacerraf 1988).

With the seminal contributions of Frei et al. (1965), Unanue and Askonas (1968), and Rosenthal and Shevach (1973) it became clear that an appropriate cellular immune response requires ACs to trap, process, and present antigen. In contrast to the humoral immune response, T lymphocytes show considerable structural restrictions in the specific reaction. Generally T lymphocytes do not react against native antigens or antigens not adequately presented by professional ACs. Although there are certain exceptions, typically antigens have to be internalized by ACs, processed, and presented to specific T lymphocytes in an MHC-restricted manner. Antigen processing consists of a distinct set of subcellular and metabolic events, which are summarized below.

The immune function carried out by professional ACs starts with a nonspecific binding of antigen to the membrane surface of the AC, a mechanism the molecular background of which has so far escaped clarification. The second step is the internalization of native antigen in a manner comparable to pinocytosis or receptor-mediated endocytosis (Fig. 1). A membrane invagination appears at the site of antigen binding, giving rise to clathrin-coated vesicles. Such endosomes move towards the interior of the cytoplasm, losing their clathrin coat. The latter has been shown to recycle back to the inner surface area of the cell membrane (Diment et al. 1988).

Endosomes containing antigenic ligands fuse with Golgi vesicles and are thus supplied with acid hydrolases such as pepstatin-sensitive protease with a membrane-anchoring moiety. In addition, it has been proposed that such cells may employ a special tool to target certain proteases such as cathepsin D to nonlysosomal vesicles. Many endosomes have been shown to contain foreign protein-mannose conjugates. Such conjugates represent adequate substrates for cathepsin D. Protone pumps localized in the membrane of the endosomes

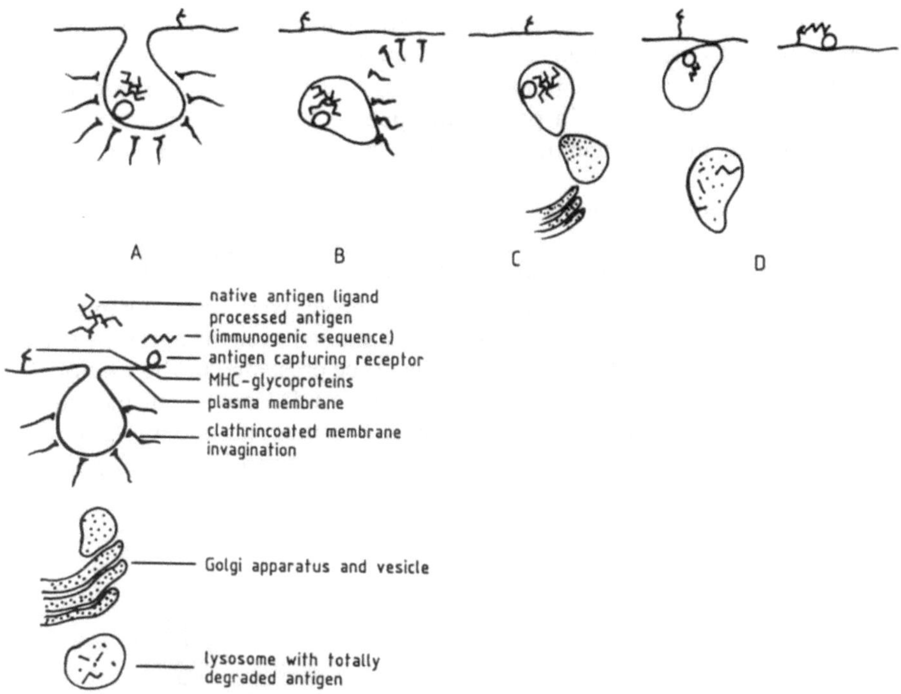

Fig. 1 A–D. Antigen processing by analogy to receptor-mediated endocytosis. **A** Plasma membrane of MHC$^+$ accessory cells carrying appropriate receptors to capture native antigenic ligands undergoes localized invagination in clathrin-equipped areas. **B** Clathrin recycles to plasma membrane and coated vesicles evolve into endosomes containing whole antigen and receptor. **C** Golgi-derived vesicles provide endosomes with proteases whereby a "selective proteolysis" is accomplished. pH reduction is maintained by the ATP-consuming protone pump localized in the vesicle membrane. Short immunogenic peptide sequences are thus resolved from the native protein antigen. **D** Remainder of protein antigen is transported to lysosomes for total degradation. Recycling of endosomal contents to plasma membrane makes possible the exposure of immunogenic sequences in conjunction with MHC glycoproteins

provide the lumen with hydrogen ions under conversion of ATP into ADP. Perhaps at this stage the dissociation of the hydrolysis products takes place. Such vesicular structures have been referred to as CURL (compartment of uncoupling of receptors and ligands). Probably some part of the smaller peptide protein sequences are recycled with the receptor back to the membrane and are conjugated with the membrane surface MHC glycoproteins over the agretope of the antigen. It has been speculated that some part of the native antigen is totally destroyed within the lysosomes.

2.1 Accessory Cells and T-Cell Activation

A wealth of literature has been published on T-cell activation in the last decade. It has been shown that during a primary immune response, virgin T lymphocytes require close cooperation with professional ACs. In contrast, T-cell response to recall antigens involving memory T cells can equally well be mediated by a large variety of nonprofessional ACs such as virus-infected cells, certain epithelial cells, and in particular specific B lymphocytes, which can present antigen most efficiently to T cells by means of their surface immunoglobulin.

Antigen presentation to virgin T lymphocytes by professional ACs is probably the initial event which activates a reaction chain culminating in blast transformation, mitogenesis, and lymphokine secretion. It has been shown that denatured antigen is subjected to selective proteolysis, resolving immunogenic sequential determinants, and then is conjugated over the agretope site of the antigen with MHC class II glycoproteins to be presented to the specifically rearranged T-cell antigen receptor, detectable as CD3 on the surface membrane of the T cells. MHC class II restricted T lymphocytes undergo a cellular clustering with ACs over CD3 and the processed antigen bridge (Fig. 2).

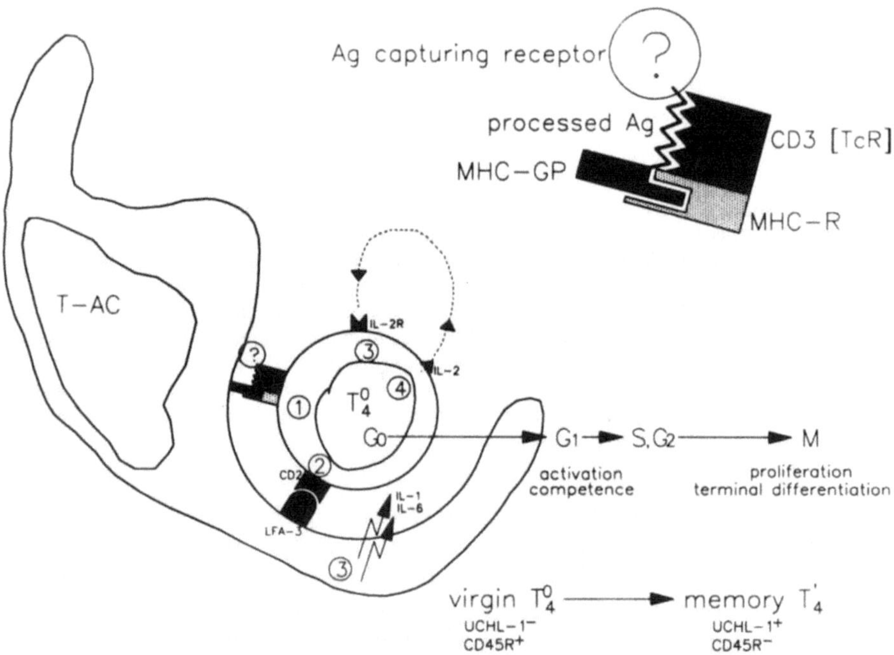

Fig. 2. Schematic survey of molecular events during accessory cell (*AC*) induction of virgin T4 lymphocytes (T°4). *Encircled items* indicate sequence of main steps preceding cell cycle progression (G_0, G_1, S, G_2, M) and terminal differentiation. *1*, Processed antigen (*Ag*) is presented as immunogenic sequences in conjunction with MHC glycoproteins (*MHC-GP*) to specifically rearranged antigen receptor (*TcR, CD3*) on MHC-restricted (*MHC-R*) T4 lymphocytes. *2*, These events are followed by the functional transformation of CD2 into LFA-3 receptors. *3*, T cells express interleukin-2 receptor (*IL-2R*); ACs produce and secrete interleukin-1 and -6 (*IL-1, IL-6*). *4*, T-cell activation is accompanied by massive secretion of interleukin-2 (*IL-2*) as an autocrine mechanism. Resting G_0 T lymphocytes progress in the cell cycle, proliferate, and show terminal differentiation, becoming UCHL-1$^+$ and CD45R$^-$ memory T helper lymphocytes capable of optimal response and massive lymphokine secretion upon recall antigen challenge

The second, closely associated, event is the formation of a receptor by CD2, which maintains an additional intercellular bridging over the leukocyte function associated antigen (LFA-3) of the AC surface membrane (SELVARAJ et al. 1987). The next step in the reaction chain is the secretion of interleukin-1 and -6 in considerable amounts by ACs (CEUPPENS et al. 1988). These factors are probably the most effective stimulators of virgin T lymphocytes, inducing them to progress from the G_0 to the G_1 phase of the cell cycle and to express surface receptor for interleukin-2. In this phase T lymphocytes acquire specific reactivity and undergo numerous metabolic changes, including enhancement of intracellular Ca^{2+}, activation of the inositol phosphate and protein kinase C system, and enhancement of mRNA within the cytoplasm. In addition, characteristically mRNA for c-*myb* is strongly transcribed during this phase of cell activation.

Interleukin-1 and -6 induction of T lymphocytes results not only in expression of interleukin-2 receptor but also in the production of interleukin-2 in addition to other lymphokines. Activated T lymphocytes develop functional competence, proliferate, and differentiate to final maturity (MALEK et al. 1985).

In cases of cytolytic T lymphocytes, which are mostly $CD8^+$ cells, the immunogenic sequential determinant is preferentially conjugated to the glycoproteins of MHC class I.

2.2 Accessory Cells and B-Cell Activation

As shown by the plaque-forming assay method, B-cell activation is closely related to the presence of ACs (MOSIER 1967). The experiments carried out by MORRISSEY et al. (1981) provided further proof of the dependency of the humoral immune reaction on MHC class II positive ACs. The antigen presented by ACs is recognized by the specifically rearranged immunoglobulin on the surface of virgin B lymphocytes, which are mostly positive for IgD. It is not clear whether a direct intercellular connection between ACs and B lymphocytes is necessary. Probably it is the binding of antigen on the surface of ACs with the specific antibody which primes ACs to secrete interleukin-1 and -6. Here again considerable subcellular and metabolic alterations in B lymphocytes take place. Among the helper functions of specific T4 lymphocytes, which also undergo intercellular binding with ACs, perhaps interleukin-2, -4, and -6, have the greatest effect upon B lymphocytes. A considerable number of subcellular and metabolic alterations are apt to result, characterizing various B-cell activation phases designated as follows: activation, competence, cell cycle, progression, proliferation, and terminal differentiation. The latter consists in the generation of memory B cells, antibody switch, immunoglobulin secretion, and production of terminally differentiated short- and long-lived plasma cells with mean half-lives of 3 days and 3 weeks, respectively. Of the large number ($\approx 10^6$/g/day) of virgin B cells generated in the bone marrow, the majority of which egress into the circulation, patrolling all probable sites of antigen presentation, only those which find their specific antigen, adequately presented by professional ACs, are privileged to survive (Fig. 3). The majority of virgin B lymphocytes are destined to die within a few hours (MACLENNAN and GRAY 1986; LORTAN et al. 1987; LIU et al. 1988; ZHANG et al. 1988).

The antigen-driven cell cycle progression and the terminal differentiation of B lymphocytes proceeds with typical alterations in their expression of receptors for Fc, complement, MHC glycoproteins, and a vast majority of other membrane molecules which make up the characteristic phenotype, of various stages of B-cell maturation and differentiation – stages starting with resting virgin B lymphocytes and progressing through activation, competence, proliferation, and terminal differentiation, giving rise to memory B cells and immunoglobulin-secreting plasma cells. These changes are paralleled by a complicated chain of molecular genetic alterations, including oncogene transcription (Fig. 3).

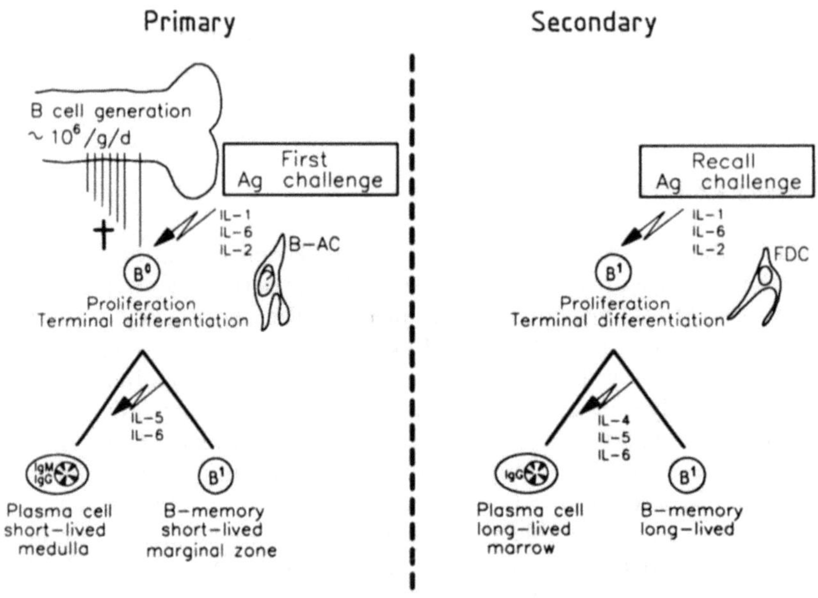

Fig. 3. The majority of newly generated (in the order of 10^6/g/d) virgin B lymphocytes (B°) are destined to die within a short time due to lack of antigen stimulation. Those induced by "specific" antigen (primary antigen challenge) are activated and traverse various functional and generational stages of differentiation, giving rise to short-lived antibody-secreting cells in the medulla and memory B lymphocytes (B^1) of the marginal zones. The latter comprise a G_0, IgD^-, IgM^+, and $IgG2c^+$ memory B-cell cohort. During secondary humoral immune response antigen is presented by the follicular dendritic (reticulum) cells (FDCs) of germinal centers. FDCs preserve native antigen in endosome-like vesicles (iccosomes). Encounter with recall native antigen initiates clonal proliferation with production of memory B cells and of long-lived antibody-secreting cells in the bone marrow. Terminal differentiation with antibody switch and secretion, like other differentiational stages, is mediated by interleukins (IL-1, -2, -4, -5, -6)

3 Accessory Cells in Normal Human and Rodent Lymph Nodes

A large variety of cells occurring in human and rodent lymph nodes have been shown to be involved in antigen binding, which is one of the major criteria of accessory cell function. Macrophages are one of the major cell types to which accessory cell function has repeatedly been ascribed. When working with particulate foreign matter or microbes such as viral, bacterial, or protozoal agents, macrophages are called for due to their phagocytic and catabolic capabilities. Nonselective lysosomal catabolism results in the complete elimination of the microbial antigens. Antigen molecules escaping phagocytic catabolism arrive at lymphoid tissue via the afferent lymph stream. A limited percentage of molecules are carried by macrophages which undergo cell demise, delivering their content to professional immune ACs, which are capable of capturing native antigens (MITCHELL and ABBOT 1965).

From studies with detectable molecules, such as those involving radioactive isotopes, enzymatic activity, or specific antibodies, it is known that intact molecules of native antigen are exclusively localized within the B-cell follicles of lymph nodes. The part of the antigen presented to T lymphocytes in the thymus-associated areas generally escapes detection due to its degradation during antigen processing. Probably major parts of the antigen presented to the T-cell system have already been processed to indetectability at the site of inoculation or during transportation within professional ACs (PERNIS et al. 1988).

In this context it is evident that ACs apparently follow the bimodal differentiation pattern of lymphocytes. T-ACs comprise a set of cells which transport antigen via afferent lymphatics into the lymph node as the so-called veiled cells and appear within the paracortical thymus-dependent areas of the lymphatic tissue as the "interdigitating (reticulum) or dendritic cells" (TEW et al. 1982). In the following we will first discuss these two cell types and then progress to dendritic ACs which bind antigen apparently in a native and unaltered form, giving B lymphocytes access to the immunogenic domains of the tertiary structure of the antigen. This group of B-ACs mainly comprises follicular dendritic cells of B-cell follicles.

Recent results may add a further cell type to this array. The findings that lining cells of lymph node sinuses bind soluble foreign proteins and share highly restricted surface antigens with other typical B-ACs indicate that these cells may also have an accessory function in humoral immunity.

3.1 Accessory Cell Involvement in Cellular Immunity (T-ACs)

Cell-mediated immunity is directed against immunogenic sequences prepared and presented by T-ACs. The primary T-cell response is induced by a large number of cells occurring in various tissue types. In addition to the functional aspects, these cells share properties such as expression of common antigens and a dendritic morphology. There is some evidence that these cells are derived

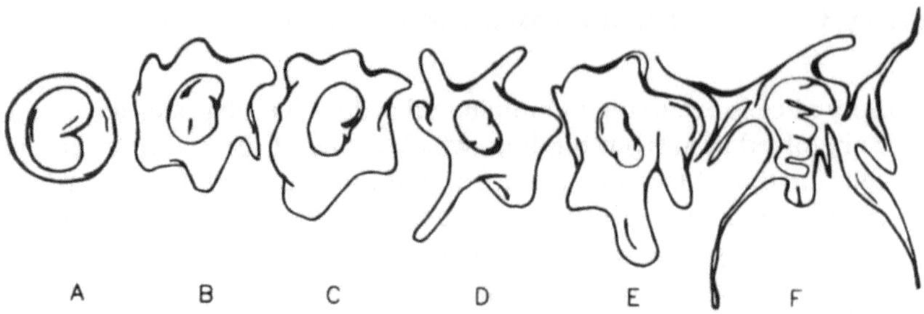

Fig. 4. Suggestive line of differentiation for T accessory cells evolving from blood monocytes (**A**) into Steinman's cells (**B**), indeterminate cells (**C**), Langerhans cells (**D**), veiled cells (**E**), and interdigitating dendritic (reticulum) cells (**F**) with increasing projections of their cytoplasmic dendrites

from a subset of blood monocytes which undergoes differentiation, with gradual acquisition of T-AC properties. On the basis of the evidence so far available, the maturation line schematically presented in Fig. 4 appears highly probable. It has been proposed that lymphoid dendritic cells of Steinman originate from a subtype of blood monocytes and may appear in subepithelial connective tissue as the indeterminate mononuclear cells which share not only CD1 and S-100 but also properties common to macrophages and the group of T-ACs such as CD11c, as shown by the monoclonal antibody Ki-M1 (RADZUN et al. 1984). Indeterminate mononuclear cells would be an appropriate candidate for the function of maintaining the recruitment of Langerhans cells within the epithelial coverings. Once pulsed with antigen, Langerhans cells appear in the afferent lymph to evolve into the terminal differentiation stage of T-ACs, the interdigitating dendritic (reticulum) cells. In the following we discuss only those cells which are regarded as regular constituents of normal human and rodent lymph nodes, excluding indeterminate cells and Langerhans cells.

3.1.1 Lymphoid Dendritic Cells (Steinman's Cells)

In cell suspensions from lymphoid organs of rodents, STEINMAN and COHN (1973) succeeded in detecting a cell type capable of presenting antigen to T lymhocytes, thus initiating a primary T-cell reaction. Steinman's cells were later shown to bind and process antigen, secrete interleukin-1, and initiate a specific T-cell reaction (STEINMAN et al. 1983; VAN VOORHIS et al. 1983; DURUM et al. 1984; KAYE et al. 1984). They have a dendritic morphology (STEINMAN and COHN 1973) and are nonphagocytic (PUGH et al. 1983; STEINMAN and COHN 1974). Though originally described in rodents, lymphoid dendritic cells have also been identified in human blood and in cell suspensions of various lymphoid organs. In all cases a close cytomorphological and immunophenotypic resemblance to Steinman's cells could be established. In addition, functional and ultrastructural findings have confirmed their close relationship to the cell types of the rodent immune system (KLINKERT et al. 1982; WONG et al. 1982; DUIJVESTIJN and BARCLAY 1984). Comparable cells in human blood and cell suspensions of lymphatic tissue were found (SPRY et al. 1980; HART and FABRE 1981; VAN VOORHIS et al. 1982; PUGH et al. 1983; FAUSTMAN et al. 1984) to stimulate a primary T-cell reaction (INABA and STEINMAN 1986) and a mixed lymphocyte culture (VAN VOORHIS et al. 1982). Despite the fact that they are nonphagocytic, lymphoid dendritic cells of Steinman seem to possess all the properties of monocytes. In the human immune system it is possible to induce a similar differentiation under special culture conditions (PETERS et al. 1987), although not all authors have been successful using this strategy.

It is widely accepted that lymphoid dendritic cells are closely related to human monocytes (VAN VOORHIS et al. 1982; KNIGHT et al. 1986) and probably represent a certain differentiation form of monocytes or a distinct subtype of these cells. This view has been strengthened by the finding that a small subtype of normal blood monocytes expresses a similar or identical phenotype regarding antigenic composition, enzyme content, ultrastructure, and functional properties. In addition, a rare type of monocytic leukemia has been described which seems to derive from this monocyte subtype in view of various cellular properties.

Under normal conditions the number of lymphoid dendritic cells is extremely low and does not exceed 0.1% of the mononuclear cells in the blood. Using monoclonal antibodies lymphoid dendritic cells are probably detectable among the CD11c$^+$ (represented by the monoclonal antibody Ki-M1) (RADZUN et al. 1984), CD1$^+$, S-100$^+$ monocyte population (VAN VOORHIS et al. 1982). A similar proportion probably exists in cell suspensions of lymphatic tissue. Lymphoid dendritic cells are nonphagocytic and weakly adherent mononuclear cells. They show moderate dendritic morphology and low specific density (KNIGHT et al. 1986; EMERY et al. 1987a, b). Most of them are positive to MHC class II glycoproteins, including HLA-DQ, -DR, and -DS. In functional terms they are potent stimulators of mixed leukocyte reaction and exceed the efficiency of separated blood monocytes or macrophages (STEINMAN et al. 1982; VAN VOORHIS et al. 1982, 1983; BJERCKE et al. 1985; SUNSHINE and MITCHELL 1985; PETERS et al. 1987). In addition to CD11c, CD1, and S-100 positivity, lymphoid dendritic cells are positive to CD45. Birbeck granules have not been found in these cells. Using adherent mononuclear cell fractions from suspensions of lymph node cells it is possible to concentrate lymphoid dendritic cells at a density of 1.055 g/ml, in contrast to other mononuclear cells, which are accumulated at higher densities.

Although it is possible to detect lymphoid dendritic cells in lymph node cell suspensions on the basis of their T-AC function and dendritic form, clear morphological visualization of these cells in corresponding sections is hardly feasible, partly due to their extreme paucity and partly due to lack of specific features.

3.1.2 Veiled Cells

The afferent lymph stream differs from efferent lymph fluid in the composition of its cellular elements. The afferent lymph stream contains a lot more nonlymphocytic cells than the efferent one (MORRIS 1972; DREXHAGE et al. 1979; HOPKINS et al. 1985). Among nonlymphoid cells, THORBECKE et al. (1980) defined a special cell type accounting for less than 1% of the afferent lymph cells. Such cells show a dendritic morphology and were designated "veiled or frilly cells." These nonphagocytic cells possess broad cytoplasmic extensions and were shown to represent Langerhans cells of the epidermis or mucosal coverings or a closely related cell type being on the way to the lymph nodes (SILBERBERG-SINAKIN et al. 1976; HOEFSMIT et al. 1982; KNIGHT 1984).

In the lymph nodes veiled cells are found within the sinuses and have been claimed to migrate into the paracortical thymus-dependent zone to evolve into interdigitating dendritic (reticulum) cells (KELLY et al. 1978; HOEFSMIT et al. 1982). The T-cell accessory function of veiled cells has been well established using the mixed leukocyte reaction assay as well as antigen-specific T-cell proliferation (EMERY et al. 1987b). In addition, veiled cells have been shown to represent potent stimulators of the T-cell-mediated B-cell differentiation into immunoglobulin-secreting cells with antibodies against antigens such as key hole limpet, hemocyanin, and ovalbumin (EMERY et al. 1987a, b). Langerhans cells of the epidermis, veiled cells, and interdigitating dendritic (reticulum) cells share the unique reactivity to the monoclonal antibodies MLDC-145 (KRAAL et al. 1986) in rodents and anti-CD1a (FITHIAN et al. 1981) as well as to antibodies recognizing S-100 antigen (TANAKA 1986) in the human immune system.

Typical veiled cells with long cytoplasmic protrusions and veils are regularly present within the sinus system of the lymph nodes, preferentially in the marginal sinus of nodes draining the skin. This has been well shown in rodents as well as humans (DREXHAGE et al. 1980). Veiled cells present in the marginal and medullary sinuses of lymph nodes draining skin or mucosa demonstrate Birbeck granules in rodents. The lymphatics draining skin in rodents may contain up to 30% veiled cells. In patients being subjected to lymphography, skin lymph was found to contain up to 18% veiled cells. On light-microscopic examinations and time-lapse cinematography of living lymph cells, veiled cells showed vigorous movements of their veils, accompanied by the appearance and disappearance of large vesicles, suggesting large volume extracellular fluid transudation (DREXHAGE et al. 1980).

In electron-microscopic studies veiled cells show long thin cytoplasmic extensions and contain a few ribosomes and a limited number of vesicles. Polyribosomes and free ribosomes are present in the remainder of the cytoplasm. Rough endoplasmic reticulum is moderately developed. Veiled cells have a moderate number of mitochondria and numerous small smooth-surfaced, clear vesicles. Microfilaments are present in all veiled cells, and some have large bundles of filaments close to the nuclear membrane. Birbeck granules have been described in veiled cells of rodent lymph (KELLY et al. 1978), especially after administration of antigen (Kamperdijk et al. 1978). The transformation of veiled cells into interdigitating dendritic (reticulum) cells (IDCs) has been concluded from the demonstration of Birbeck granules in these cells and from the finding that ligature of afferent lymphatic leads to the disappearance of IDCs (Hendriks et al. 1976). Veiled cells show considerable submicroscopic similarities to Langerhans cells and to IDCs; all three cell types share typical enzyme-cytochemical properties like membrane-bound nucleotidase, nonspecific esterase, and acid phosphatase. In functional terms all three cell types form cellular conjugates, with projections of epidermal cells or lymphocytes dipped into membrane invaginations of Langerhans cells, veiled cells, and IDCs. All three cell types have a weak glass adherence tendency, resembling the lymphoid dendritic cells in this respect. Receptors for Fc and C3 have been found for the majority of Langerhans cells and some veiled cells as well as IDCs.

3.1.3 Interdigitating Dendritic (Reticulum) Cells

On light-microscopic examination the paracortical thymus-dependent areas of human and rodent lymph nodes (Fig. 5) are regularly equipped with a distinct cell type which came to be called interdigitating cells (Veldman 1970; Veerman 1974; Hoefsmit 1975; Friess 1976) or interdigitiating reticulum cells (Kaiserling and Lennert 1974; Kaiserling 1977; Lennert et al. 1978). To exclude confusion with other dendritic cells here we use the aforementioned term interdigitating dendritic (reticulum) cells (IDCs). These cells have a broad rim of clear cytoplasm which shows interdigitating cytoplasmic projections (Kamperdijk et al. 1978; Hoefsmit et al. 1979). Even at low magnifications IDCs are easily detectable by their clear cytoplasm and their even distribution pattern within the paracortical zone. Under normal conditions they make up less than 0.1% of the cells in these areas, although their number is subject to considerable variations. The nucleus assumes a central position within the clear cytoplasm, and especially at higher magnifications shows clear deep indentations which are easily detectable due to the light tingibility of the whole nucleus. Phagosomes or particulate inclusions do not usually occur in these cells. In resin-embedded semithin sections it becomes clear that within the thymus-dependent areas of lymph nodes the T lymphocytes stay in intimate contact with the cytoplasmic projections and interdigitations of these cells. Usually five or more T lymphocytes densely surround the IDC, producing a radiate aspect.

On conventional electron-microscopic investigations (Fig. 5) IDCs reveal a broad clear cytoplasm with a small number of organelles as compared with the surface area of the cytoplasm. There are a moderate number of mitochondria, hardly any dense granules, no phagosomes, and moderate to weakly developed Golgi apparatus and ergastoplasm as well as a wealth of tubulovesicular structures with a variable number of clear vesicles which mostly resemble endosomes. The peripheral rim of the cytoplasm shows deep and

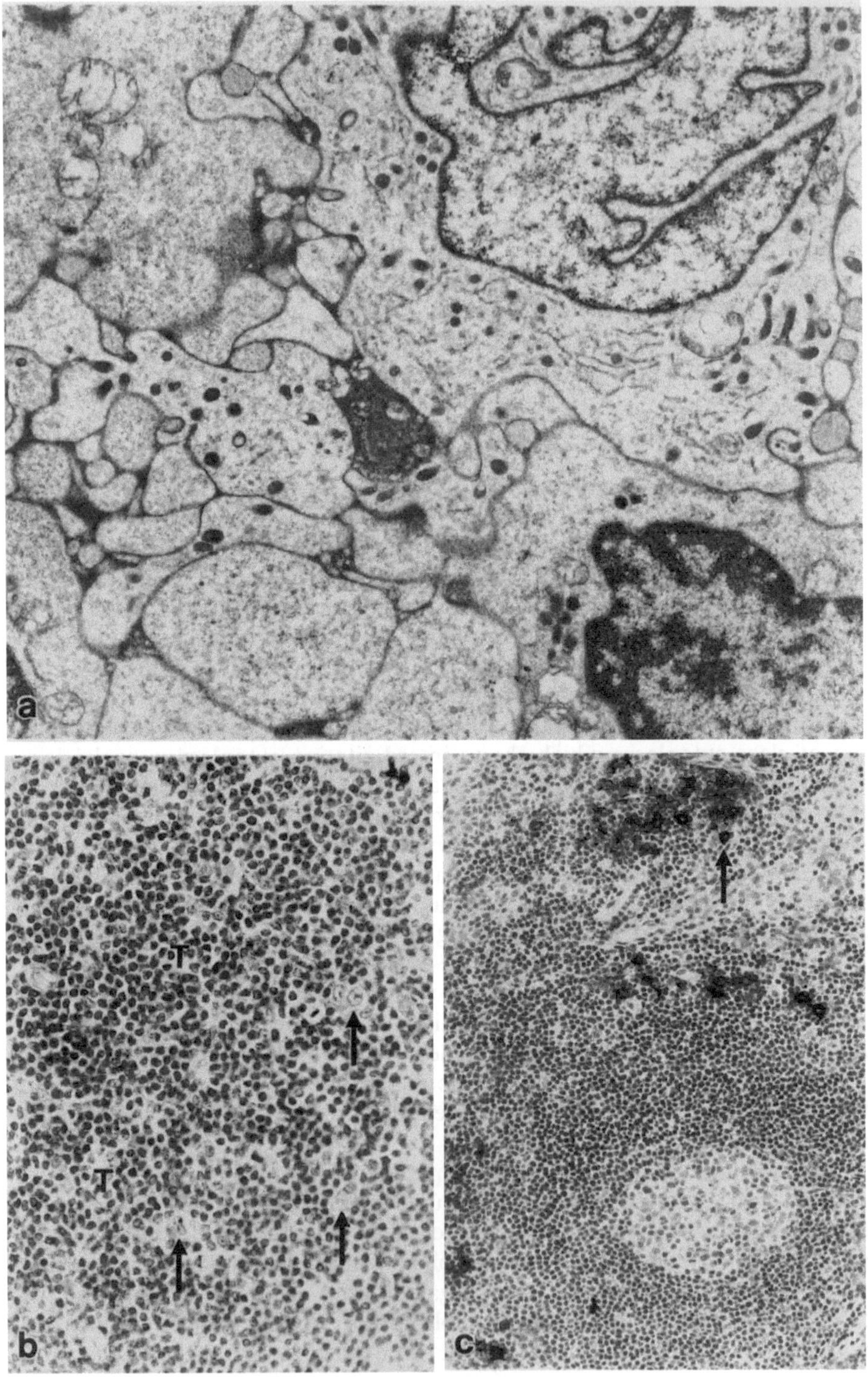
a
b
T
T
c

narrow membrane invaginations or infoldings containing stripes of projections of the neighboring T-cell cytoplasm. Such projections may be stretched to the immediate vicinity of the nuclear envelope. A small number of IDCs may possess Birbeck granules, which easily escape detection due to their extreme paucity. This is the reason why the majority of authors were unable to confirm the occurrence of Birbeck granules in these cells. Following stimulation with various antigens, preferentially after intradermal inoculation, not only the frequency of Birbeck granules increases but also the number of IDCs (KAMPERDIJK et al. 1978).

In enzyme-cytochemical studies IDCs have been shown to be weakly positive to acid phosphatase and α-naphthyl acetate esterase (KAISERLING and LENNERT 1974; VEERMAN 1974). The acid phosphatase sometimes shows a condensation in an area next to the nucleus. In addition, leucyl-β-naphthyl amidase (ELEMA and POPPEMA 1978) and adenosine triphosphatase (HEUSERMANN et al. 1974) have been described in these cells. Alkaline phosphatase and naphthol AS-D chloroacetate esterase or myeloperoxidase have been found to be negative. It has been maintained that Mg^{2+}-dependent membrane adenosyl triphosphatase distinguishes these cells from other dendritic cell types (MÜLLER-HERMELINK 1974; MÜLLER-HERMELINK et al. 1976):

Immunohistochemical (Fig. 5) studies have disclosed IDCs to be positive for complement receptor (RAUSCH et al. 1977). They are mostly positive to or can easily acquire HLA-DR, as detected by the monoclonal antibodies OKIa1 and 9.3F10. Whether they additionally express Fc and all the varieties of complement receptors is unclear. Monoclonal antibodies directed against CD1 are regularly positive with these cells, as with the other T accessory elements. Anti-CD4 shows a weak reactivity with the IDCs (BARTHÉLÉMY et al. 1986; LANDRY et al. 1988). In addition, S-100 antigen has been demonstrated in these cells (HOEFSMIT et al. 1982).

In a few careful studies ample evidence has been produced indicating that these cells represent potent activators of allogeneic mixed leukocyte reaction and stimulators of primary T-cell response (LANDRY et al. 1988). Such functional studies became possible with the ability to separate these cells from other associated cell types. Especially after exclusion of $CD3^+$ T cells, IDCs can be accumulated at a density range of 1.048–1.062 g/ml. IDCs hence are lighter than the majority of other mononuclear cells. Adequate preparations deliver a moiety of over 70% purity, which means an enormous functional potential considering the extremely high level of their inductive capabilities.

◀ **Fig. 5.** **a** Electron-microscopic image of an IDC within the paracortical T zone of a human lymph node. The nucleus is lightly stained and shows deep irregular indentations. The cytoplasm contains scattered organelles, mostly mitochondria. Elongated branched cytoplasmic projections engulf surrounding lymphocytes. The close intercellular contact implies specific functional interaction Araldite embedding, ×11 900. **b, c** A light-microscopic view of a typical paracortical T zone of a human lymph node. Note the regular distribution of IDCs (*arrows*), embedded among dense accumulations of T cells (*T*). **b** paraffin section, Giemsa staining, ×263; **c** cryostat section, immunostained for CD1, ×131

In vivo application of both soluble and particulate antigens cannot be traced to IDCs either by immunohistochemical or by enzyme-cytochemical means, and this seems also to apply to the techniques employing radioautographic methods. IDCs show no tendency to incorporate particulate matter through phagocytosis. This could be excluded by studies with latex particles and viable yeast cells. In addition experiments with sheep erythrocytes revealed identical results (LANDRY et al. 1988).

Interdigitating dendritic (reticulum) cells also occur in other tissue areas rich in lymphocytes or thymocytes in man and animals (VON GAUDECKER and MÜLLER-HERMELINK 1979). Systematic analysis along the course of the ontogeny of IDCs in developing lymphoid tissue of human fetuses shows that IDCs become detectable within full-blown T-cell areas around the 16th week of gestation.

Interdigitating dendritic (reticulum) cells are believed to be closely related to the monocyte/macrophage cell lineage and to represent, like macrophages, another parallel terminal differentiation option of blood monocytes. This has been deduced from immunohistochemical findings and observations on bone marrow chimeras as well as after ligation of afferent lymphatics, which results in a prompt reduction in the number of IDCs within individual lymph nodes (GOORDYAL and ISAACSON 1985).

3.2 Accessory Cell Involvement in Humoral Immunity (B-ACs)

Humoral immunity as represented by the appearance of antigen-specific immunoglobulins does not develop adequately unless assisted by professional ACs (MOSIER 1967; MORRISSEY et al. 1981). The question of where and by which ACs stimulation is exerted upon virgin B lymphocytes to elicit a primary humoral immune response has not yet been satisfactorily solved.

The accessory cell responsible for the secondary B-cell response is apparently a type of dendritic cell which is exclusively found within the B lymphoid follicles of lymphatic tissue. These dendritic ACs were originally described by MAXIMOW in 1927, who designated them "embryonal nonphagocytic reticulum cells." In later studies they were referred to as "dendritic reticular or reticulum cells" (NOSSAL et al. 1964) or "follicular dendritic (reticulum) cells" (FDCs). The existence of a network of dendritic cells within the B lymphoid follicles has been repeatedly confirmed by a large number of authors who have described the light- and electron-microscopic morphology of FDCs in various contributions (WHITE 1963; NOSSAL et al. 1964, 1966; MORI and LENNERT 1969; GROSCURTH 1980).

NOSSAL et al. (1968a, b) provided the first evidence for antigen binding by FDCs. Studying the microscopic distribution pattern of a detectable antigen, it was noticed that FDCs bind large amounts of the injected antigen in an apparently unaltered native form.

In morphological terms FDCs are restricted to B lymphoid follicles, irrespective of their localization. Primary follicles contain only a few FDCs. Secondary follicles with well-developed germinal centers exhibit a dense network built up by the intercommunicating long, stretched cytoplasmic dendrites of FDCs, which sometimes appear to form syncytial complexes. The widely branched cytoplasmic processes result in marked enlargement of the cell surface which serves antigen fixation and presentation (MITCHELL and ABBOT 1965; NOSSAL et al. 1968 a, b). On light-microscopic examination it is hardly possible to detect the exact outline of the cytoplasm, which possesses slender long, stretched dendrites sometimes developed only as membrane duplicatures. The cytoplasm around the nucleus consists of a narrow rim engulfing an oval nucleus of low chromatin content. The majority of FDCs possess a small, centrally located nucleolus within the pale nucleoplasm. Some of them may have two or more nuclei. Since it is difficult to detect the cytoplasmic contour of the FDC upon light microscopy, these cells are best identified on the basis of their typical nuclei (Fig. 6).

In enzyme-cytochemical studies FDCs reveal positivity to 5′-nucleotidase and probably also to nonspecific esterase. In contrast, adenosyltriphosphatase, alkaline phosphatase, myeloperoxidase, lysozyme, and naphthol AS-D chloroacetate esterase are regularly negative in these cells.

Electron-microscopic studies proved extremely helpful in elucidating the morphofunctional interrelationships. It could be shown that the ultrastructural properties of FDCs share a common pattern in rodents and human (NOSSAL et al. 1964; MITCHELL and ABBOT 1965; SZAKAL and HANNA 1968; MORI and LENNERT 1969; GROSCURTH 1980). The most striking feature is again the large number of elongated cell processes, which sometimes represent parallel strands of cytoplasmic membrane with a narrow, hardly detectable line of cytoplasm. The dendrites of several cells intertwine with each other. In the majority of cases special cell junctions can be detected between the neighboring cell processes. Desmosomes have a variable length. In such areas the cytoplasmic surface membrane is strongly thickened and shows considerable electron density. The cytoplasm under the membrane reveals a dusty distribution of electron-dense material. In other areas FDC projections closely engulf the neighboring lymphocytes, the majority of which are of the B-cell type. Within the cytoplasm of FDCs, phagosomes generally do not occur. In contrast, small clear vesicles are regularly seen, provided the cells are sufficiently preserved. Further cytoplasmic organelles include ribosomes, polyribosomes, and a scattered number of mitochondria. The Golgi apparatus and rough endoplasmic reticulum are only moderately developed. A considerable number of pinocytotic membrane invaginations or vesicles, secretory dense granules, tonofilaments, pallade bodies, and Birbeck granules are absent.

The introduction of monoclonal antibodies brought about considerable progress in our understanding of FDCs in man and animals. To our knowledge the reagent R4/23 was the first monoclonal antibody to prove reactive with human FDCs (NAIEM et al. 1983). A highly specific antibody directed against human FDCs is the mouse IgG1, designated Ki-M4 (PARWARESCH et al. 1983 a, b) and its equivalent against rat FDCs, Ki-M4R (WACKER et al. 1987). Recently, a new reagent (Ki-FDC1) was introduced in our laboratory which

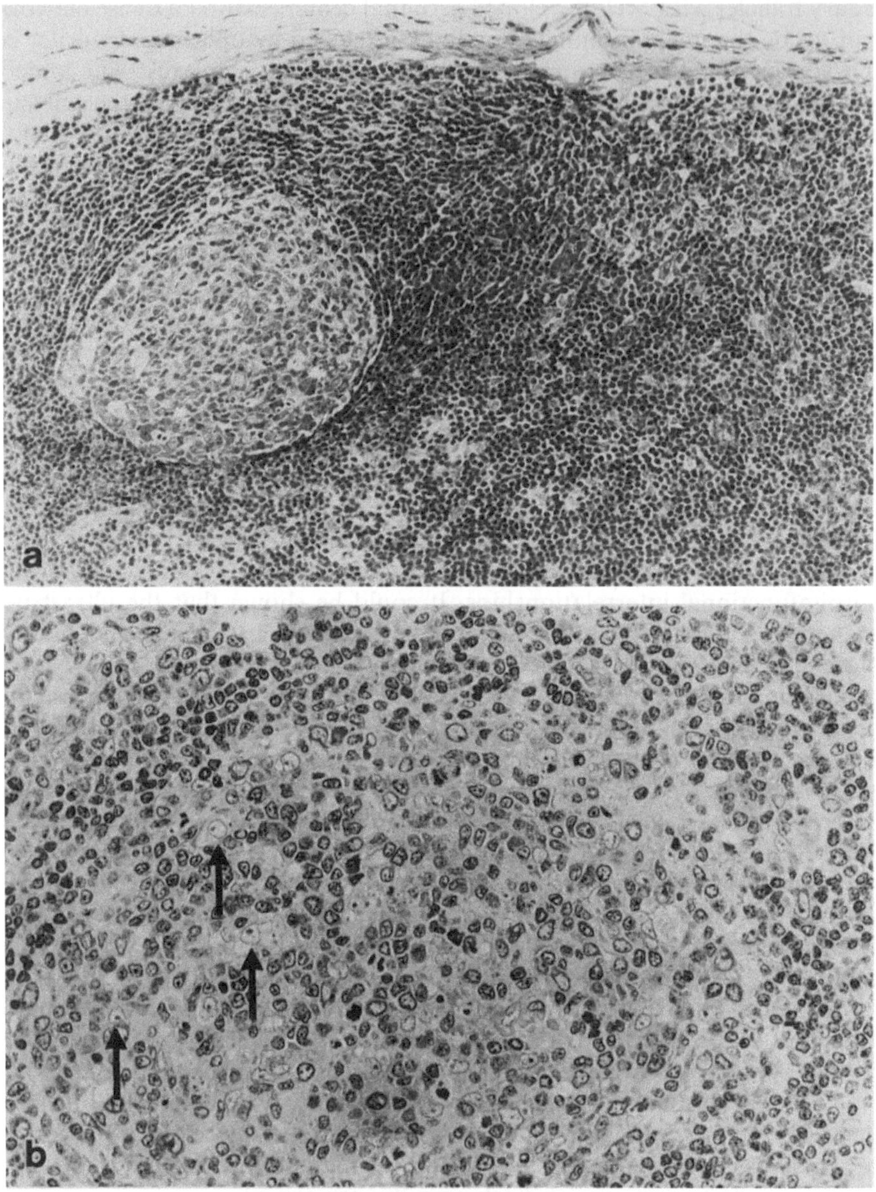

Fig. 6 a, b. Light-microscopic survey of a lymphoid follicle (**a**) of a human lymph node. At higher magnification (**b**) typical FDCs are easily detectable within the germinal center due to the light tingibility of their nuclei and the characteristic nuclear form (*arrows*). They are all closely encircled by B lymphocytes and blasts of the germinal center, designated centrocytes, centroblasts, and immunoblasts. Paraffin section, Giemsa staining, × 165 and × 330

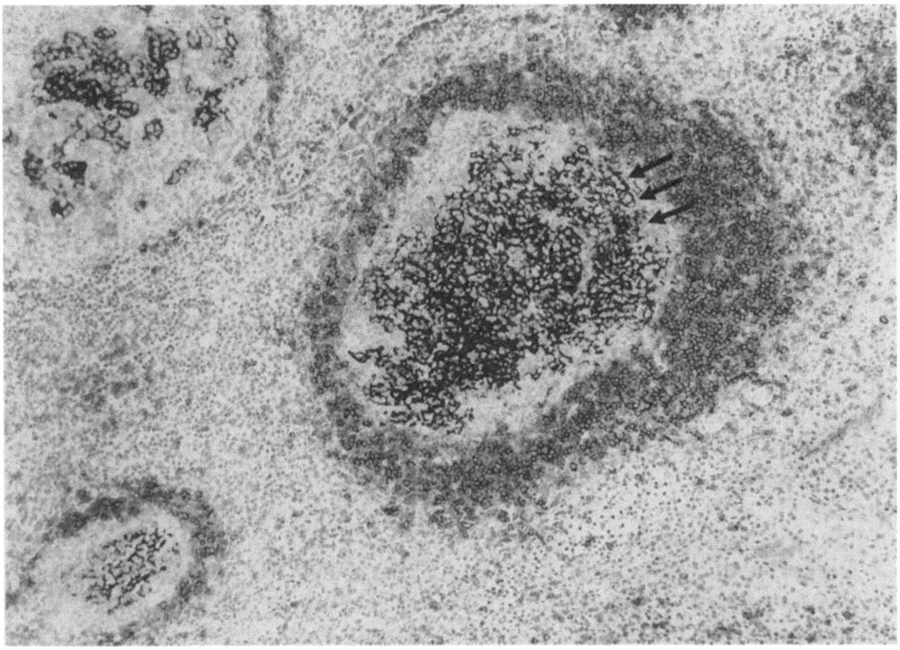

Fig. 7. Light microscopic view of a lymphoid follicle in a human lymph node. In addition to a subpopulation of follicle mantle B lymphocytes, the monoclonal antibody Ki-FDC1 immunostains the web of the FDCs (*arrows*) in routinely processed paraffin sections. ×150

makes possible immunohistological visualization of human FDCs in routinely processed formalin-fixed samples (Fig. 7).

The presence of complement receptors for C3bR and C3dR but not for C3biR can be shown on the surface membrane of human FDCs using the monoclonal antibodies CR1, CR2, and CR3. Positive results were also found with antibodies recognizing complement factors such as C1q, C4, C3c, C3d, C5, and C3b-INA. In contrast, C6, C8, C9, and C3act were not found in connection with human FDCs. Also, properdin was regularly negative. IgG, IgM, and IgA are usually detectable on human FDCs, whereas IgE and IgD are generally lacking (Imai et al. 1986).

As regards the function of FDCs, there is general agreement on their involvement in the secondary humoral immune response and the generation of B memory cells. Detectable antigens have been found to be localized at this site as immune complexes (Nossal et al. 1964; Szakal and Hanna 1968; Straus 1970; Szakal et al. 1985, 1988). In addition to Fc receptor, complement factors are believed to play a part in antigen fixation. Endotoxin or cobra venom reduces antigen binding to FDCs in lymphoid follicles.

The first evidence for possible antigen capture by lymphoid follicles was produced by Kaplan et al. (1950) and Mellors and Brzosko (1962). White (1963) drew attention to the characteristic pattern of antigen deposition, which was quite different from that of macrophages. In all these studies immunofluorescent staining techniques were applied. Using radioiodinated antigen, NOSSAL et al. (1964) were able to trace antigen localization in germinal centers with radioautographic techniques. Unequivocal evidence, however, was produced by electron-microscopic radioautography (NOSSAL et al. 1968a, b) employing different isotope-labeled antigens such as various preparations of *Salmonella adelaide*. There have been some discussions on the involvement of FDCs in the binding of tumorantigens or oncogenic viral material (SWARTZENDRUBER et al. 1967; SZAKAL and HANNA 1968; HANNA et al. 1970). Our results with in situ hybridization also indicate the occurrence of HIV and EBY genomes in FDCs.

Recall antigens have been shown to be localized on the surface membrane of FDCs as immune complexes. Most investigators seem to agree that complement and Fc receptor may play an important role in antigen binding. Since other authors have also observed antigen binding in the absence of detectable specific antibodies, it remains debatable whether the antigen binding is accomplished by Fc and C3 receptors, only. This issue has become an exciting field of research work with prospective implications for vaccination and regulation of humoral immunity.

Extensive ultrastructural studies carried out by SZAKAL et al. (1985, 1988) have shown that FDCs may have two types of dendrite. The so-called filiform projections are 0.1–0.3 µm in width and may reach a few hundred µm in length. Such dendrites are branched and may form a radiating sunburst-like pattern around the cells. Another form of dendrite shows club-shaped enlargements resembling microspheres or beads; these "beaded" dendrites range from 0.3 to 0.6 µm in diameter. Such observations became feasible after it became possible to isolate FDCs (SCHNITZLEIN et al. 1985). Having separated FDCs in cell suspensions, SZAKAL et al. (1985) succeeded in studying them with the scanning electron microscope. This technique confirmed the light-microscopic findings of a filiform and a beaded type of FDC. Other cells showed convoluted dendrites containing an amorphous material which might represent antigen-antibody complexes within and around the dendrites. Beaded dendrites showed microspheres 0.3–0.7 µm in diameter, connected together by cylindrical segments 0.02–0.05 µm in width. On transmission electron microscopy such microspheres appeared as endosome-like immune complex inclusions, designated iccosomes (SZAKAL et al. 1988). It has been convincingly demonstrated that the convoluted portion of the dendrites may, like the iccosomes, engulf native antigen or immune complexes that possibly regulate immunological memory and antibody titer during a secondary immune response.

4 Summary and Conclusion

This chapter provides a brief review of the professional accessory cells present in normal human and rodent lymph nodes. When dealing with the function of accessory cells in the immune system it has to be borne in mind that in principle all cells may possess or acquire the capability of antigen presentation, which is the decisive initiating step in the specific host defense bound to the lymphoid cells.

Professional accessory cells are arrayed at the afferent limb of the immune response. The majority of them have a typical dendritic morphology, so that the term "dendritic cells" is widely used instead of the term "accessory cells," and has replaced the traditional terms "reticulum cells" and "reticular cells." Professional accessory cells are characterized by:

1. The capability to stimulate specific T- or B-cell response following antigen pulsing
2. A dendritic morphology
3. Expression of major histocompatibility glycoproteins, complement, and Fc receptors as well as of various adhesion molecules
4. Presentation of processed or unprocessed native antigens
5. Production and secretion of interleukin-1 and interleukin-6

The bimodal differentiation of lymphocytes seems to be reflected in the occurrence of two types of dendritic accessory cell: accessory cells involved in cellular (T accessory cells) and humoral (B accessory cells) immunity.

T accessory cells of the lymph node comprise:

1. The lymphoid dendritic cell of Steinman, which probably represent a subset of blood monocytes with possible terminal differentiation into other T accessory cells
2. Veiled cells, which have been shown to represent Langerhans cells of the epidermal covering on their way to thymus-dependent areas of lymph node, probably giving rise to interdigitating dendritic (reticulum) cells
3. Interdigitating dendritic (reticulum) cells as the typical accessory cells of lymphoid T zone

The T accessory cells share morphological, ultrastructural, immunophenotypic, and functional properties, are myeloid in origin, and very probably derive from monocyte lineage. As immune stimulatory cells they present processed antigen only and initiate T-cell proliferation and differentiation by interleukin-1 and -6 secretion.

Accessory cells involved in the initiation of a primary humoral immune reaction have not been convincingly characterized. Accessory cells responsible for a secondary B-cell response, however, are the so-called follicular dendritic (reticulum) cells constituting the typical web-like structure of the primary and secondary lymphoid follicles. Unlike T accessory cells, follicular dendritic (reticulum) cells are distinguished by accentuated membrane desmosomes and extensive anastomosing branches of dendrites. Native antigen or immune complexes captured within and around the convolutions of their dendrites are prone to be involved in immunological memory and regulation of antibody titers during the secondary immune response.

References

Barthélémy H, Pelletier M, Landry D, Lafontaine M, Perreault C, Tautu C, Montplaisir S (1986) Demonstration of OKT6 antigen on human thymic dendritic cells in culture. Lab Invest 55:540–550

Benacerraf B (1988) Antigen processing and presentation. The biologic role of MHC molecules in determinant selection. J Immunol 11:17–20

Bjercke S, Braathen L, Gaudernack G, Thorsby E (1985) Relative efficiency of human Langerhans cells and blood derived dendritic cells as antigen-presenting cells. Acta Derm Venereol (Stockh) 65:374–378

Boyum A (1968) Isolation of mononuclear cells and granulocytes from human blood. Scand J Clin Lab Invest 21:77–89

Ceuppens JL, Baroja ML, Lorre K, van Damme J, Billiau A (1988) Human T cell activation with phytohemagglutinin. The function of IL-6 as an accessory signal. J Immunol 141:3868–3874

Diment S, Simmons BM, Russell JH, Stahl PD (1988) Processing of ligands in macrophage endosomes. In: Pernis B, Silverstein SC, Vogel HJ (eds) Processing and presentation of antigens. Academic, San Diego, pp 29–42

Drexhage HA, Mullink H, de Groot J, Clarke J, Balfour BM (1979) A study of cells present in peripheral lymph of pigs with special reference to a type of cell resembling the Langerhans cell. Cell Tissue Res 202:407–430

Drexhage HA, Lens JW, Cvetanov J, Kamperdijk EWA, Mullink R, Balfour BM (1980) Veiled cells resembling Langerhans cells. In: van Furth R (ed) Mononuclear phagocytes. Functional aspects, part I. Martinus Nijhoff, The Hague, pp 235–275

Duijvestijn AM, Barclay AN (1984) Identification of the bone marrow derived 1a positive cells in the rat thymus. A morphological and cytochemical study. J Leukocyte Biol 36:561–568

Durum SK, Higuchi C, Ron Y (1984) Accessory cells and the T cell activation. The relationship between two components of macrophage accessory cell function. Immunobiology 168:213–231

Elema JD, Poppema S (1978) Infantile histiocytosis X (Letterer-Siwe disease). Investigations with enzymehistochemical and sheep-erythrocyte rosetting techniques. Cancer 42:555–565

Emery DL, Dufty JH, Wood PR (1987a) An analysis of cellular proliferation and synthesis of lymphokines and specific antibody in vitro by leucocytes from immunized cattle. Vet Immunol Immunopathol 15:1–57

Emery DL, Machugh ND, Ellis JA (1987b) The properties and functional activity of non-lymphoid cells from bovine afferent (peripheral) lymph. Immunology 62:177–183

Faustman D, Steinman RM, Gebel H, Hauptfeld V, Davie J, Lacy P (1984) Prevention of rejection of murine islet allografts by pretreatment with antidendritic cell antibody. Proc Natl Acad Sci USA 81:3864–3868

Fithian E, Kung P, Goldstein G, Rubenfeld M, Fenoglio C, Edelson R (1981) Reactivity of Langerhans cells with hybridoma antibody. Proc Natl Acad Sci USA 78:2541–2544

Frei PC, Benacerraf B, Thorbecke GJ (1965) Phagocytosis of the antigen, a crucial step in the induction of the primary response. Proc Natl Acad Sci USA 53:20–23

Friess A (1976) Interdigitating reticulum cells in the popliteal lymph node of the rat. Cell Tissue Res 170:43–60

Gell PGH, Benacerraf B (1959) Studies on hypersensitivity. II. Delayed hypersensitivity to denatured proteins in guinea pigs. Immunology 2:64–70

Goordyal P, Isaacson PG (1985) Immunocytochemical characterization of monocyte colonies of human bone marrow: a clue to the origin of Langerhans cells and interdigitating reticulum cells. J Pathol 146:189–195

Groscurth P (1980) Non-lymphatic cells in the lymph node cortex of the mouse. II. Postnatal development of the interdigitating cells and the dendritic reticular cells. Pathol Res Pract 169:235–254

Hanna JR MG, Szakal AK, Tyndall RI (1970) Histoproliferative effect of Rauscher leukemia virus on lymphatic tissue: histological and ultrastructural studies of germinal centers and their relation to leukemogenesis. Cancer Res 30:1748–1763

Hart DNJ, Fabre JW (1981) Demonstration and characterization of Ia-positive dendritic cells in the interstitial connective tissues of the rat heart and other tissues, but not brain. J Exp Med 153:347–361

Hendriks HR, Eestermans IL, Hoefsmit ECM (1976) The subcutaneously sutured lymph node: a macrophage-free organ. Abstracts of the 17th Dutch Federative Meeting, Amsterdam, p 217

Heusermann U, Stutte HJ, Müller-Hermelink HK (1974) Interdigitating cells in the white pulp of human spleen. Cell Tissue Res 153:415–417

Hoefsmit ECM (1975) Mononuclear phagocytes, reticulum cells and dendritic cells in lymphoid tissues. In: van Furth R (ed) Mononuclear phagocytes in immunity, infection, and pathology. Blackwell, Oxford, pp 129–146

Hoefsmit ECM, Balfour BM, Kamperdijk EWA, Cvetanov J (1979) Cells containing Birbeck granules in the lymph and the lymph node. Adv Exp Med Biol 114:389–394

Hoefsmit ECM, Duijvestijn AM, Kamperdijk EWA (1982) Relation between Langerhans cells, veiled cells and interdigitating cells. Immunobiology 161:255–265

Hopkins J, McConnell I, Bujdoso R, Munro AJ (1985) Studies of MHC class II products on sheep peripheral and efferent lymph cells. In: Morris B, Miyasaka M (eds) Immunology of the sheep. Roche, Basel, pp 44–62

Imai Y, Yamakawa M, Masuda A, Sato T, Kasajima T (1986) Function of the follicular dendritic cell in the germinal centre of lymphoid follicles. Histol Histopathol 1:341–353

Inaba K, Steinman RM (1986) Accessory cell–T lymphocyte interactions. Antigen-dependent and -independent clustering. J Exp Med 163:247–261

Ishizaka K, Kishimoto T, Delespesse G, King TP (1974) Immunogenic properties of modified antigen E. I. Presence of specific determinants for T cells in denatured antigen and polypeptide chains. J Immunol 113:70–77

Kaiserling E (1977) Non-Hodgkin-Lymphome. Ultrastruktur and Cytogenese. (Veröffentlichungen aus der Pathologie, vol 105). Fischer, Stuttgart

Kaiserling E, Lennert K (1974) Die interdigitierende Retikulumzelle im menschlichen Lymphknoten. Eine spezifische Zelle der thymusabhängigen Region. Virchows Arch [B] 16:51–61

Kamperdijk EWA, Raaymakers EM, Deheeuw JHS, Hoefsmit ECM (1978) Lymph node macrophages and reticulum cells in the immune response. I. The primary response to paratyphoid vaccine. Cell Tissue Res 192:1–23

Kaplan MH, Coons AH, Deane HW (1950) Localization of antigen in tissue cells. III. Cellular distribution of pneumococcal polysaccharides types II and III in the mouse. J Exp Med 91:15–19

Kaye J, Gillis S, Mizel SB et al. (1984) Growth of a cloned helper T cell line by a monoclonal antibody specific for the antigen receptor: interleukin 1 is required for the expression of receptors for interleukin 2. J Immunol 133:1339–1345

Kelly RH, Balfour BM, Armstrong JA, Griffiths HJ (1978) Functional anatomy of lymph nodes. II. Peripheral lymph-borne mononuclear cells. Anat Rec 190:5–21

Klinkert WEF, LaBadie JH, Bowers WE (1982) Accessory and stimulating properties of dendritic cells and macrophages isolated from various rat tissue. J Exp Med 156:1–19

Knight SC (1984) Veiled cells – "dendritic cells" of the peripheral lymph. Immunobiology 168:349–361

Knight SC, Balfour B, O'Brien J, Buttifant L (1986) Sensitivity of veiled (dendritic) cells to cyclosporine. Transplantation 41:96–154

Kraal G, Breel M, Janse M, Bruin G (1986) Langerhans' cells, veiled cells and interdigitating cells in the mouse recognized by a monoclonal antibody. J Exp Med 163:981–997

Landry D, Lafontaine M, Cossette M, Barthélémy H, Chartraud C, Montplaisir S, Pelletier M (1988) Human thymic dendritic cells. Characterization, isolation and functional assays. Immunology 65:135–142

Lennert K, Kaiserling E, Müller-Hermelink HK (1978) Malignant lymphomas. Models of differentiation and cooperation of lymphoreticular cells. In: Clarkson B, Marks PA, Till JE (eds) Differentiation of normal and neoplastic hematopoietic cells, book B. (Cold Spring Harbor conferences on cell proliferation, vol 5). Cold Spring Harbor Laboratory, New York, pp 897–913

Liu Y-J, Oldfield S, MacLennan ICM (1988) Memory B cells in T-cell dependent antibody responses colonize the splenic marginal zones. Eur J Immunol 18:355–362

Lortan JE, Roobottom CA, Oldfield S, MacLennan ICM (1987) Newly produced virgin B cells emigrate to secondary lymphoid organs but their capacity to enter follicles is restricted. Eur J Immunol 17:1311–1316

MacLennan ICM, Gray D (1986) Antigen-derived selection of virgin and memory B cells. Immunol Rev 91:61–85

Malek TR, Schmidt JA, Shevach EM (1985) The murine Il-2 receptor. III. Cellular requirements for the induction of Il-2 receptor expression on T cell subpopulations. J Immunol 134:2405–2409

Maximow A (1927) Bindegewebe und blutbildende Gewebe. In: Möllendorf V (ed) Handbuch der mikroskopischen Anatomie des Menschen, vol 2/I. Springer, Berlin, pp 232–583

Mellors RC, Brzosko WJ (1962) Studies in molecular pathology. I. Localization and pathogenic role of heterologous immune complexes. J Exp Med 115:891–902

Mitchell J, Abbot A (1965) Ultrastructure of the antigen-retaining reticulum of lymph node follicles as shown by high-resolution autoradiography. Nature 208:500–502

Mori Y, Lennert K (1969) Electron microscopic atlas of lymph node cytology and pathology. Springer, Berlin Heidelberg New York

Morris B (1972) The cells of lymph and their role in immunological reactions. In: Meessen H (ed) Lymphgefäß-System. Springer, Berlin Heidelberg New York (Handbuch der allgemeinen Pathologie, vol 3, part 6, pp 405–456)

Morrissey PJ, Boswell HS, Scher I, Singer A (1981) Role of accessory cells in B cell activation. IV. Ia accessory cells are required for the in vitro generation of thymic independent type 2 antibody responses to polysaccharide antigens. J Immunol 127:1345–1347

Mosier DE (1967) A requirement for two cell types for antibody formation in vitro. Science 158:1573–1575

Müller-Hermelink HK (1974) Characterization of the B-cell and T-cell regions of human lymphatic tissue through enzyme histochemical demonstration of ATP-ase and 5'nucleotidase activities. Virchows Arch [B] 16:371–379

Müller-Hermelink HK, Heusermann U, Kaiserling E, Stutte HJ (1976) Human lymphatic microecology-specificity, characterization and ontogeny of different reticulum cells in the B and T cell regions. Adv Exp Med Biol 66:177–182

Naiem M, Gerdes J, Abdulaziz Z, Stein H, Mason DY (1983) Production of a monoclonal antibody reactive with human dendritic reticulum cells and its use in the immunohistological analysis of lymphoid tissue. J Clin Pathol 36:167–175

Nossal GJV, Ada GL, Austin CM (1964) Antigens in immunity. IV. Cellular localization of ^{125}I and ^{125}I-labelled flagella in lymph nodes. Aust J Exp Biol Med Sci 42:311–323

Nossal GJV, Austin CM, Pye J, Mitchell J (1966) Antigens in immunity. XII. Antigen trapping in the spleen. Int Arch Allergy Appl. Immunol 29:368–383

Nossal GJV, Abbot A, Mitchell J (1968a) Antigen immunity. XIV. Electron microscopic radioautographic studies of antigen capture in the lymph node medulla. J Exp Med 127:263–276

Nossal GJV, Abbot A, Mitchell J, Lummus Z (1968b) Antigens in immunity. XV. Ultrastructural features of antigen capture in primary and secondary lymphoid follicles. J Exp Med 127:277–290

Oppenheim JJ, Leventhal BG, Hersh EM (1968) The transformation of column-purified lymphocytes with non-specific and specific antigenic stimuli. J Immunol 101:262–270

Parwaresch MR, Radzun HJ, Feller AC, Peters KP, Hansmann M-L (1983a) Peroxidase-positive mononuclear leukocytes as possible precursors of human dendritic reticulum cells. J Immunol 131:2719–2725

Parwaresch MR, Radzun HJ, Hansmann ML, Peters KP (1983b) Monoclonal antibody Ki-M4 specifically recognizes human dendritic reticulum cells (follicular dendritic cells) and their possible precursor in blood. Blood 62:585–590

Pernis B, Silverstein SC, Vogel HJ (eds) (1988) Processing and presentation of antigens. Academic, San Diego

Peters JH, Ruhl S, Friedrichs D (1987) Veiled accessory cells deduced from monocytes. Immunobiology 176:154–166

Pugh CW, MacPherson GG, Steer HW (1983) Characterization of nonlymphoid cells derived from rat peripheral lymph. J Exp Med 157:1758–1779

Radzun HJ, Parwaresch MR, Feller AC, Hansmann M-L (1984) Monocyte/macrophage-specific monoclonal antibody Ki-M1 recognizes interdigitating reticulum cells. Am J Pathol 117:441–450

Rausch E, Kaiserling E, Goos M (1977) Langerhans cells and interdigitating reticulum cells in the thymus-dependent region in human dermatopathic lymphadenitis. Virchows Arch [B] 25:327–343

Rosenthal AS, Shevach EM (1973) Function of macrophages in antigen recognition by guinea pig T lymphocytes. J Exp Med 138:1194–1212

Schirrmacher V, Wigzell H (1974) Immune responses against native and chemically modified albumins in mice. II. Effect of electric charge and conformation on the humoral antibody response and on helper T cell responses. J Immunol 113:1635–1643

Schnizlein CT, Kosco MH, Szakal AK, Tew JG (1985) Follicular dendritic cells in suspensions: identification, enrichment and initial characterization indicating immune complex trapping and lack of adherence and phagocytic activity. J Immunol 134:1360–1368

Selvaraj P, Plunkett ML, Dustin M, Sanders ME, Shaw S, Springer TA (1987) The T lymphocyte glycoprotein (CD2) binds the cell surface ligand LFA-3. Nature 326:400–403

Silberberg-Sinakin I, Thorbecke GJ, Baer RL, Rosenthal SA, Berezowsky V (1976) Antigen-bearing Langerhans cells in skin, dermal lymphatics and in lymph nodes. Cell Immunol 25:137–151

Spry CW, Pflug AJ, Janossy G, Humphrey JH (1980) Large mononuclear (veiled) cells like "Ia-like" membrane antigens in human afferent lymph. Clin Exp Immunol 39:750–755

Steinman RM, Cohn ZA (1973) Identification of a novel cell type in peripheral lymphoid organs of mice. I. Morphology, quantitation, tissue distribution. J Exp Med 137:1142–1162

Steinman RM, Cohn ZA (1974) Identification of a novel cell type in peripheral lymphoid organs of mice. II. Functional properties in vitro. J Exp Med 139:380–397

Steinman RM, Nussenzweig MC, Austyn JM, Witmer MD, Gutchinov B, Unkeles JC, Cohn ZA (1982) Monoclonal antibody studies of mouse dendritic cells and macrophages. In: Mizuno D, Cohn ZA, Takeya K, Ishida N (eds) Self-defense mechanisms: role of macrophages. (Proc of the Naito Foundation Int Symp, Tokyo, 2–4 Nov 1981). Elsevier, Amsterdam, pp 79–112

Steinman RM, Gutchinov B, Witmer MD, Nussenzweig MC (1983) Dendritic cells are the principal stimulators of the primary mixed leukocyte reaction in mice. J Exp Med 157:613–627

Straus W (1970) Location of antibody to horseradish peroxidase in popliteal lymph nodes of rabbits during the primary and early secondary response. J Histochem Cytochem 18:120–130

Sunshine GH, Mitchell TJ (1985) Antigen presentation by spleen dendritic cells. J Invest Dermatol 85:110–114

Swartzendruber DC, Il Ma B, Murphy WH (1967) Localization of C-type virus particles in lymphoid germinal centers of C58 mice. Proc Soc Exp Biol 126:731–734

Szakal AK, Hanna Jr MG (1968) The ultrastructure of antigen localization and virus-like particles in mouse spleen germinal centers. Exp Mol Pathol 8:75–89

Szakal AK, Gieringer RL, Kosco MH, Tew JG (1985) Isolated follicular dendritic cells: cytochemical antigen localization, Normarski, SEM, and TEM morphology. J Immunol 134:1349–1359

Szakal AK, Kosco MH, Tew JG (1988) A novel in vivo follicular dendritic cell-dependent iccosome-mediated mechanism for delivery of antigen to antigen-processing cells. J Immunol 140:341–353

Tanaka Y (1986) Immunocytochemical study of human lymphoid tissues with monoclonal antibodies against S-100 protein subunits. Virchows Arch [A] 410:125–132

Tew JG, Thorbecke GJ, Steinman RM (1982) Dendritic cells in the immune response: characteristics and recommended nomenclature (a report from the Reticulo-endothelial Society Committee on Nomenclature). J Reticuloendothel Soc 31:371–380

Thorbecke GJ, Silberberg-Sinakin I, Flotte TJ (1980) Langerhans cells as macrophages in skin and lymphoid organs. J Invest Dermatol 75:32–43

Unanue ER, Askonas BA (1968) Persistence of immunogenicity of antigen after uptake by macrophages. J Exp Med 127:915–926

van Voorhis WC, Hair LS, Steinman RM, Kaplan G (1982) Human dendritic cells. Enrichment and characterization from peripheral blood. J Exp Med 155:1172–1187 van Voorhis WC, Steinman RM, Hair LS, Luban J, Wittmer MD, Koide S, Cohn ZA (1983) Specific antimononuclear phagocyte monoclonal antibody: application to the purification of dendritic cells and the tissue localization of macrophages. J Exp Med 158:126–145

Veerman AJP (1974) On the interdigitating cells in the thymus-dependent area of the rat spleen: a relation between the mononuclear phagocyte system and T-lymphocytes. Cell Tissue Res 148:247–257

Veldman JE (1970) Histophysiology and electron microscopy of the immune response. PhD Thesis, Groningen

von Gaudecker B, Müller-Hermelink HK (1979) Ontogenetic differentiation of epithelial and non-epithelial cells in the human thymus. Adv Exp Med Biol 114:19–23

Wacker H-H, Radzun HJ, Mielke V, Parwaresch MR (1987) Selective recognition of rat follicular dendritic cells (dendritic reticulum cells) by a new monoclonal antibody Ki-M4R in vitro and in vivo. J Leukocyte Biol 41:70–77

Waldron JA, Horn RG, Rosenthal AS (1973) Antigen-induced proliferation of guinea pig lymphocytes in vitro: obligatory role of macrophages in the recognition of antigen by immune T-lymphocytes. J Immunol 111:58–64

White RG (1963) Functional recognition of immunologically competent cells by means of the fluorescent antibody technique. In: Wolstenholme GEW, Knight J (eds) Immunologically competent cells. (CIBA Foundation Study Group). Churchill Livingstone, London, pp 6

Wong TW, Klinkert WEF, Bowers WE (1982) Immunological properties of thymic cell subpopulations: rat thymic dendritic cells are potent accessory cells and stimulators in a mixed leukocyte culture. Immunobiology 160:413–423

Zhang J, Liu Y-J, MacLennan ICM, Gray D, Lane PJL (1988) B cell memory to thymus-independent antigens type 1 and type 2: the role of lipopolysaccharide in B memory induction. Eur J Immunol 18:1417–1424

Macrophages in Different Compartments of the Non-neoplastic Lymph Node

E. W. A. Kamperdijk, E. B. J. van Nieuwkerk, M. A. M. Verdaasdonk, and E. C. M. Hoefsmit

1 The Normal Lymph Node

1.1 The Different Compartments of the Lymph Node and Their Immunological Function

Lymph nodes are encapsulated, commonly kidney-shaped, organs which filter tissue fluid supplied by afferent lymph vessels. In most species these vessels pierce the capsule on the convex surface and open into the subcapsular sinus, which is ultimately integrated with the medullary sinuses in the concavity of the hilus of the organ. The lymph is filtered in the fine meshes of the reticulo-endothelial tissue (stroma) which supports the sinuses and the compact lymphatic tissue of the node. After filtration the lymph leaves at the hilus via the efferent lymphatic vessels, which usually follow the route of the larger veins and may either join a large collecting lymphatic duct or link with another lymph node as afferent vessels. Finally all lymph is collected in large lymphatic ducts which join the bloodstream at the base of the neck in the subclavian veins. All lymph vessels possess small valves to force the lymph stream in one direction.

In lymph nodes a cortex and medulla can be distinguished. The cortex, which is compact in appearance, can be subdivided into an outer cortex com-

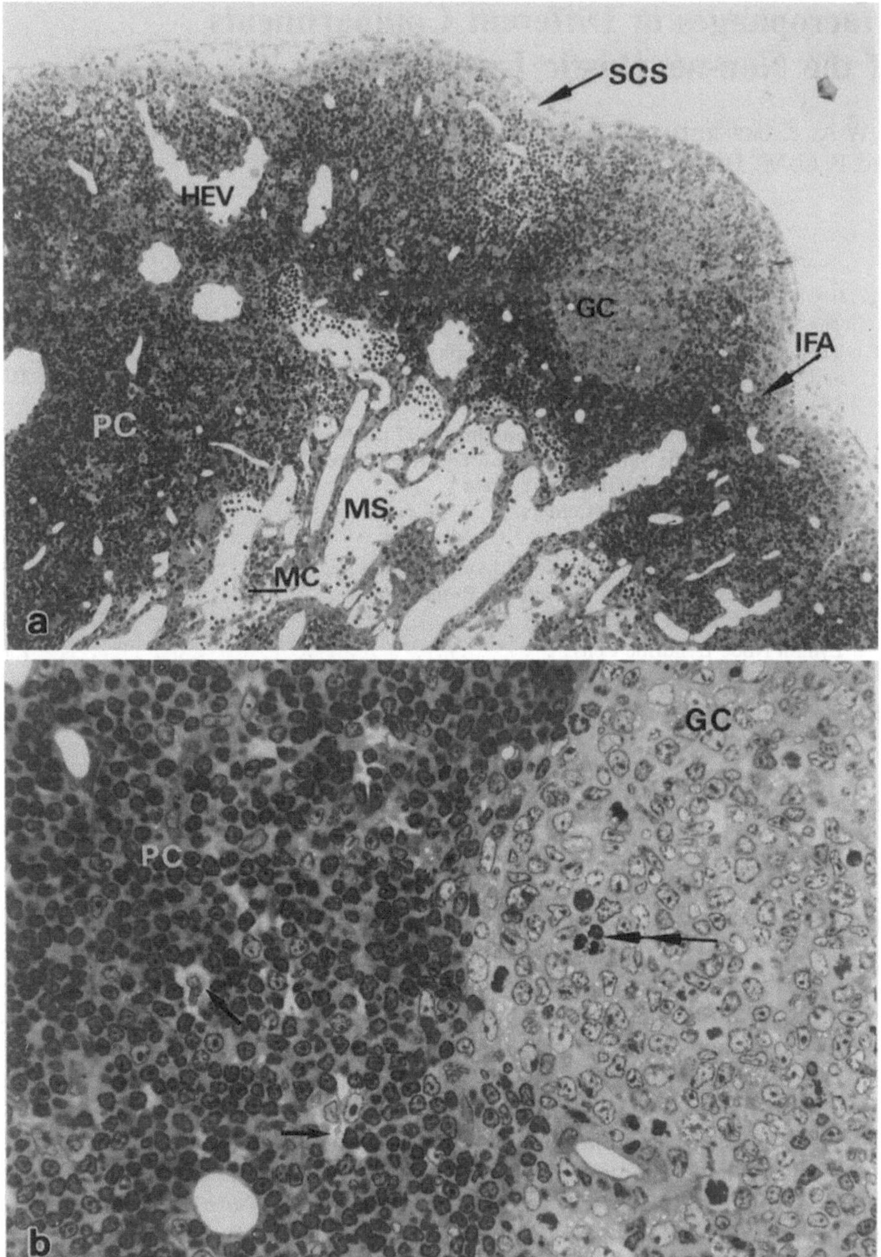

Fig. 1. a Histological section of a rat popliteal lymph node. *SCS*, subcapsular sinus; *IFA*, interfollicular area; *GC*, germinal center; *PC*, paracortex; *HEV*, high endothelial venule; *MC*, medullary cord; *MS*, medullary sinus. Perfusion fixation, 1 μm Epon section, stained with toluidine blue. ×90. **b** Histological section with paracortex (*PC*) and germinal center (*GC*) of a popliteal lymph node. In the paracortex interdigitating cells can easily be recognized by their lucent cytoplasm (*arrow*). The germinal center contains tingible body macrophages (*double arrow*) surrounded by many blast cells. ×425

prising the follicles and the interfollicular areas and an inner cortex. This inner part is also designated the paracortex (GUTMAN and WEISSMAN 1972), paracortical areas (FOSSUM 1980), or deep cortex (BÉLISLE and SAINTE-MARIE 1981 a; Chap. 2 in this volume) (Fig. 1). It has been shown, using careful tridimensional studies (BÉLISLE and SAINTE-MARIE 1981 b), that this area consists of several basic "units." Each of these units is supplied by its own afferent lymph vessel (BÉLISLE and SAINTE-MARIE 1981 b; SAINTE-MARIE et al. 1982). The medulla is open in structure and consists of a network of compact lymphatic tissue, forming the medullary cords which traverse the medullary sinuses. In the hilus blood vessels enter the node and divide into arterioles in the connective tissue. The vessels penetrate the inner and outer cortex and branch into a capillary network which rejoins via the high endothelial venules and veins running back towards the hilus. Although there are variations between the lymph nodes of different species (HEATH et al. 1986; MERIGHI et al. 1986; HEATH and SPALDING 1987), the structure of the human lymph node resembles the structure just described. The lymph node is not only a filter organ, but also an organ responsive to antigenic stimulation. Because this function is crucial to the survival of the individual, lymph nodes are present throughout the body and are especially numerous in areas draining organs with environmental contact.

It has been demonstrated that the outer cortex, comprising the follicles and interfollicular areas, is mainly populated by B lymphocytes (HOWARD et al. 1972), whereas the parocortex is mainly a T-cell compartment. Both cell populations enter the node via the high endothelial venules in the paracortex (NIEUWENHUIS and FORD 1976). From this area B cells migrate to the outer cortex (HOWARD et al. 1972) but T cells remain in the paracortex. Both populations ultimately migrate to the medulla and finally leave the node via the efferent lymph vessels. Only a small proportion of the lymphocytes enter the node by way of the afferent lymphatics (SAINTE-MARIE and PENG 1979).

The lymph follicles can be distinguished into primary and secondary follicles. The primary follicles consist of compact aggregations of small lymphocytes, whereas secondary follicles contain a distinct germinal center, in which lymphoblasts predominate. The germinal centers are covered by a crescent-shaped cap or corona containing relatively small lymphocytes, which belong to the recirculating pool of B cells.

It is evident that the lymph node contains several compartments, each with its own immunological function. In the paracortex the specific cellular response takes place, expanding the pool of antigen-specific T cells (and probably memory T cells); in the interfollicular areas the humoral immune response is induced, finally resulting in the secretion of antibody by plasma cells in the medullary cords; and the germinal centers are involved in the generation of memory B cells (KEUNING 1972).

2 Macrophages

Macrophages form a heterogeneous population as expressed by differences in characteristics such as morphology, enzyme activity, cell surface properties, and functional capacities. Together these characteristics determine the phenotypic appearance of these cells, which depends on environmental circumstances such as state of activity (COHN 1978; BEELEN et al. 1978), the developmental stage of the individual macrophage (COHN and BENSON 1964), and the localization in different tissues (FLOTTE et al. 1982) and compartments (HOEFSMIT 1975).

A major function of these cells is to digest material endocytosed by pinocytosis or phagocytosis. According to the mononuclear phagocyte system (VAN FURTH et al. 1972), they originate in the bone marrow and have a long life span. In contrast to polymorphonuclear leukocytes, they have the ability to adapt their lysosomal enzymes to the requirements of the environment (ASLINE and COHN 1970). They have Fc and C3 receptors.

Macrophages also have important functions in the regulation of the immune response (UNANUE et al. 1984). Since they are mobile cells, they can concentrate antigens, transport them to distant sites, and finally present them to immunocompetent T cells. For activation of these T cells macrophages have to express Ia antigens, the determinants encoded for the I region of the MHC complex.

2.1 Macrophages in the Different Compartments of the Normal Lymph Node

It has been shown at the light and electron-microscopic levels, that it is possible in lymph nodes to distinguish between cells forming the stroma (i.e., reticulum and endothelial cells) and the mononuclear phagocytes (HOEFSMIT 1975; HOEFSMIT et al. 1980). It appeared that each of the compartments of the node contains its own characteristic macrophage (Table 1).

Table 1. Macrophages in the different compartments of the lymph node

Compartment	Mononuclear phagocytes
Subcapsular sinus	Sinus macrophages
Interfollicular area	Large actively phagocytic macrophages
Follicle center	Tingible body macrophages
Paracortex	Interdigitating cells
Medullary sinus	Large actively phagocytic macrophages

2.1.1 *Macrophages in the Subcapsular and Medullary Sinuses*

In these areas, which are in open communication, the filter function predominates. Macrophages are free in the sinuses or apposed to the reticulum cells in the rat. Many of them can be recognized by the macrophage-specific monoclonal antibodies ED3 (Dijkstra et al. 1985) and TRPM-3 (Takeya et al. 1987). Different developmental stages can be distinguished, ranging from small monocyte-like cells measuring about 8–12 µm to large macrophages with a diameter of 35 µm or more. The nucleocytoplasmic ratio of the small macrophages is about 1:2, while the large macrophages may have ratios ranging from 1:4 up to 1:8.

The relatively small cells usually show a ruffled membrane and sometimes finger-like cell processes. Almost all of them have a central spot of acid phosphatase activity, and are strongly Ia positive. Electron-microscopic studies reveal that the irregularly shaped nucleus is surrounded by bundles of microfilaments interspersed with mitochondria. Active micropinocytosis and large phagolysosomes are usually absent, indicating no distinct phagocytic activity. The Golgi area is located in the nuclear hof and contains a variable number of small coated vesicles measuring 50–70 nm, which are presumably primary lysosomes. Sometimes larger vesicles which vary in diameter are also present in this area. The membrane of these vesicles is normally separated from its contents by a clear halo with a constant thickness of about 10 nm. These vesicles contain heterogeneous material of variable electron density representing secondary lysosomes or phagolysosomes (Daems et al. 1969).

The larger macrophage is irregularly shaped with blunt-ended cell processes. The nucleus is slightly indented or bilobate with one or more well-developed nucleoli. Acid phosphatase activity is present throughout the whole cytoplasm, while only some of these cells are Ia positive.

The surrounding microfilaments are, in comparison to the small monocyte-like cells, less prominent. Mitochondria interspersed with numerous strands of rough endoplasmatic reticulum surround the nucleus and the extensive Golgi area. The cells frequently have large phagolysosomes, containing heterogeneous material of variable electron density and sometimes recognizable cellular debris. Especially in the medullary sinuses they are present in large numbers, sometimes forming cell clusters with lymphocytes (Farr and DeBruyn 1975). It is clear that these cells are more mature than the relatively small cells.

2.1.2 *Macrophages in the Interfollicular Areas*

Immediately under the subcapsular sinus an almost continuous layer of macrophages is present. This layer is two to four cells thick in the interfollicular area and diminishes gradually towards the periphery of the primary and secondary follicles (Hendriks et al. 1980). They have acid phosphatase activity throughout the whole cytoplasm and may selectively ingest and retain hydroxy starch or Ficoll (HUMPHREY and GRENNAN 1981), by which they can be distinguished from other macrophage populations.

The large, actively phagocytic cells are usually rounded; the plasma membrane is very irregular and ruffled with vacuoles near the surface. The nucleocytoplasmic ratio is maximally 1:2. The cytoplasm contains Golgi stacks and many dense bodies, which are located along microtubules radiating from the cytocenter. These cells may ingest all types of necrotic leukocytes; granulocytes, mast cells, lymphocytes, and even plasma cells can be distinguished inside a phagolysosome (Fig. 2).

Deeper in the cortex macrophages are sometimes present which show large numbers of incompletely digested necrotic cells, by virtue of which they are very similar with the tingible body macrophages characteristic for the germinal center. They can also be found between the large phagocytic cells bordering the subcapsular sinus, and in primary follicles.

2.1.3 Macrophages in Germinal Centers

The characteristic germinal center macrophage is the tingible body macrophage (TBM, FLEMMING 1885). TBMs have a relatively smooth surface and are more or less polygonal. They all show strong acid phosphatase activity in the whole cytoplasm. Their nucleus is commonly eccentrically localized, and they contain lymphocytes in all stages of degradation and other recognizable cellular debris (Fig. 3). Most probably they are unable to synthesize the lysosomal enzymes needed to digest all material which they have phagocytosed and as a result they themselves have become degenerate. This should explain the presence of aggregation of large effete macrophages filled with residual bodies and myelin figures.

In mouse lymph node follicles TBMs appeared to be positive not only for F4/80 (which is a differentiation marker for macrophages) and Ia antigen but also for Thy-1, which is associated with ribosomes and endoplasmic reticulum as well as their plasma membrane. This means that germinal center TBMs represent a unique, vigorously phagocytic subset of mature macrophages, which express both macrophage and thymocyte markers (SMITH et al. 1988). TBMs are not confined to germinal centers but can be found elsewhere in the outer cortex. SWARTZENDRUBER and CONGDON (1963) clearly demonstrated that TBMs are nonselective; they phagocytose not only lymphocytes but also plasma cells, erythrocytes, and even granulocytes. Since erythrocytes and granulocytes are not usually present in germinal centers, they must have been phagocytosed elsewhere in the outer cortex and transported into the germinal center. In an attempt to follow the migration of the pre-TBMs into germinal centres, carbon was injected into rat footpads (HOEFSMIT et al. 1980). One week later there was strong endocytosis of these particles, not only by medullary macrophages but also by the large, actively phagocytosing macrophages bordering the subcapsular sinus. During the following weeks the number of carbon-containing macrophages diminished but the amount of carbon per cell

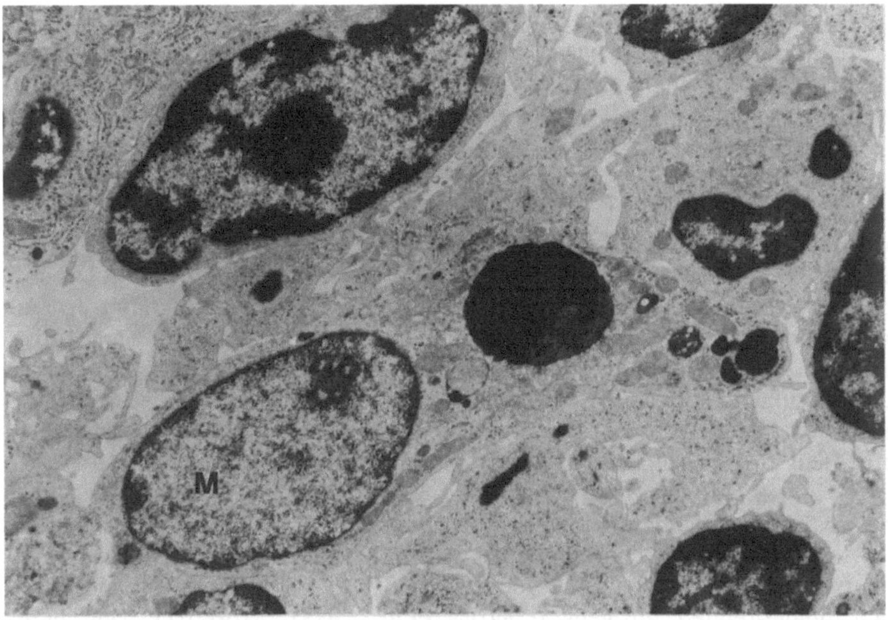

Fig. 2. Large actively phagocytic macrophage (*M*) in the interfollicular area. The cytoplasm contains a necrotic lymphocyte. ×12 150

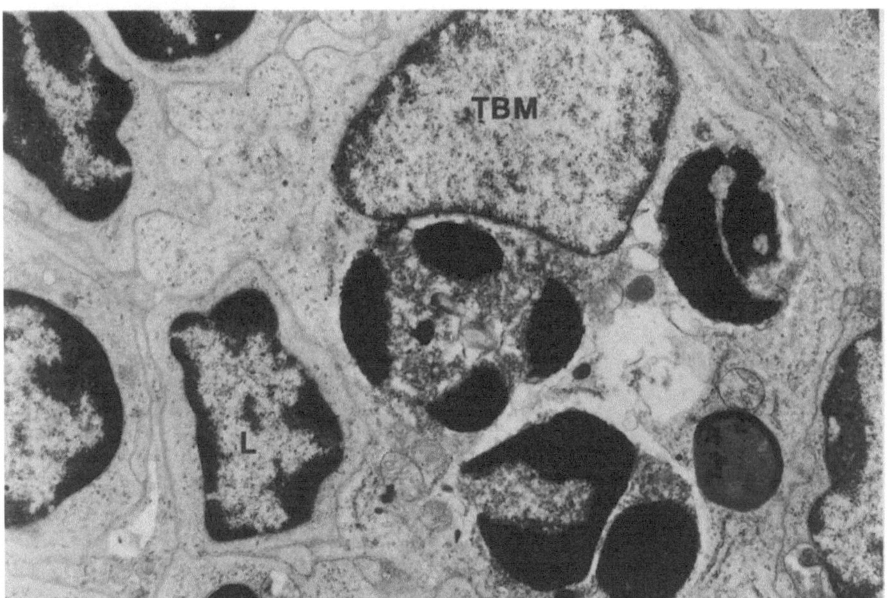

Fig. 3. A TBM in a germinal center. The cytoplasm contains phagolysosomes with lymphocytes in different stages of degradation. *L*, small lymphocyte. ×9500

increased and these carbon-laden cells were found in the deeper parts of the cortex. After 3 weeks all TBMs in the germinal centers were filled with carbon. In the outer cortex the reticulum cells still contained small amounts of carbon, whereas the macrophages in this area were free of carbon. Most probably macrophages endocytose carbon, then die and are themselves phagocytosed by other macrophages.

Another nonlymphoid cell which is characteristic for the germinal center is the follicular dendritic cell (FDC, NOSSAL et al. 1968). This cell has also been designated as the dendritic reticulum cell, but since the origin of the cell is still under discussion this name seems less appropriate. These cells may trap and retain immune complexes. They have slender cell processes, forming a web-like structure. The nuclei have a euchromatic structure and appear triangular or quadrangular in section. The cytoplasm consists of a thin layer surrounding the nucleus, with extensions forming the cell processes. These cell processes are embedded in electron-dense material, probably immune complexes (HOEFSMIT 1975; CHEN et al. 1978) (Fig. 4). It has been suggested that these cells are immigrating cells which belong to the mononuclear phagocyte system since they share phenotypic characteristics with cells of the monocyte/macrophage lineage such as Fc and C3 receptors, MHC class II antigens, and some macrophage-related antigens (GERDES et al. 1983). Moreover TEW et al. (1984), in an ultrastructural study, suggested that in the subcapsular sinus of

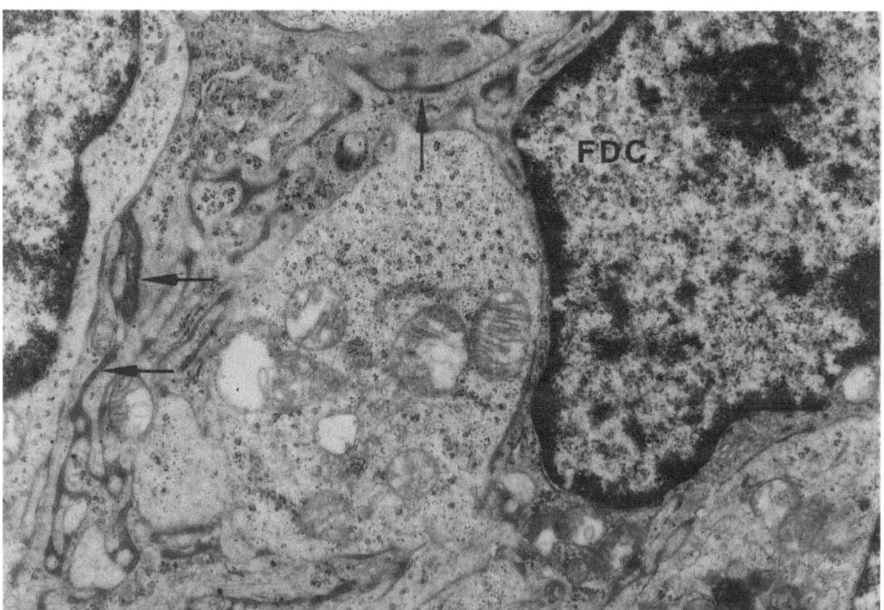

Fig. 4. Part of a FDC in a germinal center. The cytoplasm shows many fine ramifications. Electron-dense material, probably an antigen–antibody complex, is present in the intercellular space (*arrows*). *L*, lymphocyte. ×31 000

mouse lymph nodes, immune complexes are trapped by dendritic cells (DCs; STEINMAN and COHN 1973; TEW et al. 1982) and transported to follicular regions (SZAKAL et al. 1983). The mechanism of transport might involve migration of these pre-FDCs with a concomitant maturation into FDCs. However, it has been shown that, in contrast to DCs, FDCs are not bone marrow derived (HUMPHREY et al. 1984) and do not demonstrate acid phosphatase activity (EIKELENBOOM 1978).

It has been demonstrated that not only FDCs in germinal centers but also fibroblastic reticulum cells (FRCs) in primary follicles trap immune complexes (DIJKSTRA et al. 1984; KAMPERDIJK et al. 1987a). This observation, together with the existence of transitional forms between the two cell types during ontogenic development (GROSCURTH 1980; HEUSERMANN et al. 1980; VILLENA et al. 1983), indicates that FDCs represent a specialized reticulum cell, characteristic for germinal centers. There are now strong indications that DCs belong to the cell lineage Langerhans cell, veiled cell, and interdigitating cell (see Sects. 3.1 and 3.2).

2.1.4 Macrophages in the Paracortex

The interdigitating cell (IDC), first described by VELDMAN (1970), is the characteristic type of macrophage of the paracortex (HOEFSMIT 1975). Similar cells are also present in other lymphoid tissues such as spleen periarteriolar lymphocyte sheath (VEERMAN and VAN EWIJK 1975) and thymus medulla (DUIJVESTIJN and HOEFSMIT 1981). Enzyme- and immunohistochemical studies show that they have an acid phosphatase spot of varying intensity located centrally, and that all of them are persistently Ia positive. The cytoplasm of these cells is strikingly lucent (Fig. 1 b) and forms blunt processes which interdigitate with finger-like extensions of adjacent lymphocytes, mainly of the T helper phenotype (Fig. 5). IDCs vary in size but are usually large cells, 20–30 µm in diameter, excluding the cell processes. The nucleus is irregularly shaped and usually in an eccentric position. The cell membrane shows tubular invaginations. In the cytoplasm well-developed Golgi complexes are located around a cytocenter. Many relatively small lysosomes with heterogeneous electron-dense material are arranged along microtubules which radiate from a pair of centrioles. Relatively small mitochondria, variable in number, and large numbers of small, smooth vesicles, closely packed together, are frequently observed in other parts of the cytoplasm. VEERMAN and VAN EWIJK (1975) describewd these structures as a vesicular complex, which should be distinguished from the tubulovesicular system described by VELDMAN (1970) (see Fig. 6). The cell was first described as an interdigitating reticulum cell by VELDMAN (1970) in the paracortex of the rabbit lymph node. He suggested that the lysosomal complex together with the tubular invaginations of the cell membrane form a secretory tubulovesicular system responsible for the synthesis of glycoproteins and for transporting them from the Golgi apparatus, via the tubulovesicular system, to the cell membrane. VELDMAN was unable to

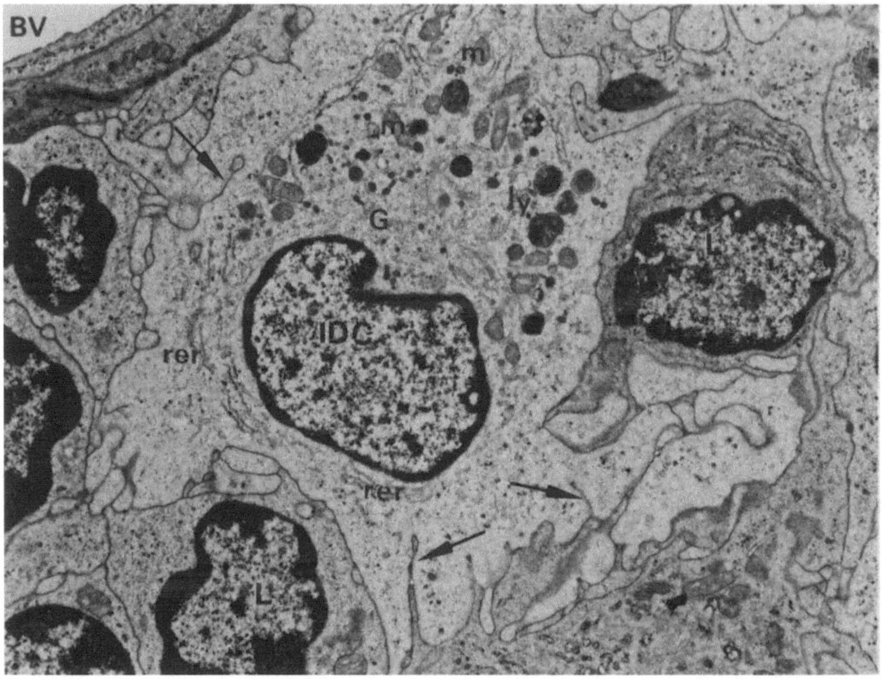

Fig. 5. Ultrastructure of an IDC of a normal rat. The cytoplasm is electron-lucent and contains Golgi cisterns (*G*), rough endoplasmic reticulum (*rer*), mitochondria (*m*), and lysosomes (*ly*). The cell membrane shows tubular invaginations (*arrows*). *L*, lymphocyte; *BV*, blood vessel. ×7900

detect distinct signs of phagocytic activity and therefore classified them as nonphagocytic reticular cells (KAISERLING and LENNERT 1974; RAUSCH et al. 1977), i.e., cells which belong to the stroma. Since it is clear that these cells represent mobile cells (KAMPERDIJK et al. 1978; HOEFSMIT et al. 1982) originating in the bone marrow (DUIJVESTIJN and BARCLAY 1984) which can phagocytose under certain circumstances (KAMPERDIJK et al. 1982; FOSSUM and VAALAND 1983), we prefer the term interdigitating cell to interdigitating reticulum cell.

3 Macrophages in Antigen-Stimulated Lymph Nodes

After antigenic stimulation lymph nodes are involved in the immune response, a process of cooperation between lymph node macrophages and different lymphocyte subsets. To study the reactivity of the different macrophage populations in the course of the immune response, rat lymph nodes were stimulated with different types of antigen: (a) antigens which give rise to a humoral

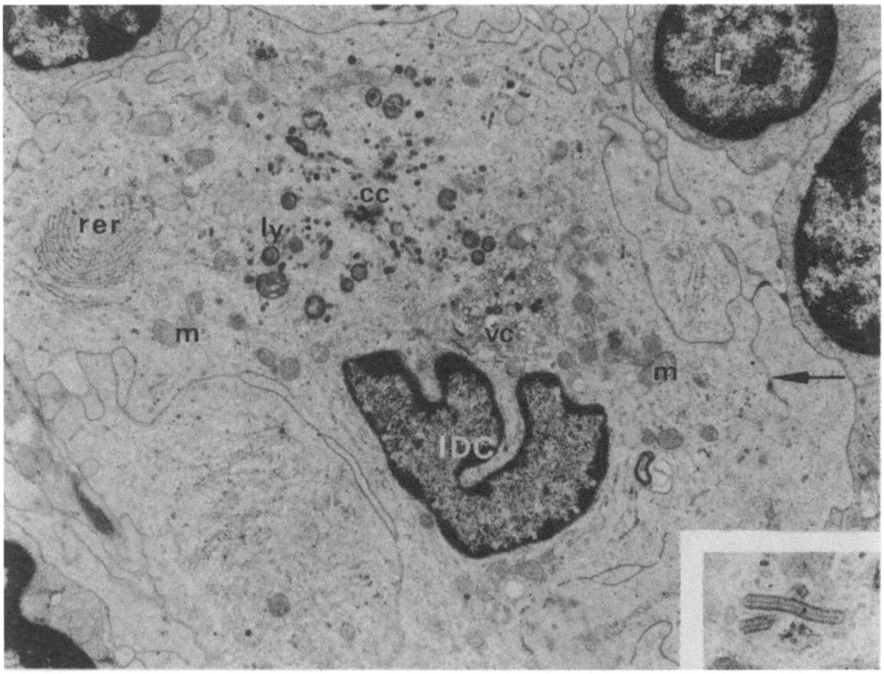

Fig. 6. An IDC in the paracortex, 1 day after administration of PTV. The cytoplasm contains a cytocenter (*cc*), mitochondria (*m*), a vesicular complex (*vc*), lysosomes (*ly*), rough endoplasmic reticulum (*rer*), and Birbeck granules (*inset*). The cell membrane shows tubular invaginations (*arrow*). *L*, lymphocyte. ×7900

immune response (paratyphoid vaccine) and (b) antigens which provoke a specific T-cell reaction (viable *Listeria monocytogenes*).

3.1 Macrophages in the Humoral Immune Response

A series of male Wistar rats were given 0.1 ml paratyphoid vaccine (PTV), containing 5×10^9 formol-killed microorganisms/ml, in one footpad, i.e., an ectodermal environment. Whole organisms were used, which provoked a thymus-dependent as well as a thymus-independent immune response. The draining popliteal lymph nodes were examined at the light and electron-microscopic levels at different time intervals ranging from 6 h to 6 weeks. The secondary response was studied too in animals boosted 6 weeks after primary immunization. In the primary response the first lymphoblasts appeared in the outer and inner cortex 9 h after stimulation. After 2 days many lymphoblasts and mitotic lymphocytes were present in the enlarged paracortex. One day later many plasmablasts appeared in the corticomedullary region and after 4 days many well-developed plasma cells populated the medullary cords. The germinal cen-

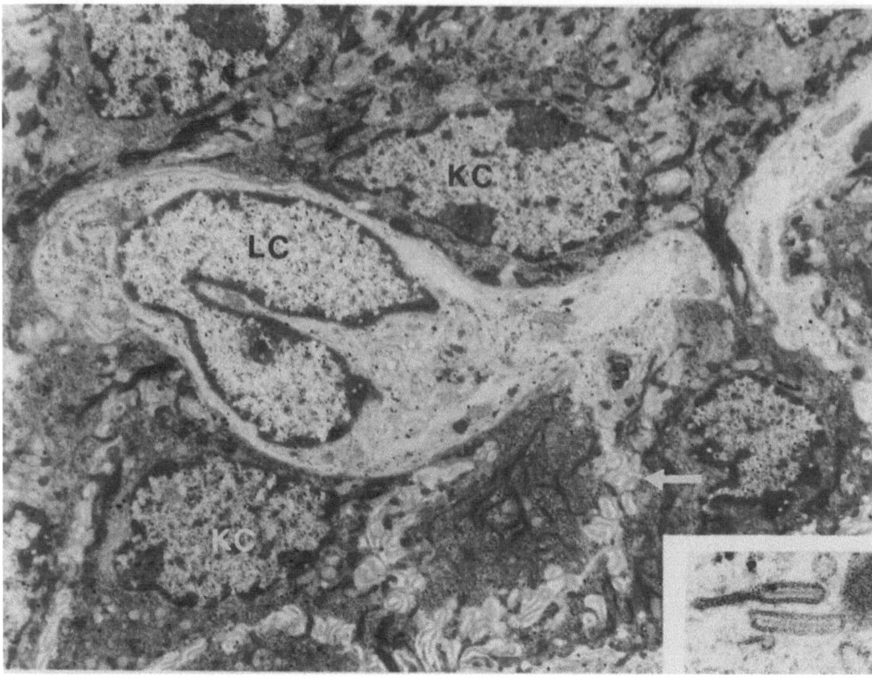

Fig. 7. Langerhans cell (*LC*) in the epidermis of a normal rat. The cytoplasm is electron-lucent. *Arrow* indicates cytoplasmic protrusions. *KC*, keratinocyte. × 6900. *Inset*: Birbeck granules

ter reaction started at day 2 with the appearance of groups of lymphoblasts in the outer cortex beneath the large macrophages bordering the subcapsular sinus. A maximum was reached after 8 days, at the same time as the highest number of TBMs was present. Circulating antibody was first detected 3 days after stimulation. One day later the maximum level of antibody was detected, followed by a gradual decrease during the next days. These different observations reflect three phases in the immune response:

1. The induction phase: up to 1 day. The immunocompetent B and T cells were stimulated in the outer cortex and the paracortex, respectively.
2. The proliferation phase between the 1st and 4th days after stimulation. Many lymphoblasts and mitotic lymphoid cells populated both the outer cortex and the paracortex, as did many plasmablasts. Moreover T cell–B cell interaction occurred in this phase.
3. The memory phase from the 4th day onwards, when the immune response gradually diminished and the germinal center reaction became prominent.

During these phases of the immune response none of the reticulum cells in the inner cortex and the paracortex, except for the FRCs in the follicle center which transformed into well-developed FDCs (KAMPERDIJK et al. 1978), showed any distinct morphological change. However, the behavior of the different macrophage populations was strikingly different. The induction phase was characterized by an influx of monocyte-like exudate macrophages from the subcapsular sinus into the interfollicular area and paracortex (KAMPERDIJK et al. 1978, 1984). They commonly showed an indented or irregularly shaped euchromatic nucleus and a high nucleocytoplasmic ratio. The cytoplasm was moderately electron-dense and contained some relatively small phagolysosomes in the center of the cell. In the paracortex transitional forms between these cells and IDCs were seen. In the subcapsular sinus a minority of these cells showed characteristic long veils like the veiled cells described in the afferent lymph of the rabbit and the pig (KELLY et al. 1978; DREXHAGE et al. 1980; LENS et al. 1983).

Six hours and 1 day after stimulation (i.e., in the induction phase) these newly arrived macrophages, transitional forms, and mature IDCs sometimes contained Birbeck granules (Fig. 6), the characteristic cell organelle of the epidermal Langerhans cell (BIRBECK et al. 1961) (Fig. 7), whereas the large, actively phagocytic macrophages characteristic for the interfollicular area and the medullary macrophages never contained Birbeck granules.

During the proliferation phase in the subcapsular sinus, the monocyte-like exudate cells were largely replaced by larger, actively phagocytosing cells. In the paracortex many intermediate forms between the newly arrived monocyte-like exudate macrophages and IDCs were still present (Fig. 8). In the memory

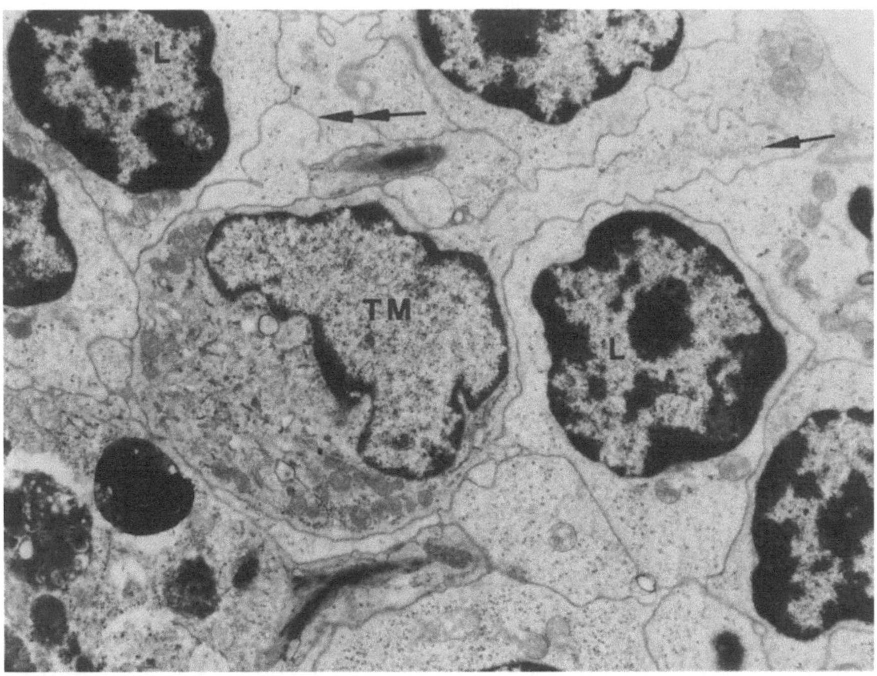

Fig. 8. Transitional macrophage (*TM*) in the paracortex, 2 days after PTV administration. Electron-lucent cytoplasmic processes, characteristic for IDCs are already present (*arrow*). *Double arrow* indicates tubular invaginations. *L*, lymphocyte. ×10 500

phase the number of newly arrived macrophages and transitional forms gradually decreased and the paracortex was repopulated by large numbers of well-developed IDCs (Fig. 9). No Birbeck granule could be found in any macrophages after the 1st day after stimulation.

In the secondary response the immunological reactions were much more pronounced. The proliferation phase overlapped the induction phase and the first plasma cells were seen earlier in the medullary cords. Moreover the transformation of newly arrived exudate macrophages (including veiled cells) into IDCs occurred faster. Birbeck granule containing cells were also only observed in the induction phase. In the proliferation phase many transitional cells were seen in close relationship with surrounding lymphoblasts. In the memory phase the blast reaction gradually diminished and the number of IDCs was increased. Some of them were engaged in active phagocytosis (KAMPERDIJK et al. 1982). They frequently contained phagolysosomes with recognizable necrotic cellular and sometimes nuclear material (Fig. 10), thus resembling TBMs of the germinal center in this respect.

These experiments show that in each phase of the humoral immune response a morphologically different type of cell predominates in the lymph node: the newly arrived macrophage in the induction phase, a transitional macrophage in the proliferation phase, and the IDC in the memory phase.

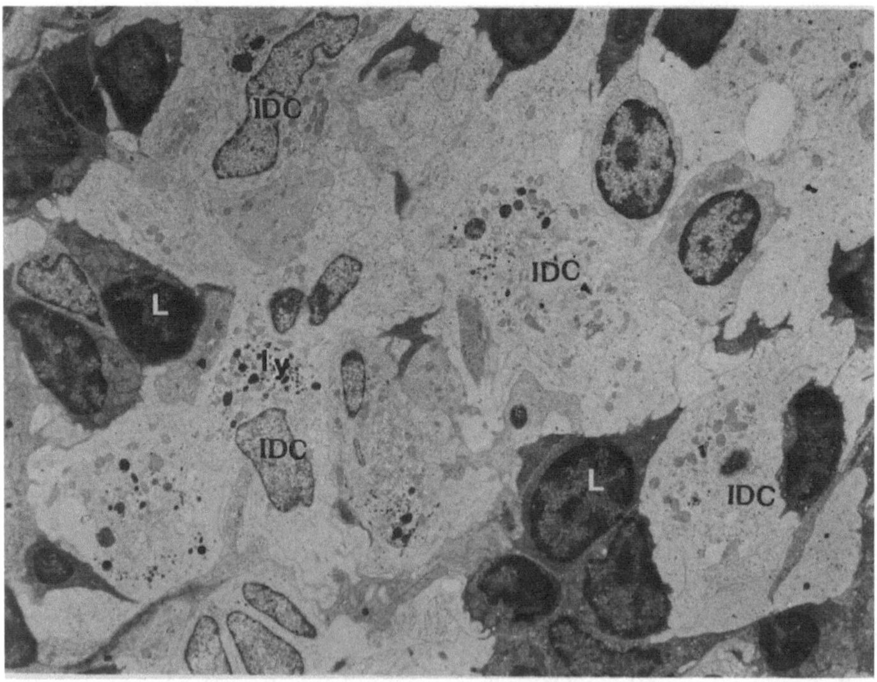

Fig. 9. Large numbers of IDCs in the paracortex, 2 weeks after PTV stimulation. Lysosomes (*ly*) are present in a central area of the cell. *L*, lymphocyte. ×3100

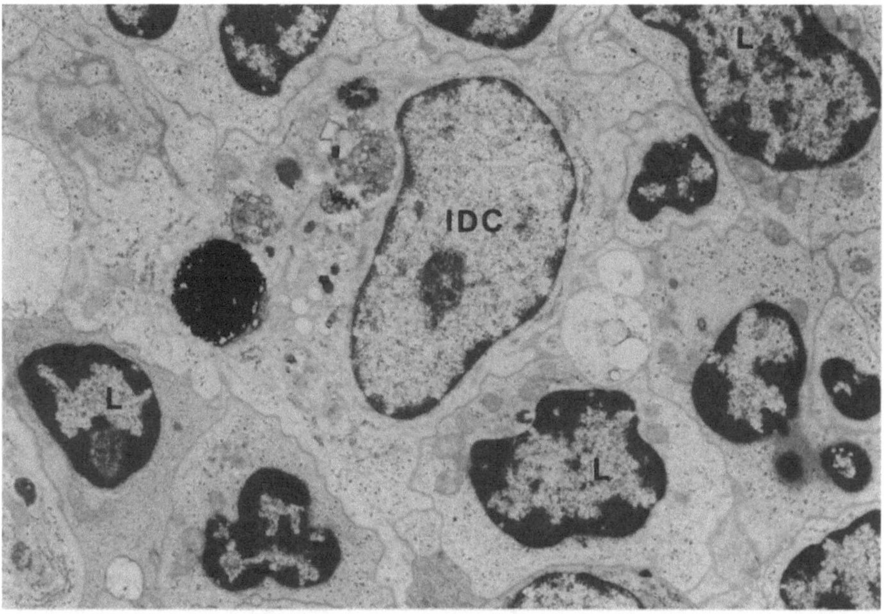

Fig. 10. An IDC containing a necrotic lymphocyte, 2 weeks after PTV stimulation in a preimmunized rat. *L*, lymphocyte. ×7100

Exclusively in the induction phase the newly arrived macrophages (including veiled cells) and IDCs may contain Birbeck granules, suggesting a sequence: Langerhans cell in the epidermis, veiled cell in the afferent lymph, and IDC in the paracortex.

To evaluate the immunological significance of the Birbeck granules in these cells, PTV was also injected in the rat peritoneal cavity and the immune response studied in the draining parathymic lymph node (Yoffey and Courtice 1956). It appeared that these reactions showed a very close resemblance to the reactions observed in the popliteal lymph node. However, the population of newly arrived macrophages, including transitional forms and IDCs, characteristic for the induction phase, never contained Birbeck granules (Kamperdijk et al. 1984) (Fig. 11).

These observations clearly show that: (a) the occurrence of Birbeck granules depends on the site of exudate provocation (i.e., the area in which the antigen is injected) and (b) these cell organelles are not obligatory for lymphocyte stimulation; they only can be used as a marker for morphologically different cell populations.

3.2 The Specific T-Cell Reaction

To study the reactivity of lymph node macrophages in a specific T-cell reaction a series of rats were inoculated with *Listeria* in one footpad. Each animal

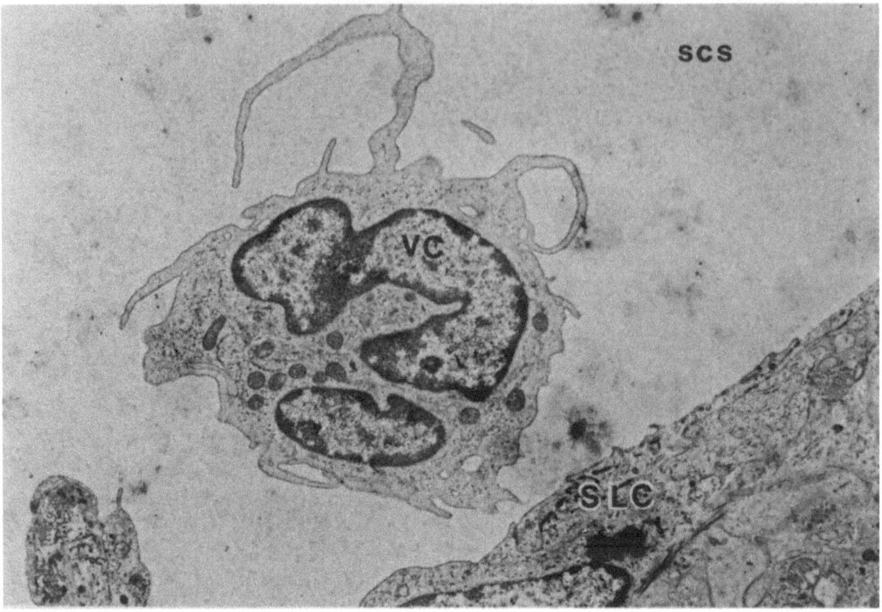

Fig. 11. Veiled cell (*VC*) in the subcapsular sinus (*SCS*) of a parathymic lymph node, 6 h after stimulation. Birbeck granules are absent. *SLC*, sinus lining cell. ×6700

received 0.1 ml of a saline suspension containing 5×10^7 viable parasites/ml. After different time intervals, ranging from 1 h to 6 weeks, the draining popliteal lymph nodes were investigated both light and electron microscopically.

During the first days after inoculation we observed only a T-cell response. After 2 weeks a plasma cellular reaction and germinal center reaction were also seen. The first generalized lymphoblast reaction was detected in the paracortex 1 day after stimulation. During the following days the number of lymphoblasts increased steadily, reaching a maximum on the 4th day. This coincides with maximal extension of the paracortex. During the subsequent increase, there was no development of plasma cells. The blast cells showed no rough endoplasmic reticulum in the cytoplasm and thus did not represent plasmablasts. Hereafter the lymphoblasts generated a population of antigen-sensitized small T lymphocytes (MCGREGOR and LOGIE 1975). This T-cell reaction could also be roughly divided into an induction phase (which precedes the first blast reaction), proliferation phase (proliferation of lymphocytes, reaching its maximum at day 4), and memory phase (blast reaction decreases again, adding a circulating pool of antigen-sensitized small T cells). The kinetics of the macrophages in the induction phase showed some similarities with those in the corresponding period of the humoral immune response: a heterogeneous population of small monocyte-like macrophages and large, actively phagocytosing macrophages penetrated the outer cortex via the subcapsular sinus (Fig. 12).

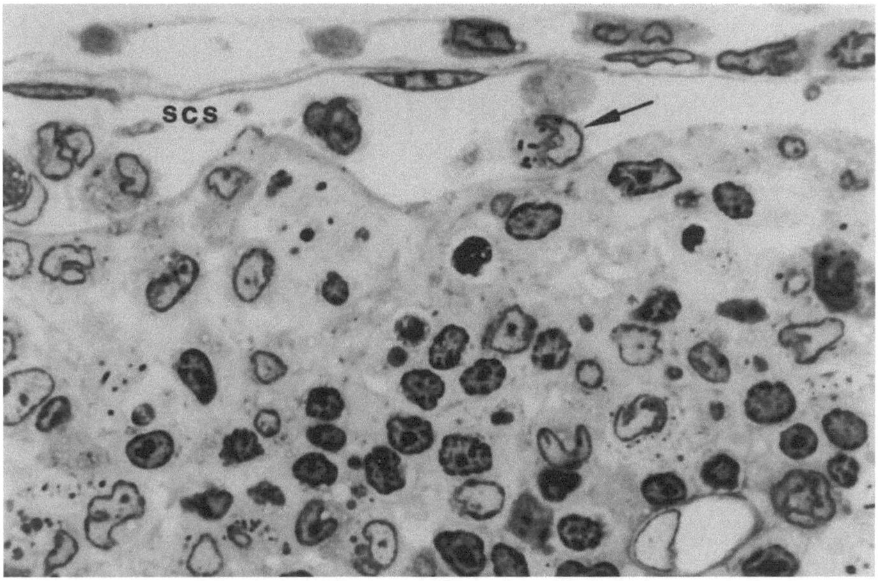

Fig. 12. Light microscopy: macrophage containing several bacteria (*arrow*) in the subcapsular sinus (*SCS*), 1 day after stimulation. ×1120

About 40% of these cells showed characteristic long veils, and some of them contained Birbeck granules. The monocyte-like exudate macrophages sometimes contained cellular debris and also intact bacteria, present in phagosomes or even freely in the cytoplasm. Most probably the microorganisms were attacked by these macrophages at the injection site. At the same time intact bacteria were also seen in the large, actively phagocytosing macrophages bordering the subcapsular sinus and in IDCs in the paracortex. In these cells *Listeria* survived and were able to multiply in the cytoplasm of all of these macrophages. They may penetrate into the nucleus and cause necrosis of these cells (Fig. 13), finally resulting in the total disappearance of all macrophages bordering the subcapsular sinus (Fig. 14). The newly arrived macrophages, intermingled with polymorphonuclear leukocytes and lymphocytes, formed aggregates at several sites in the outermost layer of the cortex.

In the proliferation phase, the correlation of the development of these aggregates of macrophages with the inability of the macrophages, including IDCs, to kill these bacteria was most prominent. The aggregates increased in size as long as the mononuclear phagocytes were unable to digest *Listeria*. However, it appeared that they decreased again as soon as the macrophages/IDCs eliminated the bacteria, suggesting that the development of these cellular infiltrates is caused by the inability of macrophages to digest *Listeria*.

The memory phase was characterized by the appearance of large numbers of well-developed IDCs in the paracortex and the disappearance of the con-

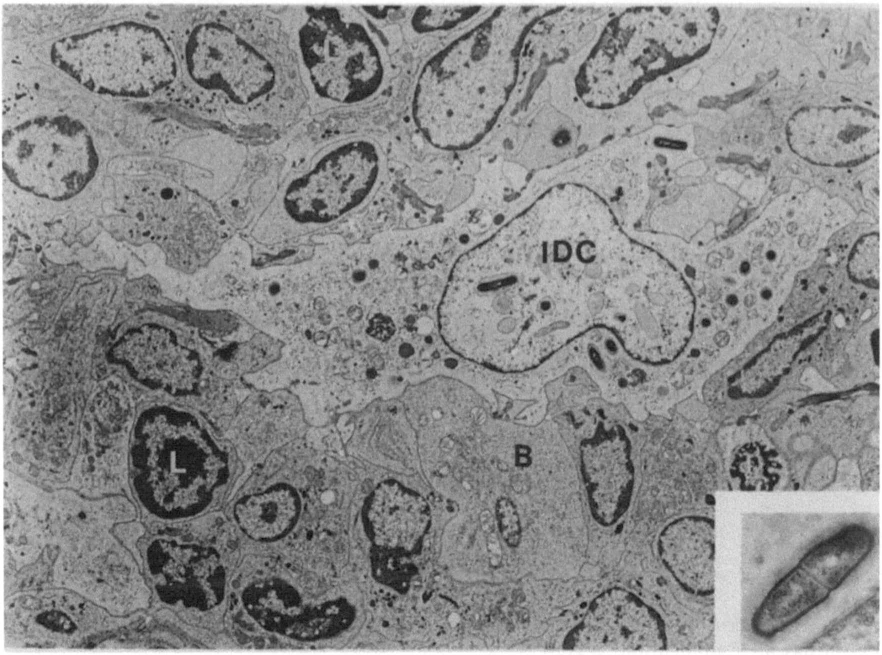

Fig. 13. An IDC containing both intracytoplasmic and intranuclear bacteria, 2 days after injection of *Listeria monocytogenes*. *B*, lymphoblast; *L*, lymphocyte. × 3500. *Inset*: dividing bacterium, which is embedded in the cytoplasm without an enclosing membrane. × 18 200

glomerates of macrophages. Some IDCs showed digestion of *Listeria* (Fig. 15) and even necrotic cells (Fig. 16), demonstrating again that they have the abilities of "professional" macrophages. They never showed mitotic activity. As far as the role of macrophages in the immune response is concerned, our results strongly suggest a relationship between the different populations of macrophages and the different stages of the primary specific T-cell response: the macrophages which induce the immune response are clearly different from the (immune) macrophages which are able to kill and digest the "facultative parasites." The monocyte-like macrophages, including veiled cells, predominate during the induction of the response. After antigenic stimulation veiled cells in the afferent lymph (HOEFSMIT et al. 1979; DREXHAGE et al. 1980; BALFOUR et al. 1981) and transitional cells and IDCs in the paracortex (KAMPERDIJK and HOEFSMIT 1978; KAMPERDIJK et al. 1978, 1982) may show Birbeck granules, characteristic for epidermal Langerhans cells. This suggests that these morphologically different cells are different developmental stages of the cell and that they transform their morphology depending on the microenvironment. Only the first developmental stages of these newly arrived macrophages are involved in stimulation of the immunocompetent lymphocytes (see also SILBERBERG-SINAKIN et al. 1976).

Our results show a correlation between the presence of many lymphoblasts and the generated sensitized T cells in the paracortex and the ability of lymph

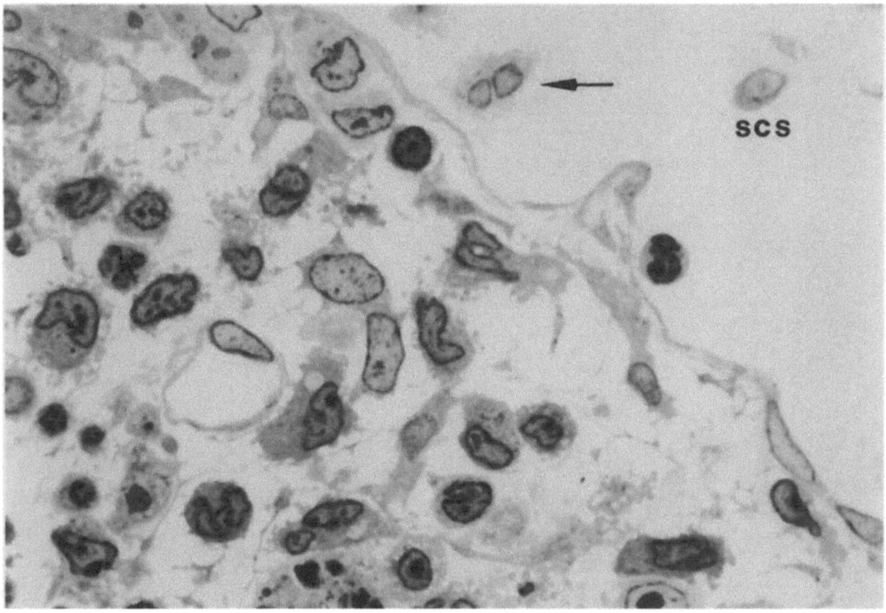

Fig. 14. Interfollicular area, almost completely depleted from the characteristic type of macrophage, 2 days after stimulation. *Arrow* indicates a veiled cell present in the subcapsular sinus (*SCS*). ×1310

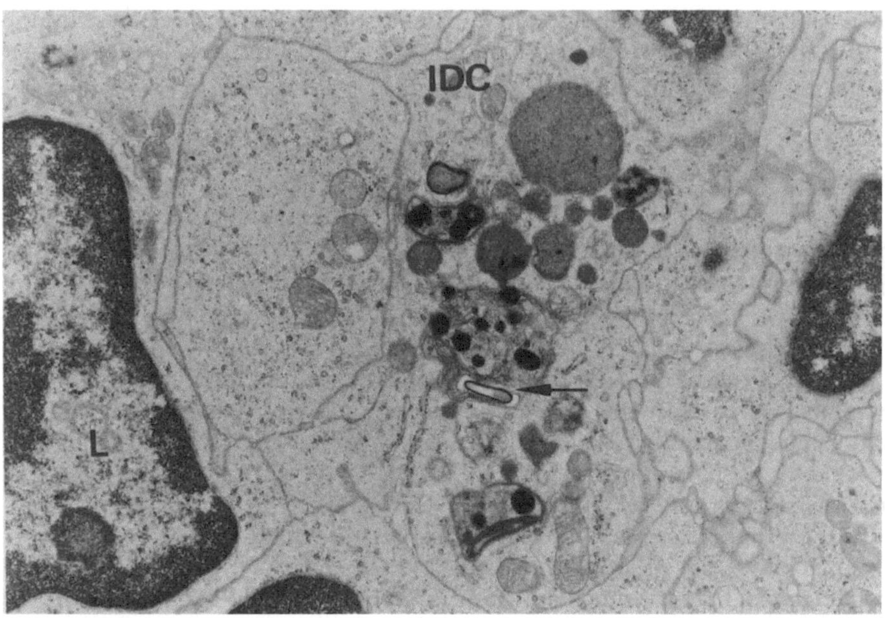

Fig. 15. An IDC with a digested bacterium (*arrow*) in the paracortex 6 days after stimulation. *L*, lymphocyte. ×11 000

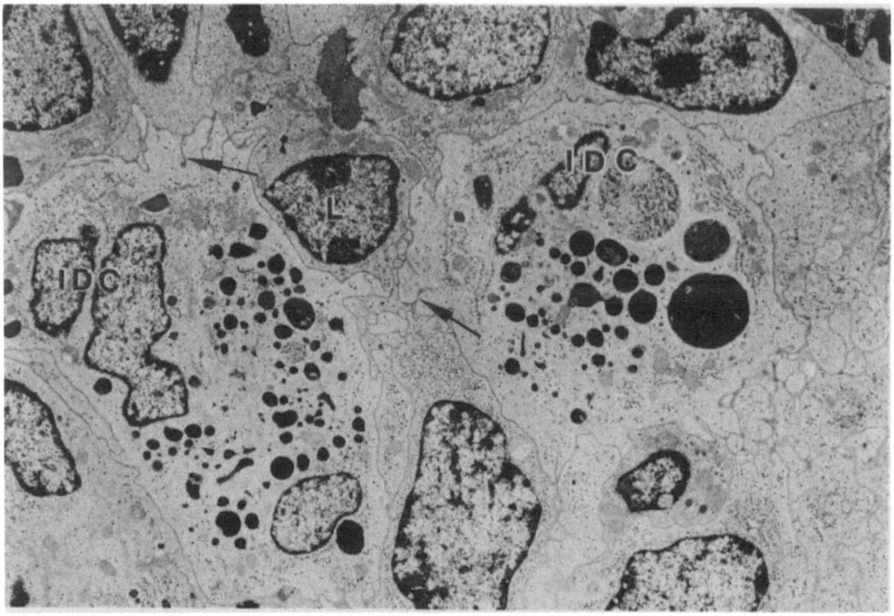

Fig. 16. Characteristic IDC with partly digested lymphocytes 6 days after injection of *Listeria monocytogenes*. The cytoplasm is electron-lucent, and the cell membrane possesses tubular invaginations (*arrows*). *L*, lymphocyte. × 5900

node macrophages to kill LISTERIA. Most probably factors released by the sensitized cells activate the macrophages/IDCs to kill the parasites (BLANDEN and LANGMAN 1972; COLLINS 1978).

4 Lymph Node Dendritic Cells

Dendritic cells (DCs, TEW et al. 1982) were originally described by STEINMAN and COHN (1973) in mice as nonlymphoid cells that could be isolated from lymphoid organs. Similar cells have now been obtained from lymphoid tissues of other species. It has been demonstrated that these Fc receptor negative, bone marrow derived cells (KLINKERT 1984; BOWERS and BERKOWITZ 1986) are extremely potent accessory cells, particularly involved in the induction of T cell-dependent responses. It has been suggested that in contrast to other cells which may present antigen, such as macrophages (UNANUE et al. 1984), B cells, endothelial cells, and even megakaryocytes, these cells are particularly important in a primary response (INABA and STEINMAN 1986).

To identify the in situ equivalent of these cells, DCs were isolated and characterized from normal and antigen-stimulated rat lymph nodes in the different phases of the immune response (see also KAMPERDIJK et al. 1985, 1987b).

The (skin draining) popliteal lymph nodes were stimulated in the same way and with the same antigen (PTV) as already described in Sect. 3.1. The animals were killed by decapitation after 1 day (induction phase) or after 2 weeks (memory phase). The control rats were given 0.1 ml 0.9% NaCl and killed after 1 day (normal lymph nodes). After removal, the lymph nodes were cut into small pieces, which were gently pressed through a nylon gauze to bring the cells into suspension. Low density cells, obtained by flotation at 1000 *g* on Ficoll-metrizoate (P = 1.084 g/ml) were irradiated at 1000 rad and cultured for 18 h. After this procedure most of the lymphocytes were necrotic. After removal of these cells by centrifugation on Ficoll-metrizoate, the nonlymphoid cell population was separated into Fc receptor negative and Fc receptor positive cells by EA rosetting, followed by centrifugation on Ficoll-metrizoate. The floating, non-EA-rosetting fraction contained the purified dendritic cells, the EA-rosetting fraction the macrophages.

It appeared that the number of DCs isolated from lymph nodes in the induction phase was much higher than the number of these cells obtained from normal lymph nodes or lymph nodes in the memory phase. Enzyme- and immunecytochemistry revealed that all DCs had acid phosphatase in a central spot near the lobulated nucleus and were persistently Ia positive. At the ultrastructural level they had an irregular outline; some of them showed blunt pseudopodia, others moderate veils, thus resembling veiled cells from skin draining lymph (LENS et al. 1983; DABROWSKI et al. 1989), the precursor cells of the IDCs. They also showed morphological aspects of the large mononuclear cells demonstrated in the thoracic duct lymph of normal (PUGH et al. 1983) and congenitally athymic nude rats (FOSSUM 1984) after mesenteric lymphadenectomy. Although the central area frequently contained small and medium-sized phagolysosomes, these cells never showed endocytosis of recognizable extracellular material. Only DCs obtained from lymph nodes in the induction phase may contain Birbeck granules (Fig. 17).

Interdigitating cells and their precursors in situ show almost the same characteristics: they have an irregularly shaped nucleus, an acid phosphatase spot in a juxtanuclear position, and Ia antigen on their cell membrane. Moreover these cells may contain Birbeck granules in the induction phase of the provoked immune response. However, it has been shown that in contrast to DCs, IDCs may display phagocytic activity not only in lymph nodes (see also FOSSUM and VAALAND 1983; FOSSUM et al. 1984, FOSSUM and ROLSTAD 1986) but also in spleen (LEVINE et al. 1983) and thymus (DUIJVESTIJN et al. 1982). This indicates that DCs isolated from lymph nodes of the rat are the in vitro equivalents of the non-actively phagocytosing population of IDCs. These findings were confirmed by BREEL et al. (1987) in the mouse using the monoclonal antibodies MIDC-8 and NLDC-145 (KRAAL et al. 1986). Moreover these studies again suggested a relationship between the epidermal Langerhans cells in the skin, veiled cells in the afferent lymph, and IDCs in the skin draining lymph node (HOEFSMIT et al. 1982). Recently FOSSUM (1988) collected MHC class II positive dendritic leukocytes (DCs) with veiled cell morphology from the throacic duct of rats. After reinjection into veins or footpads they only entered

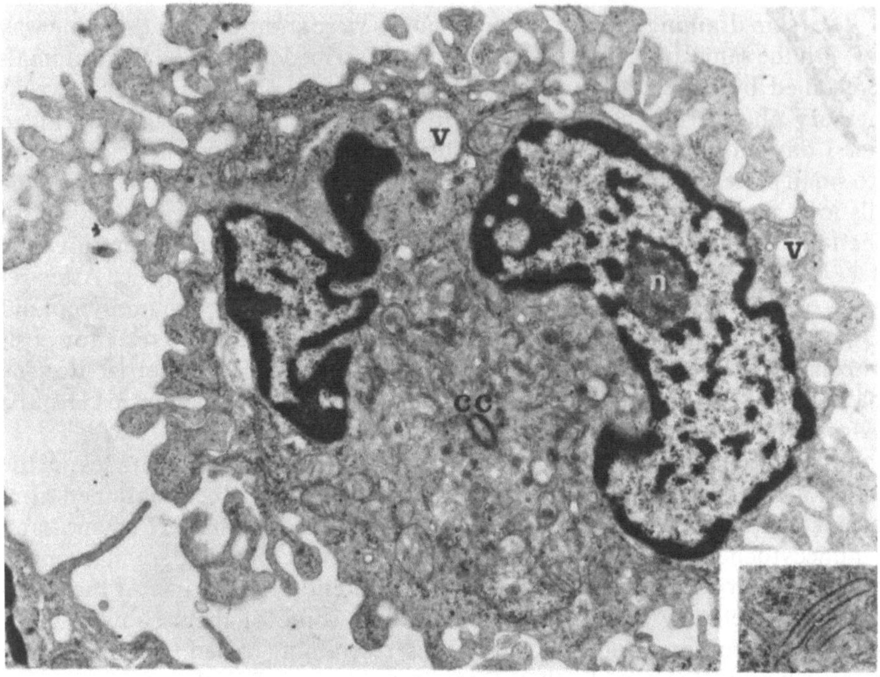

Fig. 17. Dendritic cell, isolated 1 day after PTV stimulation. The cytoplasm is rather electron-dense and extends blunt pseudopodia. The eccentrically localized nucleus is reniform and has a nucleus (*n*). Vacuoles (*v*) are present near the plasma membrane. Birbeck granules (*inset*) are frequently present. *cc*, cytocenter. ×6100

the lymph node by way of the afferent lymphatics, localizing in the paracortex and acquiring the morphology of mature IDCs.

5 Concluding Remarks

In this chapter the characteristic macrophages in the different compartments of the lymph node have been described. The reactivity of these cells was followed after antigenic stimulation. In the induction phase veiled cells enter the node via the afferent lymphatics and predominate in the outer and inner cortex; in the proliferative phase these cells transform into IDCs, which predominate in the memory phase. Our observations suggest that Langerhans cells in the skin can pick up antigen and transport it as veiled cells by way of the afferent lymphatics and subcapsular sinus into the outer cortex, followed by stimulation of the immunocompetent T cells in the paracortex. IDCs function as effector cells rather than inducer cells. They never show mitotic activity, and may probably be considered as end cells.

We described these DC-related cells (veiled cells, including IDCs) as members of the mononuclear phagocyte system. This justified not only by their origin and morphological aspects (Hoefsmit 1975; Balfour et al. 1981) but also by their migration properties and phagocytic capacity in both a primary (Kamperdijk et al. 1978; Kamperdijk and Hoefsmit 1979) and a secondary immune response (Kamperdijk et al. 1982). Moreover after activation they may digest *Listeria monocytogenes,* as macrophages do (Kamperdijk and Hoefsmit 1979). However, in the literature it is still an open question whether the cells of the DC familly (Langerhans cells, veiled cells, and IDCs) belong to the mononuclear phagocyte system (van Furth et al. 1972) or represent a separate cell line which originates in the bone marrow (Klinkert 1984).

As reviewed by Steinman and Inaba (1985), phenotypically and functionally differences exist between DCs and monocytes/macrophages. It has been shown that DCs are much more potent than monocytes/macrophages in T-cell proliferative responses to alloantigen and concanavalin A (Young and Steinman 1988). In a primary mixed leukocyte reaction (MLR) allogeneic DCs form multicellular aggregates with responsive T cells, while B cells and monocytes in an MLR do not form such structures within 2 days (Flechner et al. 1988). Moreover ontogenic studies using different monoclonal antibodies suggest that DCs and macrophages have a separate origin (Janossy et al. 1986). However, the DC family seems to be closely related to the monocytes/macrophages. Thus it has been shown that Langerhans cells share Fc receptors and CR1 with macrophages and express macrophage-specific markers, whereas CR1 decreases in epidermal Langerhans cells during maturation into DCs (Schuler et al. 1988). Recent observations show that partially purified blood monocytes transform into DCs during culture in serum-free medium (Peters et al. 1987). This does not, however, exclude the possibility that there is some differentiation at the stem cell level or at the level of early precursors in the bone marrow or blood. Alternatively precursors may differentiate into a DC or macrophage depending on environmental factors. There is also the question of the irreversibility of differentiation and whether DCs can subsequently become classical macrophages. Monoclonal antibodies may provide a tool to obtain pure cell populations by which these questions can be answered.

References

Axline SG, Cohn ZA (1970) In vitro induction of lysosomal enzymes by phagocytosis. J Exp Med 131:1239–1252

Balfour BM, Drexhage HA, Kamperdijk EWA, Hoefsmit ECM (1981) Antigen presenting cells, including Langerhans cells, veiled cells and interdigitating cells. In: Porter R, Whelan J (eds) Micro-environments in haemopoietic and lymphoid differentiation. Pitman Medical, London, pp 281–301

Beelen RHJ, Broekhuis-Fluitsma DM, Korn C, Hoefsmit ECM (1978) Identification of exudate resident macrophages on the basis of peroxidatic activity. J Reticuloendothelial Soc 23:103–110

Bélisle C, Sainte-Marie G (1981 a) Tridimensional study of the deep cortex of the rat lymph node. I. Topography of the deep cortex. Anat Rec 199:45–59

Bélisle C, Sainte-Marie G (1981 b) Tridimensional study of the deep cortex of the rat lymph node. II. Relation of deep cortex units to afferent lymphatic vessels. Anat Rec 199:61–72

Birbeck MS, Breathnach AS, Everall JD (1961) An electron microscopical study of basal melanocytes and high-level clear cells (Langerhans cells) in vitiligo. J Invest Dermatol 37:51–64

Blanden RV, Langman RE (1972) Cell-mediated immunity to bacterial infection in the mouse. Thymus-derived cells as effectors of acquired resistance to *Listeria monocytogenes*. Scand J Immunol 1:379–388

Bowers WE, Berkowitz MR (1986) Differentiation of dendritic cells in cultures of rat bone marrow cells. J Exp Med 163:872–883

Breel M, Mebius RE, Kraal G (1987) Dendritic cells of the mouse recognized by two monoclonal antibodies. Eur J Immunol 17:1555–1559

Chen LL, Adams JC, Steinman RM (1978) Anatomy of germinal centres in mouse spleen with special reference to follicular dendritic cells. J Cell Biol 77:148–164

Cohn ZA (1978) The activation of mononuclear phagocytes: fact, fancy and future. J Immunol 121:813–816

Cohn ZA, Benson B (1964) The differentiation of mononuclear phagocytes. Morphology, cytochemistry and biochemistry. J Exp Med 121:153–166

Collins FM (1978) Cellular antimicrobial immunity. Crit Rev Microbiol 7:27–91

Daems WT, Wisse E, Brederoo P (1969) Electron microscopy of the vacuolar apparatus. In: Dingle JT, Fell HB (eds) Lysosomes in biology and pathology, vol 1. North Holland, Amsterdam, pp 64–112

Dabrowski MI, Galkowska H, Olszewski WL (1989) Functional characteristics of veiled cells from canine prenodal lymph. Immunobiology 178:316–328

Dijkstra CD, Kamperdijk EWA, Döpp EA (1984) The ontogenetic development of the follicular dendritic cell. An ultrastructural study by means of intravenously injected horse radish peroxidase (HRP)-anti HRP complexes as marker. Cell Tissue Res 236:203–206

Dijkstra CD, Döpp EA, Joling P, Kraal G (1985) The heterogeneity of mononuclear phagocytes in lymphoid organs: distinct macrophage subpopulations in the rat recognized by monoclonal antibodies ED1, ED2 and ED3. Immunology 54:589–599

Drexhage HA, Lens JW, Cvetanov J, Kamperdijk EWA, Mullink R, Balfour BM (1980) Veiled cells, resembling Langerhans cells. In: von Furth R (ed) Mononuclear phagocytes, functional aspects. Martinus Nijhoff, The Hague, pp 235–272

Duijvestijn AM, Hoefsmit ECM (1981) Ultrastructure of the rat thymus: the micro-environment of T lymphocyte maturation. Cell Tissue Res 218:279–292

Duijvestijn AM, Barclay AN (1984) Identification of bone marrow derived Ia positive cells in the rat thymus. A morphological and cytochemical study. J Leukocyte Biol 36:561–568

Duijvestijn AM, Köhler YG, Hoefsmit ECM (1982) Interdigitating cells and macrophages in the acute involuting rat thymus. An electronmicroscopical study on phagocytic activity and population development. Cell Tissue Res 224:291–301

Eikelenboom P (1978) Dendritic cells in the rat spleen follicles. A combined immuno- and enzyme histochemical study. Cell Tissue Res 190:79–87

Farr AG, De Bruyn PPH (1975) Macrophage-lymphocyte clusters in lymph nodes: a possible substrate for cellular interactions in the immune response. Am J Anat 144:209–231

Flechner ER, Freudenthal PS, Kaplan G, Steinman RM (1988) Antigen-specific T-lymphocytes efficiently cluster with dendritic cells in the human primary mixed leucocyte reaction. Cell Immunol 111:183–195

Flemming W (1885) Studien über Regeneration der Gewerbe. Arch Mikrosk Anat 24:50–92

Flotte TJ, Springer TA, Thorbecke GJ (1982) Dendritic cell and macrophage staining by monoclonal antibodies in tissue sections and epidermal sheets. Am J Pathol 111:112–124

Fossum S (1980) The architecture of rat lymph nodes. II. Lymph node compartments. Scand J Immunol 12:411–420

Fossum S (1984) Characterization of Ia^+ non-lymphoid cells in peripheral lymph from congenitally athymic nude rats. Scand J Immunol 19:49–61

Fossum S (1988) Lymph borne dendritic leucocytes do not recirculate, but enter the lymph node paracortex to become interdigitating cells. Scand J Immunol 27:97–105

Fossum S, Rolstad B (1986) The roles of interdigitating cells and natural killer cells in the rapid injection of allogenic lymphocytes. Eur J Immunol 16:440–450

Fossum S, Vaaland JL (1983) The architecture of rat lymph nodes. I. Combined light and electron microscopy of lymph node cell types. Anat Embryol 167:229–246

Fossum S, Rolstad B, Ford WL (1984) Thymus independence, kinetics and phagocytic ability of interdigitating cells. Immunobiology 168:403–413

Gerdes J, Stein H, Mason DY, Ziegler A (1983) Human dendritic reticulum cells of lymphoid follicles: their antigenic profile and their identification as multinucleated giant cells. Virchows Arch [B] 42:161–172

Groscurth P (1980) Nonlymphatic cells in the lymph node cortex of the mouse. II. Postnatal development of the interdigitating cells and the dendritic reticular cells. Pathol Res Pract 169:235–254

Gutman GA, Weissman IL (1972) Lymphoid tissue architecture. Experimental analysis of the origin and distribution of T cells and B cells. Immunology 23:465–479

Heath TJ, Spalding HJ (1987) Pathways of lymph flow to and from the medulla of lymph nodes in sheep. J Anat 155:177–188

Heath TJ, Kerlin RL, Spalding HJ (1986) Afferent pathways of lymph flow within the popliteal node in sheep. J Anat 149:65–75

Hendriks HR, Eestermans IL, Hoefsmit ECM (1980) Depletion of macrophages and disappearance of postcapillary high endothelial venules in lymph nodes deprived of afferent lymphatic vessels. Cell Tissue Res 211:375–389

Heusermann U, Zurborn KH, Schroeder L, Stutte MJ (1980) The origin of the dendritic reticulum cell. An experimental enzyme-histochemical and electron microscopic study on the rabbit spleen. Cell Tissue Res 209:279–294

Hoefsmit ECM (1975) Mononuclear phagocytes, reticulum cells and dendritic cells in lymphoid tissues. In: van Furth R (ed) Mononuclear phagocytes in immunity, infection and pathology. Blackwell Scientific, Oxford, pp 129–146

Hoefsmit ECM, Balfour BM, Kamperdijk EWA, Cvetanov J (1979) Cells containing Birbeck granules in the lymph and the lymph node. Adv Exp Med Biol 114:389–395

Hoefsmit ECM, Kamperdijk EWA, Balfour BM (1980) Lymph node macrophages and reticulum cells in the immune response. In: van Furth R (ed) Mononuclear phagocytes, functional aspects. Martinus Nijhoff, The Hague, pp 1809–1835

Hoefsmit ECM, Duijvestijn AM, Kamperdijk EWA (1982) Relation between Langerhans cells, veiled cells and interdigitating cells. Immunobiology 161:255–265

Howard JG, Hunt SV, Gowans JL (1972) Identification of marrow-derived and thymus-derived small lymphocytes in the lymphoid tissues and thoracic duct lymph of normal rats. J Exp Med 135:200–219

Humphrey JH, Grennan D (1981) Different macrophage populations distinguished by means of fluorescent polysaccharides. Recognition and properties of marginal zone macrophages. Eur J Immunol 11:221–228

Humphrey JH, Grennan D, Sundaram V (1984) The origin of the follicular dendritic cells in the mouse and the mechanism of trapping immune complexes on them. Eur J Immunol 14:859–864

Inaba K, Steinman RM (1986) Accesory cell–T lymphocyte interactions. Antigen-dependent and -independent clustering. J Exp Med 163:247–261

Janossy G, Rofill M, Poulter LW et al. (1986) Separate ontogeny of two macrophage-like accessory cell populations in the human fetus. J Immunol 136:4354–4361

Kaiserling E, Lennert K (1974) Die interdigitierenden Reticulumzellen in menschlichen Lymphknoten. Virchows Arch [B] 16:51–61

Kamperdijk EWA, Hoefsmit ECM (1978) Birbeck granules in lymph-node macrophages. Ultramicroscopy 3:137

Kamperdijk EWA, Hoefsmit ECM (1979) The reaction of lymph node macrophages upon *Listeria monocytogenes*. Ultramicroscopy 4:160

Kamperdijk EWA, Raaymakers EM, de Leeuw JHS, Hoefsmit ECM (1978) Lymph node macrophages and reticulum cells in the immune response. I. The primary response to paratyphoid vaccine. Cell Tissue Res 192:1–23

Kamperdijk EWA, de Leeuw JHS, Hoefsmit ECM (1982) Lymph node macrophages and reticulum cells in the immune response. The secondary response to paratyphoid vaccine. Cell Tissue Res 227:277–290

Kamperdijk EWA, van den Berg M, Hoefsmit ECM (1984) Lymph node accessory cells in the immune response. The primary response to parathyphoid vaccine in rat parathymic lymph nodes. Cell Tissue Res 237:39–42

Kamperdijk EWA, Kapsenberg ML, van den Berg M, Hoefsmit ECM (1985) Characterisation of dendritic cells, isolated from normal and stimulated lymph-nodes of the rat. Cell Tissue Res 242:469–474

Kamperdijk EWA, Dijkstra CD, Döpp EA (1987a) Transport of immune complexes from the subscapular sinus into lymph node follicles of the rat. Immunobiol 174:395–405

Kamperdijk EWA, Verdaasdonk MAM, Beelen RHJ (1987b) Visual and functional expression of Ia antigen on macrophages and dendritic cells in ACI/MaI rats. Transplant Proc XIX:3024–3028

Kelly RH, Balfour BM, Armstrong JA, Griffiths S (1978) Functional anatomy of lymph nodes. II. Peripheral lymph-borne mononuclear cells. Anat Rec 190:5–22

Keuning FJ (1972) Dynamics of immunoglobulin forming cells and their precursors. In: Ballieux RE, Gruber M, Seyen HG (eds) Immunoglobulins. North Holland, Amsterdam, pp 1–14

Klinkert WEF (1984) Rat bone marrow precursors develop into dendritic accessory cells under the influence of a conditioned medium. Immunobiology 168:414–424

Kraal G, Breel M, Janse M, Bruin G (1986) Langerhans cells, veiled cells and interdigitating cells in the mouse recognized by a monoclonal antibody. J Exp Med 163:981–997

Lens JW, Drexhage HA, Benson W, Balfour BM (1983) A study of cells present in lymph draining from a contact allergic reaction in pigs sensititzed to DNFB. Immunology 49:415–422

Levine S, Cacho P, Sowinski R, Thelmo WL (1983) Depletion of lymphoid tissues by tilorone. Ultrastructure and synergistic interaction with anti lymphocyte serum. Am J Pathol 111:174–183

McGregor DD, Logie PS (1975) Macrophage–lymphocyte interactions in infection immunity. In: van Furth R (ed) Mononuclear phagocytes in immunity, infection and pathology. Blackwell Scientific, Oxford, pp 631–649

Merighi A, Galloni M, Gobetto A (1986) Architecture of swine lymph node: light and scanning electron microscopical studies. Exp Biol 46:101–110

Nieuwenhuis P, Ford WL (1976) Comparative migration of B and T lymphocytes in the rat spleen and lymph nodes. Cell Immunol 23:254–267

Nossal GJV, Abbot A, Mitchell J, Lummus Z (1968) Antigens in immunity. XV. Ultrastructural features of antigen capture in primary and secondary lymphoid follicles. J Exp Med 172:277–290

Peters JH, Ruhl S, Friedrichs D (1987) Veiled accessory cells deduced from monocytes. Immunobiology 176:154–166

Pugh CW, MacPherson GG, Steer HW (1983) Characterization of non-lymphoid cells derived from rat peripheral lymph. J Exp Med 157:1758–1779

Rausch E, Kaiserling E, Goos M (1977) Langerhans cells and interdigitating reticulum cells in the thymus dependent region in human dermatopathic lymphadenitis. Virchows Arch [B] 25:327–343

Sainte-Marie G, Peng FS (1979) Morphology of the extrafollicular zone and pseudo-follicles of the rat lymph node and their role in lymphocyte traffic. Adv Exp Med Biol 114:59–64

Sainte-Marie G, Peng FS, Bélisle C (1982) Overall architecture and pattern of lymph flow in the rat lymph node. Am J Anat 164:275–309

Schuler G, Inaba K, Witmer M, Steinman R (1988) The immunologic properties of epidermal Langerhans cells. In: Permis B, Silverstein SC, Vogel HJ (eds) Processing and presentation of antigens. Academic, New York, pp 179–185

Silberberg-Sinakin I, Thorbecke GJ, Baer RL, Rosenthal SA, Berezowsky V (1976) Antigen-bearing Langerhans cells in skin, dermal lymphatics and in lymph nodes. Cell Immunol 25:137–151

Smith JP, Kosco MH, Tew JG, Szakal AK (1988) Thy-1 positive tingible body macrophages (TBM) in mouse lymph nodes. Anat Rec 222:380–390
Spector WG, Reichhold N, Ryan GB (1970) Degradation of granuloma inducing micro-organisms by macrophages. J Pathol 101:339–354
Steinman RM, Cohn ZA (1973) Identification of a novel cell type in peripheral lymphoid organs of mice. I. Morphology, quantitation, tissue distribution. J Exp Med 137:1142–1162
Steinman RM, Inaba K (1985) Stimulation of the primary mixed leucocyte reaction. Crit Rev Immunol 5:331–338
Swartzendruber DC, Congdon CC (1963) Electron microscope observations on tingible body macrophages in mouse spleen. J Cell Biol 19:641–649
Szakal AK, Holmes KL, Tew JG (1983) Transport of immune complexes from the subcapsular sinus to lymph node follicles on the surface of nonphagocytic cells, including cells with dendritic morphology. J Immunol 131:1714–1727
Takeya M, Hsiao L, Takahashi K (1987) A new monoclonal antibody, TRPM-3, binds specifically to certain rat macrophage populations: immunohistochemical and immunoelectron microscopic analysis. J Leukocyte Biol 41:187–195
Tew JG, Thorbecke GJ, Steinman RM (1982) Dendritic cells in the immune response. Characteristics and recommended nomenclature. J Reticuloendothel Soc 31:371–380
Tew JG, Mandel TE, Phipps RP, Szakal AK (1984) Tissue localization and retention of antigen in relation to the immune response. Am J Anat 170:407–420
Unanue ER, Beller DI, Lu CY, Allen PM (1984) Antigen presentation: comments on its regulation and mechanism. J Immunol 132:1–5
van Furth R, Cohn ZA, Hirsch JG, Humphrey JH, Spector WG, Langevoort HL (1972) The mononuclear phagocyte system: a new classification of macrophages, monocytes and their precursor cells. Bull WHO 46:845–852
Veerman AJP, van Ewijk W (1975) White pulp compartments in the spleen of rats and mice. Cell Tissue Res 156:416–441
Veldman JE (1970) Histophysiology and electron microscopy of the immune system. Acad. Thesis, Groningen, The Netherlands
Villena A, Zapata A, Rivera-Pomar JM, Barrutia MG, Fongua J (1983) Structure of the non-lymphoid cells during the postnatal development of the rat lymph nodes, fibroblastic reticulum cells and interdigitating cells. Cell Tissue Res 229:219–232
Yoffey JM, Courtice FC (1956) Lymphatics, lymph and lymphoid tissue. Edward Arnold, London, p 177
Young JW, Steinman RM (1988) Accessory cell requirements for the mixed-leukocyte reaction and polyclonal mitogens as studied with a new technique for enriching blood dendritic cells. Cell Immunol 111:167–182

Phenotypic Characterization of Macrophages in Non-neoplastic Lymph Nodes

S. BÖDEWADT-RADZUN, H.-H. WACKER, H. J. RADZUN, and M. R. PARWARESCH

1 Introduction

Lymphatic tissue in general, and lymph nodes in particular, are the physiological sites of the specific immune response to soluble and particulate foreign matter, where close interaction between macrophages, accessory cells, and immunocompetent lymphocytes is required. At least two types of antigen arrive at lymph nodes, where they are trapped, processed, and presented to the specific immunocompetent lymphocytes. The soluble molecules are conveyed by the lymph stream and can be directly bound by the accessory cells. In the case of complex or particulate antigens, preparatory digestion is necessary in order to resolve at least one part of the components and soluble molecules following the usual path of phagocytosis accomplished by the typical macrophages. A considerable fraction of the antigens is destroyed by lytic processes. Soluble fragments are bound by the accessory cells. This means that macrophages may be relevant to the development of a specific immune response (UNANUE and ASKONAS 1968; BENACERRAF 1988) and constitute a regular cellular component of normal and reactive lymph nodes. Nevertheless, in the absence of particulate antigens macrophages do not seem to be indispensable for the establishment of the specific immune response. From this it may be concluded that although macrophages do occur within lymphatic tissue and lymph nodes subjected to everyday antigenic stimulation, their appearance in notable quantities indicates a special situation which excedes the boundaries of a usual immune response. Indeed, in contrast to general expectations, the number of professional macrophages in lymph nodes is limited and is far below that in the spleen, where macrophages represent constant constituents of the red pulp. This means either that phagocytosis does not occur within normal lymph nodes, or that lymph nodes do not represent a preferential site of filtration of particulate matter. One way to analyze lymph node macrophages is to follow the morphofunctional compartments liable to be populated by the cells of the monocyte/macrophage system subsumed under the term "macrophages." This is the approach taken within this chapter: first the normal situation is considered, followed by the lymph node responses to microbial or other primers of an inflammatory reaction (lymphadenitis).

2 Macrophages of Normal Lymph Nodes and in Lymphadenitis

2.1 Lymph Node Capsule

2.1.1 Macrophages of Normal Lymph Node Capsule

Like other connective tissue sites, the lymph node capsule is equipped with a resident type of macrophage randomly distributed throughout the tissue. Under normal noninflammatory conditions these macrophages generally show no signs of phagocytosis or functional activity. They are only detectable when stained with specific immune reagents. The majority of these macrophages have a fusiform structure with long, stretched cytoplasm, and are closely packed among dense bundles of collagenous fibers. Such monocyte-derived potential phagocytes have been referred to as "histiocytes" or "resident macrophages." They are a constant cellular constituent of connective tissue in practically every organ. These cells reveal positivity for nonspecific acid esterase, acid phosphatase, and lysozyme. Using antibodies against lysozyme or monocyte-derived acid esterase, an identical immunohistochemical pattern is produced.

Resident macrophages of connective tissue have an extremely low mitotic rate and are hardly ever positive to the proliferation nuclear antigen detectable with the monoclonal antibody Ki-67 (GERDES et al. 1984), indicating the immediate terminal differentiation. The immunophenotype (Tables 1, 2) of such monocyte-derived cells in lymph node capsule under physiological conditions can be given as positive to CD11c (Ki-M1), Ki-M2, Ki-M3, Ki-M5, Ki-M6, Ki-M7, Ki-M8, OKM1, and Mono1, and as negative to Ki-M4, R4/23, Ki-M9, CD1, CD4, and S-100 (Fig. 1). Antigens expressed by these cells are

Table 1. Monoclonal antibodies and polyclonal antisera[a] used for the immunophenotyping of the monocyte/macrophage system within lymphatic tissue

Antibody	Major specificities	Source
Ki-M1 (CD11c)	Mononuclear phagocytes, IDCs	Behring, own lab.
Ki-M2	Mononuclear phagocytes	Behring, own lab.
Ki-M3	Mononuclear phagocytes	Own laboratory
Ki-M4	FDCs	Behring, own lab.
Ki-M5	Mononuclear phagocytes, granulocytes	Behring, own lab.
Ki-M6 (CD68)	Mononuclear phagocytes	Behring, own lab.
Ki-M7 (CD68)	Mononuclear phagocytes, granulocytes	Behring, own lab.
Ki-M8	Mononuclear phagocytes	Behring, own lab.
Ki-M9	Sinus-lining cells	Own laboratory
OKM1 (CD11b)	Mononuclear phagocytes, granulocytes	Ortho
Mono1	Mononuclear phagocytes, granulocytes	Coulter
R4/23	FDCs	Dakopatts
OKT4 (CD4)	Helper/inducer T cells	Ortho
OKT6 (CD1a)	Cortical thymocytes, IDCs	Ortho
Mac387	Mononuclear phagocytes, granulocytes	Dakopatts
Anti-S-100[a]	IDCs	Dakopatts
Anti-lysozyme[a]	Mononuclear phagocytes, granulocytes	Dakopatts

FDCs, follicular dendritic (reticulum) cells; IDCs, interdigitating dendritic (reticulum) cells

Table 2. Immunophenotype of cells of the monocyte/macrophage system in lymphatic tissue

Antibody	Capsule M_ϕ	Sinus M_ϕ	Medullary pulp M_ϕ	T zone		B follicle	
				M_ϕ	IDCs	M_ϕ	FDCs
Ki-M1	+	+	+	+	+	+	–
Ki-M2	+	+	+	+	–	–	–
Ki-M3	+	+	–	–	–	+	–
Ki-M4	–	–	–	–	–	–	+
Ki-M5	+	+	+	+	–	+	–
Ki-M6	+	+	+	+	–	+	–
Ki-M7	+	+	+	+	–	+	–
Ki-M8	+	+	+	+	–	–	–
Ki-M9	–	–	–	–	–	–	–
OKM1	+	+	–	–	–	+	–
Mono1	+	+	–	+	–	–	+
R4/23	–	–	–	–	–	–	+
OKT4	(+)	(+)	(+)	–	–	(+)	–
OKT6	–	–	–	–	+	–	–
Mac387	+	+	+	+	–	+	–
Anti-S-100	–	–	–	–	+	–	–
Anti-lysozyme	+	+	+	+	–	+	–

M_ϕ, macrophages; IDCs, interdigitating dendritic (reticulum) cells; FDCs, follicular dendritic (reticulum) cells

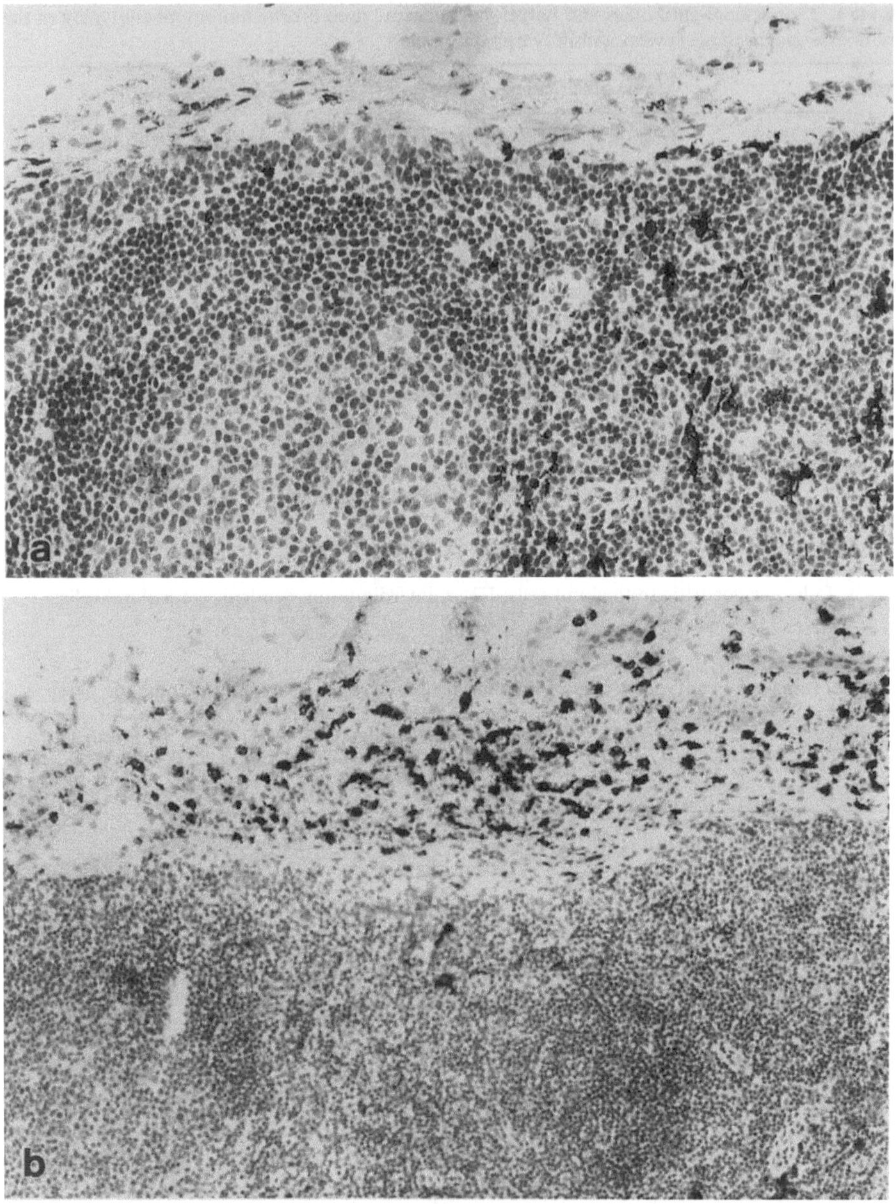

Fig. 1 a, b. Macrophages of lymph node capsule under physiological conditions (**a** ×176) and in a case of perilymphadenitis (**b** ×88). Cryostat section of lymph node, immunoperoxidase staining with Ki-M8

localized on cytoplasmic membrane. Exceptions are the monoclonal antibodies Ki-M6, Ki-M7, and Ki-M8, which recognize intracytoplasmic antigens.

2.1.2 Macrophages in Perilymphadenitis

Inflammatory processes involving lymph node capsule are common (Fig. 1) and do not differ from inflammatory processes at other tissue sites. The chemotactic stimulation exerted upon blood monocytes gives rise to enhanced immigration of blood monocytes into the tissue, where they constitute the tissue compartment of exudate macrophages (BEELEN et al. 1977). Typical inflammatory-type macrophages are rounded and have a broad cytoplasm and an oval or kidney-shaped nucleus of low chromatin content. They are richly equipped with lysosomes or phagosomes and have a high content of acid hydrolases such as nonspecific acid esterase, acid phosphatase, and lysozyme. Inflammatory macrophages reveal a strong positivity to the antigens recognizable by the monoclonal antibodies CD11c (Ki-M1), Ki-M2, Ki-M5, OKM1, and Mono1. In addition to these membrane-bound antigens, a few intracytoplasmic antigens are detectable with Ki-M6, Ki-M7, and Ki-M8, as well as with Mac387. A negative reaction is encountereed for the monoclonal antibodies CD1, CD4, Ki-M4, R4/23, Ki-M9, and S-100. Under inflammatory conditions not only abundant full-blown macrophages are detectable, but also a good number of recently immigrated blood monocytes which show the typical immunophenotype of blood monocytes as described by RADZUN (1985) and RADZUN et al. (1988).

2.2 Lymphatic Sinuses

2.2.1 Macrophages of Normal Lymphatic Sinuses

Under noninflammatory conditions, lymph node sinuses contain no or only a few professional macrophages. They may, however, be densely populated by mononuclear cells consisting of lymphocytes, dendritic cells, and a few macrophages. The overwhelming majority of cells present within the sinuses of normal human and rodent lymph nodes are the sinus-lining cells and the underlying myofibroblasts, which belong to the structural constituents of the sinus. None of these cells can be considered as macrophages or histiocytes since they are nonphagocytic and lack phenotypic markers of professional phagocytes.

Single macrophages do occur in some normal lymph node sinuses. Their macrophage nature is documented by signs of phagocytosis, a high content of lysosomal acid phosphatase and β-glucuronidase, and their strong activity for nonspecific acid esterase. Such macrophages reveal positivity to CD11c (Ki-M1), Ki-M2, Ki-M3, Ki-M5, Ki-M6, Ki-M7, Ki-M8, OKM1, and Mono1. They are regularly negative to Ki-M4, Ki-M9, R4/23, CD1, and S-100.

2.2.2 *Sinus Macrophages in Lymphadenitis*

In cases of *nonspecific lymphadenitis,* lymph node sinuses are partly filled with monocyte-derived cells, preferentially with exudate macrophages. These cells are densely packed among the structural constituents of the sinus. Such macrophages have a rounded clear cytoplasm, and a centrally located, slightly indented, and weakly stained nucleus. The majority of the exudate macrophages within the sinuses are positive for nonspecific acid esterase, β-glucuronidase, acid phosphatase, and lysozyme.

Despite the enormous diversity of the macrophages the reaction pattern of these cells within the lymphatic sinuses remains more or less identical throughout the various forms of reactive alteration, with so-called simple sinus histiocytosis (LENNERT 1961; SYMMERS 1978). In inflammatory processes such as chronic nonspecific lymphadenitis there are also a large number of newly immigrated monocytes within the dilated sinuses. These cells are positive to CD11c (Ki-M1), Ki-M2, Ki-M3, Ki-M5, Ki-M6, Ki-M7, Ki-M8, OKM1, and Mono1. In contrast the monoclonal antibodies recognizing CD1 and S-100 give a negative reaction in these cells.

True macrophages of sinuses seen in various forms of lymphadenitis have to be strictly distinguished from cells seen in *immature sinus histiocytosis* and in *sinus catarrh.* The former cells are positive to antibodies recognizing CD19 (Immature B lymphocytes), Ki-B3, and Ki-B5 (pan-B cell reagents) and to immunoglobulins (Fig. 2). They are mostly IgG positive and IgM negative and have been clearly classified as mature B lymphocytes (STEIN et al. 1984). Myelomonocytic or macrophage-specific antigens are not detectable on these cells. In cases of sinus catarrh there may be a loosely intermingled small number of macrophages, but the overwhelming majority of the cells filling the dilated sinuses are sinus-lining cells. They are regularly negative to the above-mentioned antibodies, including anti-lysozyme, and other typical markers of macrophages. They are easily discernible due to their specific reactivity with the monoclonal antibody Ki-M9 and to some extent also Ki-M4. In addition, antibodies recognizing desmoplakin are reactive with these cells. Except for follicular dendritic (reticulum) cells, sinus-lining cells are the only lymph node cell type with membrane desmosomes.

Although epithelioid cells, as a specialized form of blood monocyte, occur in a wide range of reactive lymph node disorders such as Piringer-type lymphadenitis, tuberculosis, sarcoidosis, brucellosis, and syphilis, the occurrence of such cells within sinuses is rare. They are sometimes present in tuberculosis, small groups being observed within the sinuses.

An interesting although incompletely understood entity is the lesion variously called giant cell sinus reticulosis (ROBB-SMITH 1947), hemophagocytic lymphadenopathy, or sinus histiocytosis with massive lymphadenopathy (ROSAI and DORFMAN 1969). Sinuses are dilated and partly populated by a variable accumulation of cells generally regarded as macrophages, together with a large number of lymphocytes, erythrocytes, and other blood cells. The immunophenotype of these cells is still unclear. It is, however, known that they reveal an

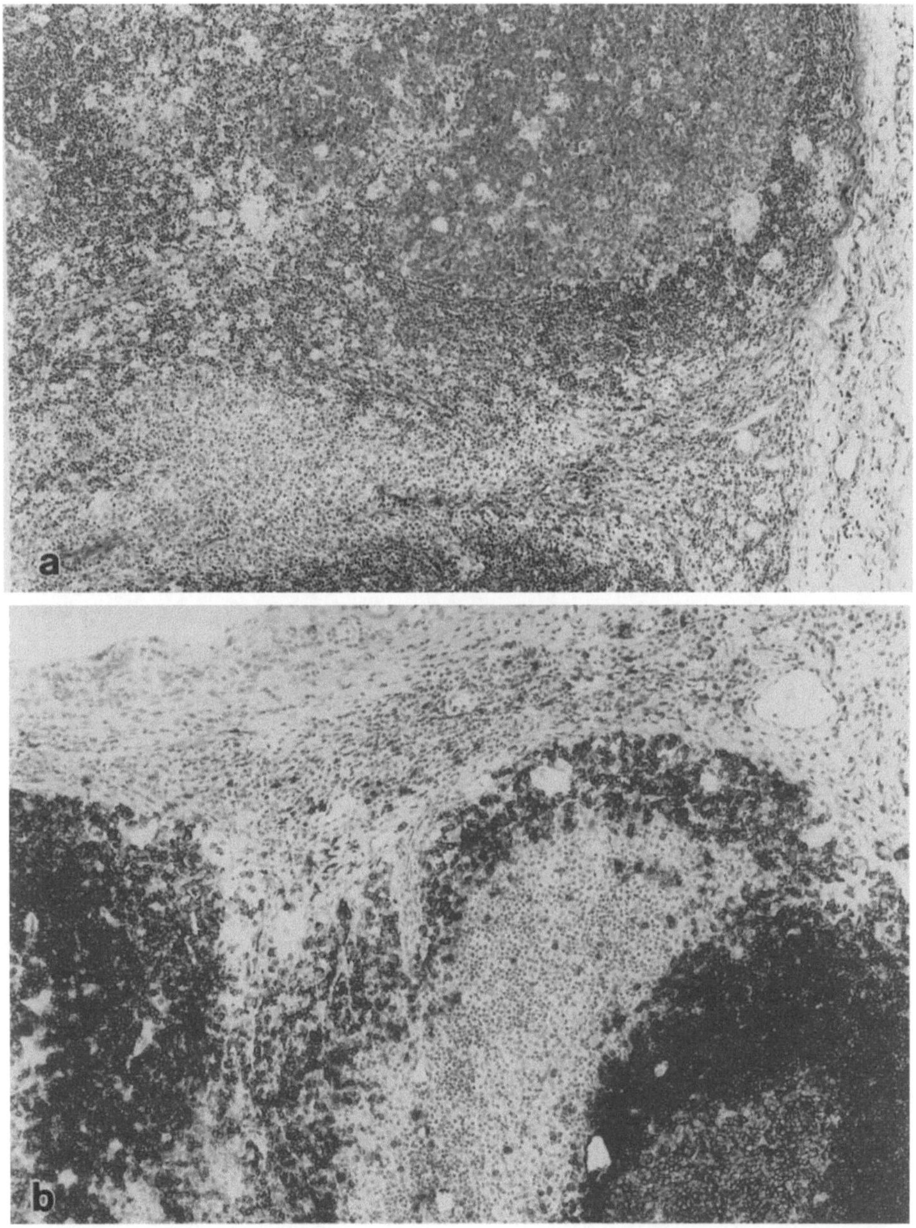

Fig. 2 a, b. Immature sinus histiocytosis in a case of Piringer's lymphadenitis with monocytoid B lymphocytes in paratrabecular and marginal sinuses. **a** paraffin section of lymph node, Giemsa staining, ×44. **b** cryostat section of lymph node, immunoperoxidase staining with CD22 (B lymphocyte specific), ×88

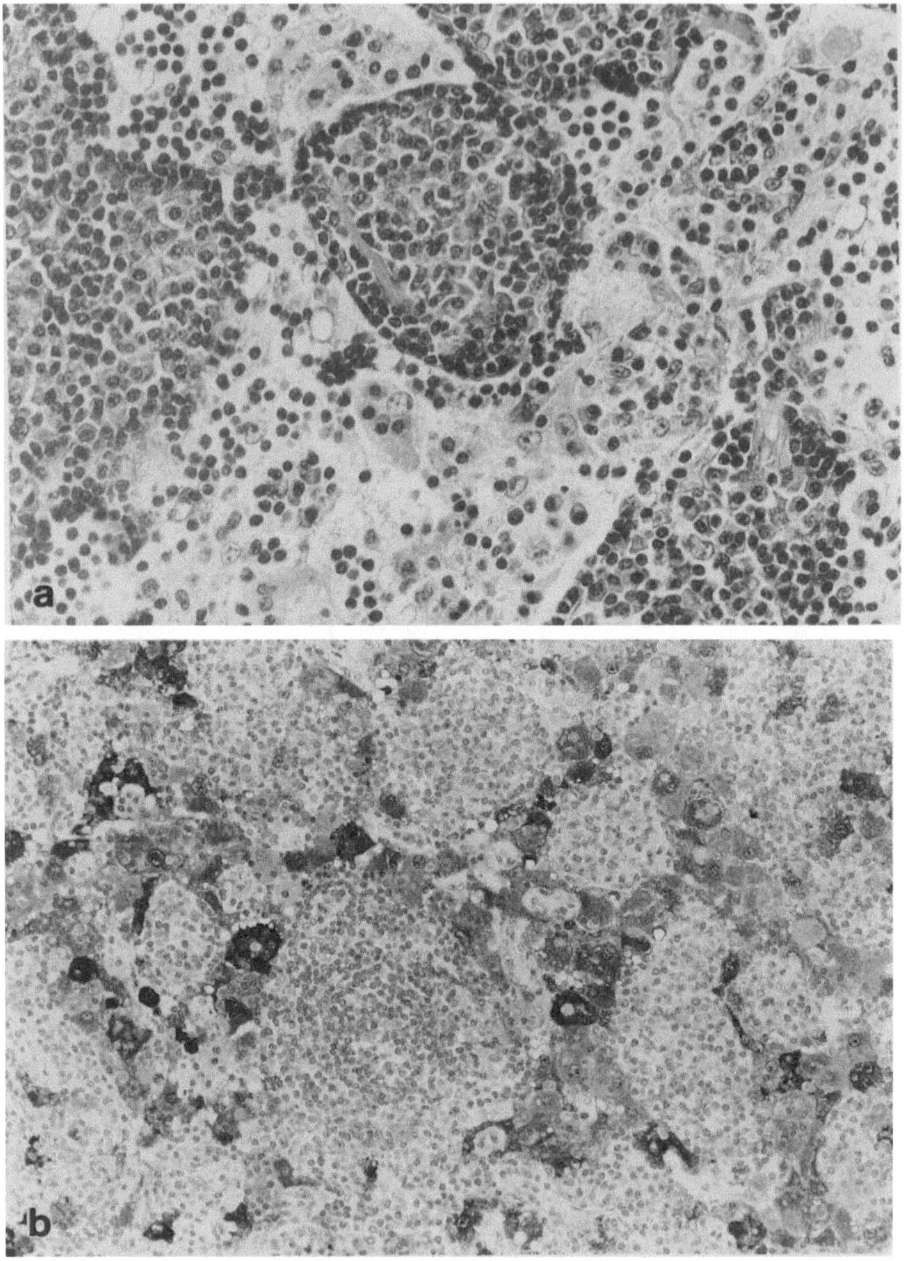

Fig. 3 a, b. Rosai-Dorfman lymphadenopathy with S-100 positive cells showing lymphophagocytosis within sinuses. **a** paraffin section of lymph node, Giemsa staining, × 352. **b** cryostat section of lymph node, immunoperoxidase staining, × 88

unexpected reactivity to S-100. This antibody reacts with the phagocytosing cells of Rosai-Dorfman lymphadenopathy (Fig. 3).

In Whipple's disease, pneumatosis of the lymph node, cholegranulomatous lymphadenitis, and lymphadenopathy secondary to lymphangiography using iodized oil (Robb-Smith 1947), a large number of macrophages accumulate in the sinuses. In addition, lymphadenopathy rich in macrophages is observed after administration of polyvinylpyrrolidone (povidone) and following inoculation of polymeric organosilicone compounds in cosmetic surgery or for the moulding of prosthetic joints. These macrophages express major histocompatibility class II antigens, complement receptor, CD4, lysozyme, and anti-α-1 antitrypsin. In addition, they are reactive with CD11c (Ki-M1), Ki-M2, Ki-M3, Ki-M5, Ki-M6, Ki-M7, Ki-M8, OKM1, and Mac387.

2.3 Medullary Pulp

2.3.1 Macrophages of Normal Medullary Pulp

Under normal steady state conditions the perisinusoidal medullary pulp cords consist of small lymphocytes, plasma cells, and a small number of macrophages. Such phagocytes display the usual phenotype of professional macrophages, being positive to CD11c (Ki-M1), Ki-M2, Ki-M5, and especially Ki-M8 (Fig. 4). Among other macrophage-specific markers Mac387,

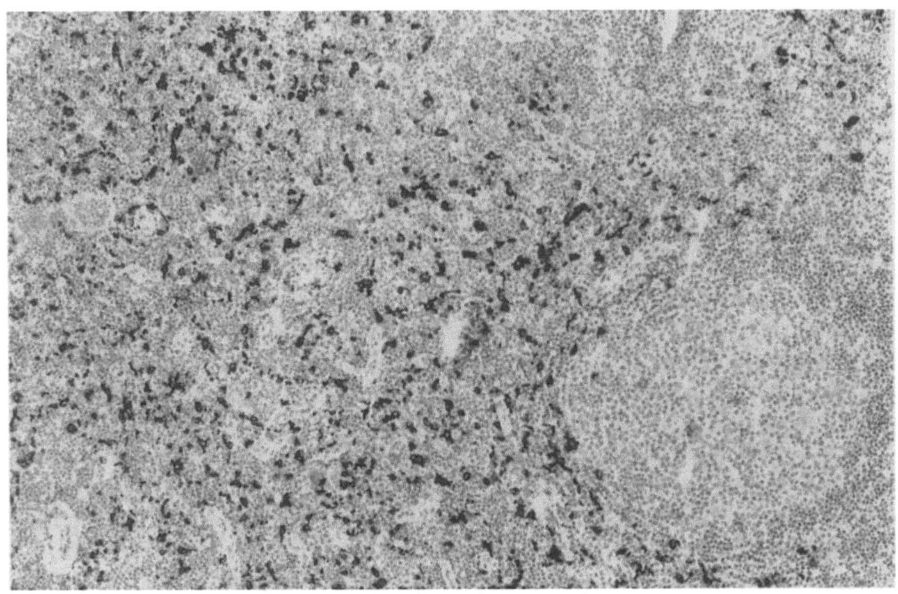

Fig. 4. Macrophages of normal medullary pulp immunostained with the monoclonal antibody Ki-M8. Cryostat section of lymph node, immunoperoxidase staining, ×88

lysozyme, nonspecific acid esterase, acid phosphatase, and β-glucuronidase are also positive. Monoclonal antibodies Ki-M4, OKM1, Mono1, S-100, and CD1 are regularly negative.

Under normal conditions typical dendritic (reticulum) cells are not detectable in this area. This applies to both the B-accessory and the T-accessory type of dendritic cell.

2.3.2 Macrophages of Medullary Pulp in Lymphadenitis

Assuming that a notable antigen influx into the lymph node may cause alterations that can be subsumed under the designation lymphadenitis, a modest variation is to be expected in the macrophage composition of the medullary pulp. This consists of a mild increase in the density and distribution of professional phagocytes positive to CD11c (Ki-M1), Ki-M2, Ki-M5, and Ki-M8. In addition, there is typically an increase in the number of dendritic cells, which are in charge of antigen transport from the sinus to the functional compartments of the lymphatic tissue. In adequately selected samples a minor number of dendritic cells with positivity for Ki-M4, R4/23, Ki-B1p [recognizing follicle mantle lymphocytes and follicular dendritic (reticulum) cells in paraffin-embedded tissue], and Ki-M9 may be detectable. In addition, these cells are positive to HLA-DR, Fc receptor, and complement receptors.

As evidence of the enhancement of antigen presentation to the T lymphocytes, a restricted number of dendritic cells positive to CD1, S-100, and CD11c (Ki-M1) may be observed.

In sinus histiocytosis with massive lymphadenopathy as described by Rosai and Dorfman (1969), an entity that may represent a reactive lymph node disease, there is an immense increase in S-100 reactive cells within the pulp cords (Fig. 5), mostly lacking any signs of phagocytosis. Cells with an identical immunophenotype but having incorporated large numbers of blood cells (preferentially lymphocytes and erythrocytes) are detectable within the sinuses, which are only partly preserved, being partly replaced by fibrotic areas or collapsed.

Cases of lymphadenitis caused by application of oils, polyvinylpyrrolidone, silicone, or various types of infectious agent are regularly associated with a massive accumulation of macrophage-type cells within the pulp cords. In the case of foreign substances, particulate matter, and indigestible agents, the majority of these cells are professional macrophages positive to CD11c (Ki-M1), Ki-M5, and Ki-M8 as well as lysozyme and Mac387; acid hydrolases are also positive in these cells.

Some infections, such as tuberculosis, sarcoidosis, Piringer's lymphadenitis, leprosy, and syphilis may be associated with epithelioid cells. The underlying specific immunological mechanisms leading to the evolution of epithelioid cells from monocytes are only poorly understood. It is, however, known that specific T-cell clones are significantly involved in the generation of epithelioid cells. Small epithelioid cell clusters occur in cases of Piringer's lymphadenitis, which is usually caused by toxoplasmosis or infectious mononucleosis.

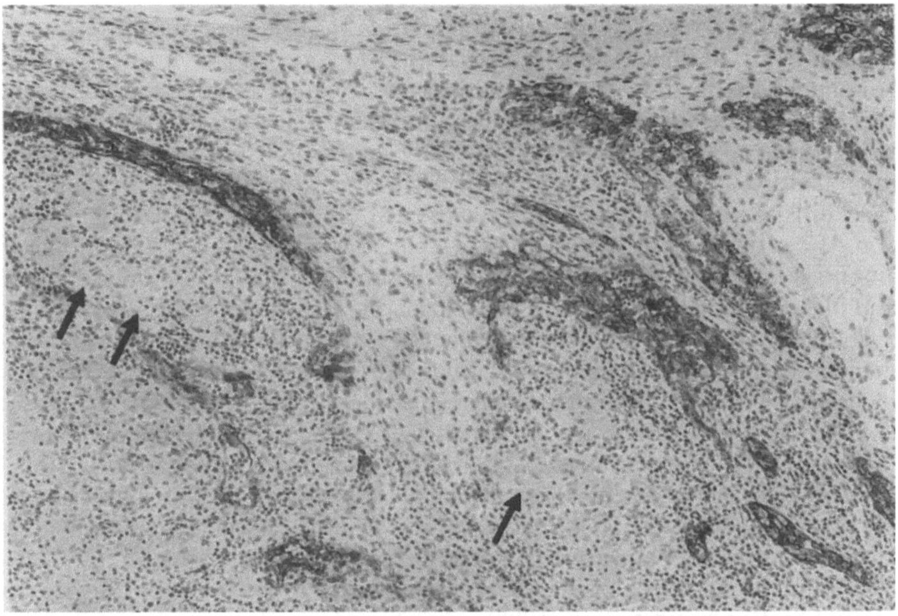

Fig. 5. Rosai-Dorfman lymphadenopathy showing an increase in phagocytosing cells (*arrows*) within the medullary pulp displaying Ki-M9 positive sinus structures. Cryostat section of lymph node, immunoperoxidase staining, × 88

Epithelioid cell granulomas with or without caseation may be caused by tuberculosis, sarcoidosis, berylliosis, syphilis, tuberculoid leprosy, and Hodgkin's disease. Similar reactions may be present in lymph nodes draining carcinomas or even within the tumor tissue itself, preferentially in seminomas and lymphoepithelial carcinomas of the larynx.

The immunophenotypes of the cluster-type and the granuloma-type epithelioid cell reaction are essentially the same. The main cell surface antigens expressed by these cells are detectable by the monoclonal antibodies Ki-M1, Ki-M6, and Mono1. As compared with professional macrophages the activity for nonspecific acid esterase is strongly diminished. Such cells develop a specific isoenzyme of acid phosphatase which is not inhibitible by the addition of tartrate.

Another type of lymph node inflammation that has a vast variety of causes is so-called necrotizing granulomatous lymphadenitis. The characteristic necrotizing nontuberculous inflammatory alterations are seen in yersinial mesenteric lymphadenitis and in tularemia. They are characterized by a central necrosis which mostly contains a scattered number of neutrophils and monocytes and is closely surrounded by macrophges. In contrast to epithelioid cells, these macrophages are not negative but strongly positive to Ki-M8. Like epithelioid cells, they are positive to Mono1. The reactivity of Ki-M8 is a useful differential diagnostic aid in separating epithelioid cell type from granulomatous necrotizing forms of lymphadenitis.

A special type of necrotizing lymphadenitis has been described by KIKUCHI et al. (1977). In this lesion, which is accompanied by a mostly cervical lymphadenopathy in young women, there are irregular necrotic foci within the lymph nodes, mostly surrounded by macrophages. In contrast to other necrotizing types of lymphadenitis, hardly any neutrophils are present. Another main feature of this type of lymphadenitis is the presence of foci of mononuclear cells recently identified as derivatives of the monocyte/macrophage system (FACCHETTI et al. 1988). These cells, originally called lymphoblasts (LENNERT and REMMELE 1958) and later designated T-associated plasma cells and plasmacytoid T cells (MÜLLER-HERMELINK et al. 1973, 1983; FELLER et al. 1983; HORNY et al. 1986), are best called plasmacytoid monocytes, as recommended by FACCHETTI et al. (1988). Such cells have been repeatedly observed in various types of myeloproliferative disorder. Even in cases in which the lymph nodes were not clearly involved, there were a considerable number of these foci. The differentiation of plasmacytoid monocytes from professional macrophages may present some problems. However, whereas macrophages are positive to CD11c (Ki-M1), Ki-M8, and Mono1, plasmacytoid monocytes lack these properties and are positive, in contrast, to CD4, Ki-M2, and Ki-M6. The immunophenotype of plasmacytoid monocytes has been thoroughly described by FACCHETTTI et al. (1988). They have been shown to be positive for the monoclonal antibodies LN2 (B lymphocytes and mononuclear phagocytes), MT1 (T lymphocytes, mononuclear phagocytes, and granulocytes), OKM5 (monocytes and platelets), EBM11 (mononuclear phagocytes), Y1-82A (mononuclear phagocytes), Ki-M6, Ki-M7, KP1 (mononuclear phagocytes), and Leu-M1 (granulocytes and endothelia), and to express HLA class II antigens. In addition, the monoclonal antibody OKT9, which recognizes transferrin receptor, is positive. This is also the case for the monoclonal antibodies which recognize CD45, the leukocyte common antigen.

2.4 T Zone

2.4.1 Macrophages of Normal Lymphatic T Zone

The paracortical area of lymph nodes is populated by dense accumulations of T lymphocytes containing a small number of macrophages, while the majority of the nonphagocytosing myelomonocytic cell types are so-called interdigitating dendritic (reticulum) cells which are closely surrounded by rosetting T cells (Fig. 6). These interdigitating dendritic (reticulum) cells are distinguished by their typical reactivity for CD1 and S-100. The majority of them also react positively to CD11c (Ki-M1). Professional macrophages positive to CD11c (Ki-M1), Ki-M8, and Mono1 may be present in limited numbers within the T zone under normal conditions.

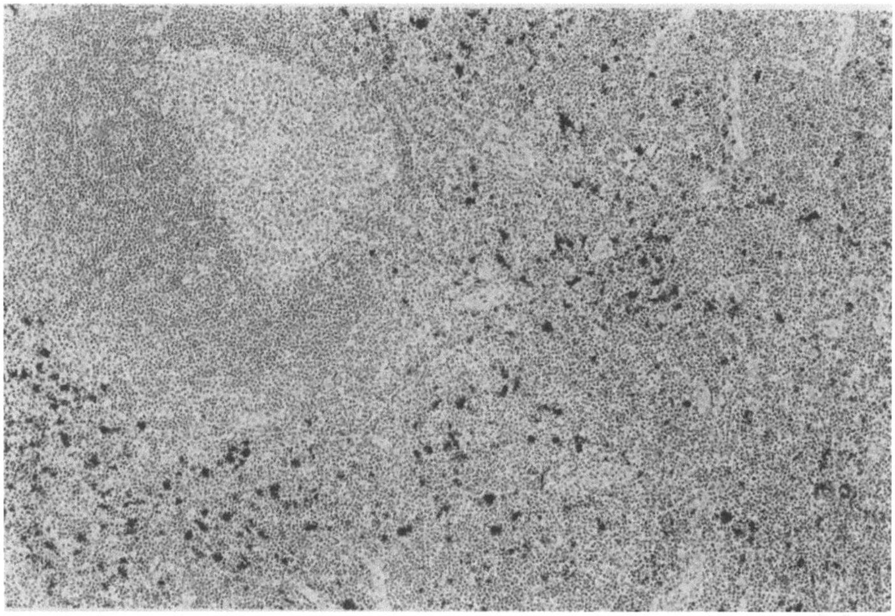

Fig. 6. Interdigitating dendritic (reticulum) cells immunostained with the polyclonal S-100 antiserum within the paracortical T zone. Paraffin section of lymph node, immunoperoxidase staining, ×44

2.4.2 T Zone Macrophages in Lymphadenitis

An exaggerated influx into lymph nodes of antigen-presenting cells for cellular immunity is a common finding in skin diseases. The diagnostic histological picture in such diseases has been designated dermatopathic lymphadenitis (Fig. 7). In characteristic cases the subcapsular and peritrabecular sinuses are dilated and contain a large number of mononuclear cells, mostly veiled cells, and a small number of Langerhans cells. In addition, some professional macrophages may be present. Such cells extend into the pulp. The most striking finding is the accentuation of the T zone, which is often sharply demarcated against the surrounding areas. Within the T zone there are clusters of interdigitating dendritic (reticulum) cells closely surrounded by rosetting T lymphocytes. The broad and clear cytoplasm of interdigitating dendritic (reticulum) cells render them visible even at low magnification. In addition, scattered professional macrophages are encountered, of which some contain melanin and hemosiderin in their typical phagosomes. This is also reflected by the immunohistochemical findings. On the one hand there are clusters of cells positive to CD1, CD11c (Ki-M1), and S-100. On the other hand there are typical macrophages positive to CD11c (Ki-M1), Ki-M2, Ki-M5, Ki-M6, Ki-M7, and Ki-M8. In addition, these macrophages possess large amounts of hydrolytic enzymes and lysozyme. The professional macrophages are distinguished by a strong reactivity to Mac387.

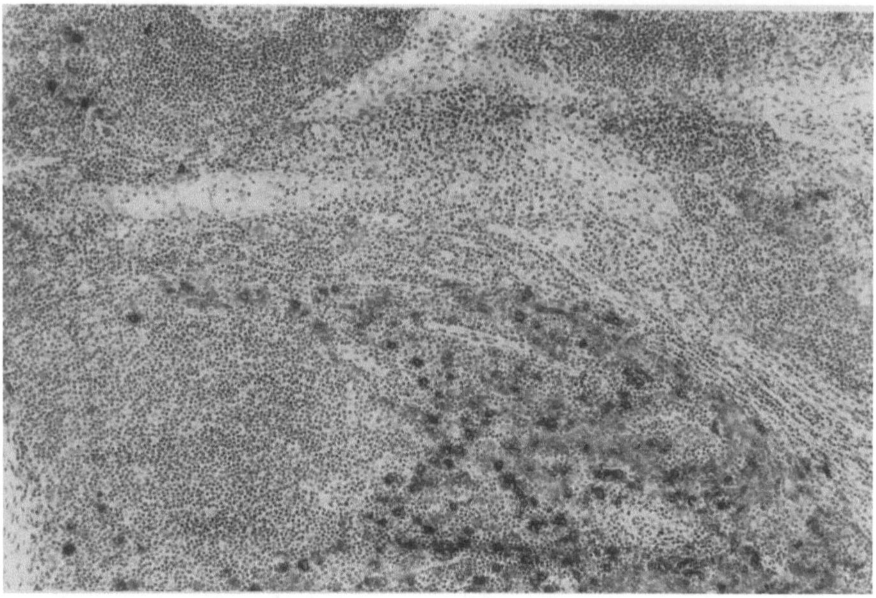

Fig. 7. Dermatopathic lymphadenitis showing an increase in antigen-presenting cells for cellular immunity immunostained with the monoclonal antibody OKT6. Cryostat section of lymph node, immunoperoxidase staining, × 88

Given that less than 1% of the interdigitating dendritic (reticulum) cells and the typical macrophages found in such cases of dermatopathic lymphadenitis are positive to the proliferation-associated nuclear antigen Ki-67, the increase in such cells must be explained by enhanced influx, most probably via afferent lymphatics. Local proliferation may occur but can hardly account for the large number of dendritic cells and macrophages (PARWARESCH and WACKER 1984; FOSSUM 1988).

The T zone is also involved in more or less all other types of lymphadenitis, including Piringer's type, necrotizing granulomatous, and tuberculous lymphadenitis. The immunophenotype of monocyte/macrophage-derived cells in such cases is identical to that of those found in other sites of the pulp.

2.5 B Follicles

2.5.1 Macrophages of Normal Lymphatic B Follicles

Primary follicles usually lack phagocytosing cells, though a small number of follicular dendritic (reticulum) cells can be detected in these structures. Secondary follicles may contain a considerable number of nonlymphocytic cells, including professional macrophages and follicular dendritic (reticulum) cells. The macrophages found within the germinal centers have been referred to as

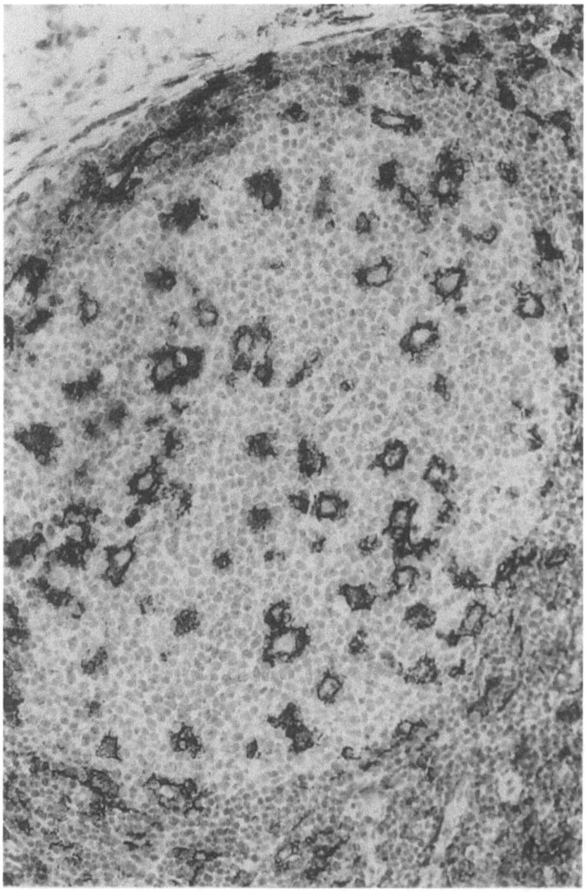

Fig. 8. Starry-sky macrophages of normal lymphatic B follicles immunostained with the monoclonal antibody Ki-M1. Cryostat section of lymph node, immunoperoxidase staining, ×176

tingible body macrophages or starry-sky macrophages (Fig. 8). Immunohistochemically these cells are distinguished by a strong reactivity to CD11c (Ki-M1) and Ki-M6, whereas they are regularly negative to Ki-M2, Ki-M5, and Ki-M8 as well as CD1, CD4, and Mono1.

Clearly distinct from the professional macrophages of germinal centers are the so-called follicular dendritic (reticulum) cells, which form a dense network via the desmosomal junctions of their cytoplasmic processes. These cells ensure the immune stimulation of B lymphocytes during secondary immune reaction to recall antigen (TEW et al. 1979; SZAKAL et al. 1983; UNANUE 1984). They are not involved in phagocytosis. CD11c (Ki-M1), Ki-M2, Ki-M5, Ki-M6, Ki-M7, and Ki-M8 are regularly negative in these cells. Considering these properties, it should not prove at all difficult to discern follicular dendritic (reticulum) cells from other elements of the monocyte/macrophage system.

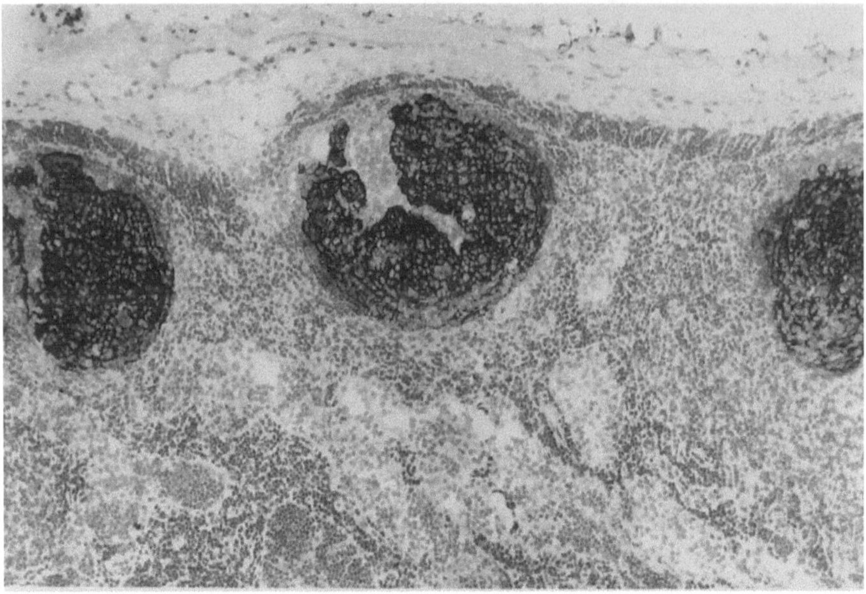

Fig. 9. Follicular dendritic (reticulum) cells immunostained with the monoclonal antibody Ki-M4. Cryostat section of lymph node, immunoperoxidase staining, × 88

Ki-M4 and R3/24 are two monoclonal antibodies which specifically recognize follicular dendritic (reticulum) cells (Fig. 9) – all other cell types are regularly negative to these antibodies. Mono1 is the only monocyte/macrophage reactive antibody which immunostains follicular dendritic (reticulum) cells (NAIEM et al. 1983; PARWARESCH et al. 1983a, b).

2.5.2 Follicular Macrophages in Lymphadenitis

In cases of acute or chronic nonspecific lymphadenitis, follicular hyperplasia may be observed without any substantial change in the major features of the nonlymphoid cells of germinal centers. The necrotizing and granulomatous types of lymphadenitis may involve all or parts of the B follicles. A fairly typical finding are the small clusters of epithelioid cells within the germinal centers or parts of B follicles which are often seen with the so-called PIRINGER-KUCHINKA type of lymphadenitis, described in 1953. The main cause is probably toxoplasmosis, though an identical picture may be caused by various other infectious agents. Epithelioid cells within the B follicles are common in Crohn's disease. The immunophenotype of epithelioid cells in this particular site does not differ from that described in other areas of the lymph node.

3 Concluding Remarks

Although the objective of this chapter was to describe the differential phenotypic features of macrophages using a set of fairly specific reagents, reference had to be made to the classification and certain other features of macrophages. The term "macrophage" was applied in a generic way, covering all monocyte-derived differentiation forms irrespective of their phagocytic capabilities. The data presented indicate that it is well possible to distinguish between professional phagocytes and nonphagocytic dendritic (or reticulum) cells specialized to process and present antigen. Immunohistochemical methods proved especially efficient in disclosing the bimodal differentiation of these cells, reflecting their functional engagement in cellular or humoral immunity, as well as the typical features of professional phagocytes.

References

Beelen RHC, Broekhuis-Fluitsma DM, Korn C, Hoefsmit ECM (1977) Identification of exudate-resident macrophages on the basis of peroxidatic activity. J Reticuloendothel Soc 23:103–110

Benacerraf B (1988) Antigen processing and presentation. The biologic role of MHC molecules in determinant selection. J Immunol 141:17–20

Facchetti F, De Wolf-Peeters C, Mason DY, Pulford K, van den Oord JJ, Desmet VJ (1988) Plasmacytoid T cells. Immunohistochemical evidence for their monocyte/macrophage origin. Am J Pathol 133:15–21

Feller AC, Lennert K, Stein H, Bruhn HD, Wuthe HH (1983) Immunohistology and aetiology of histiocytic necrotizing lymphadenitis. Report of three instructive cases. Histopathology 7:825–839

Fossum S (1988) Lymph-borne dendritic leucocytes do not recirculate, but enter the lymph node paracortex to become interdigitating cells. Scand J Immunol 27:97–105

Gerdes J, Lemke H, Baisch H, Wacker H-H, Schwab V, Stein H (1984) Cell cycle analysis of a cell proliferation-associated human nuclear antigen defined by the monoclonal antibody Ki67. J Immunol 133:1710–1715

Horny HP, Feller AC, Horst HA, Lennert K (1986) Immunocytology of plasmacytoid T-cells: marker analysis indicates a unique phenotype of this enigmatic cell. Hum Pathol 18:28–32

Kikuchi M, Yoshizumi T, Nakamura H (1977) Necrotizing lymphadenitis: possible acute toxoplasmic infection. Virchows Arch [A] 376:247–253

Lennert K (1961) Lymphknoten. Diagnostik in Schnitt und Ausstrich. Bandteil A: Cytologie und Lymphadenitis. In: Lubarsch O, Henke F, Rössler R, Uehlinger E (eds) Handbuch der speziellen pathologischen Anatomie und Histologie, vol I/3 A. Springer, Berlin Heidelberg New York

Lennert K, Remmele W (1958) Aryometrische Untersuchungen an Lymphknotenzellen des Menschen. I. Mitt. Germinoblasten, Lymphoblasten und Lymphocyten. Acta Haematol (Basel) 19:99–113

Müller-Hermelink HK, Kaiserling E, Lennert K (1973) Pseudofollikuläre Nester von Plasmazellen (eines besonderen Typs) in der paracorticalen Pulpa menschlicher Lymphknoten. Virchows Arch [B] 14:47–56

Müller-Hermelink HK, Steinmann G, Stein H, Lennert K (1983) Malignant lymphoma of plasmacytoid T-cells. Morphologic and immunologic studies characterizing a special type of T-cell. Am J Surg Pathol 7:849–862

Naiem M, Gerdes J, Abdulaziz Z, Stein H, Mason DY (1983) Production of a monoclonal antibody reactive with human dendritic reticulum cells and its use in the immunohistological analysis of lymphoid tissue. J Clin Pathol 36:167–175

Parwaresch MR, Wacker H-H (1984) Origin and kinetics of resident tissue macrophages. Parabiosis studies with radiolabelled leucocytes. Cell Tissue Kinet 17:25–39

Parwaresch MR, Radzun HJ, Feller AC, Peters K-P, Hansmann ML (1983a) Peroxidase-positive mononuclear leukocytes as possible precursors of human dendritic reticulum cells. J Immunol 131:2719–2725

Parwaresch MR, Radzun HJ, Hansmann M-L, Peters K-P (1983b) Monoclonal antibody Ki-M4 specifically recognizes human dendritic reticulum cells (follicular dendritic cells) and their possible precursors in blood. Blood 62:585–590

Piringer-Kuchinka A (1953) Eigenartiger mikroskopischer Befund an excidierten Lymphknoten. Verh Dtsch Ges Pathol 36:352–362

Radzun HJ (1985) Immunhistochemie des menschlichen mononukleär-phagozytischen Systems. Fischer, Stuttgart (Progress in pathology, vol 124)

Radzun HJ, Kreipe H, Zavazava N, Hansmann ML, Parwaresch MR (1988) Diversity of the human monocyte/macrophage system as detected by monoclonal antibodies. J Leukocyte Biol 43:41–50

Robb-Smith AHT (1947) The lymph node biopsy. In: Recent advances in clinical pathology. J&A Churchill, London, pp 350–370

Rosai J, Dorfman RF (1969) Sinus histiocytosis with massive lymphadenopathy: a newly recognized benign clinicopathological entity. Arch Pathol 87:63–70

Stein H, Lennert K, Mason DY, Lingru S, Ziegler A (1984) Immature sinus histiocytes. Their identification as a novel B-cell population. Am J Pathol 117:44–52

Symmers WStC (1978) The lymphoreticular system. In: Symmers WStC (ed) Systemic pathology, vol 2. Churchill Livingstone, Edingburgh, pp 504–892

Szakal AK, Homes KL, Tew JG (1983) Transport of immune complexes from the subcapsular sinus to lymph node follicles on the surface of nonphagocytic cells, including cells with dendritic morphology. J Immunol 131:1714–1727

Tew JG, Mandel TE, Burgess AW (1979) Retention of intact HSA for prolonged periods in the popliteal lymph nodes of specifically immunized mice. Cell Immunol 45:207–212

Unanue ER (1984) Antigen-presenting function of the macrophage. Ann Rev Immunol 2:395–428

Unanue ER, Askonas BA (1968) Persistence of immunogenicity of antigen after uptake by macrophages. J Exp Med 127:915–926

Immunoelectron-microscopic Investigations of Lymph Nodes

M.-L. HANSMANN and H.-H. WACKER

1 Introduction

The conventional morphological techniques applied in the investigation of lymphoid tissue have been given an additional dimension by the introduction of monoclonal antibodies (mAbs), (KÖHLER and MILSTEIN 1975) into immunohistochemical procedures. The broad range of the antibodies already available and the diversity of the theoretically achievable reagents reflect the potential of these procedures.

The detection of antigenic sites by certain mAbs makes possible clear characterization of individual structures in lymphoid tissue. A set of new reagents has been directed against lymphocyte subtypes, monocytes, and macrophages as well as dendritic reticulum cells (4th International Conference on Human Leukocyte Differentiation Antigens, Vienna, 1989). Other antibodies have been utilized to selectively visualize fiber architecture, vascular cells, and/or other elements of supportive tissue. The application of these reagents to neoplasms of lymphoid tissue is providing a wealth of new information. The diversity of non-Hodgkin's lymphomas, for example, has been further elucidated according to their B- or T-cell origin (STANSFELD et al. 1988).

Despite the numerous possibilities for identifying various cell types in lymphoid tissue by means of immunohistochemistry using mAbs, there still remain major shortcomings. The disadvantage of most of these antibodies is their inability to detect the target antigen in routinely processed sections. Frozen sections are not available in the majority of cases. In addition, the structural preservation is poor in such tissue samples. In such cases we think the application of immunoelectron microscopy would be appropriate and beneficial.

2 B Cells

Using conventional electron microscopy B lymphocytes are characterized by round to slightly irregularly shaped nuclei with dense chromatin, small nucleoli, and a narrow rim of cytoplasm. The cytoplasm contains a number of scattered organelles such as mitochondria, a few lysosomes, and occasionally short profiles of rough endoplasmic reticulum. The ability of B lymphocytes to produce immunoglobulins has its correlate in varying amounts of rough endoplasmic reticulum, which is considerably enhanced in lymphoplasmacytoid cells and in full-blown plasma cells. The majority of germinal center cells are of B-cell lineage, as shown by various techniques (for literature see Müller-Hermelink and Lennert 1978; Stein et al. 1982; Peters et al. 1987). The B-lymphoid cells in the germinal centers have been designated as centrocytes, centroblasts, and immunoblasts. The centroblasts are medium-sized to large cells with round to ovoid nuclei and a moderately condensed heterochromatin. These cells usually contain medium-sized nucleoli which are most often located in the immediate vicinity of the nuclear membrane. Centroblasts have medium-sized to broad cytoplasm which contains a variable amount of rough endoplasmic reticulum. The centrocytes are smaller than centroblasts. Their nuclei are irregularly shaped and the heterochromatin is usually condensed at the nuclear membrane. The cytoplasm of the centrocytes contains only a few organelles. The B-cell nature of these cells has been established through the detection of immunoglobulins with immunoelectron-microscopic techniques (Tsunoda et al. 1978; Dobashi et al. 1982). On the electron-microscopic level immunoglobulins could be demonstrated not only in the ergastoplasm but also on polyribosomes and within the nuclear envelope. It was possible to localize the exact subcellular compartments, such as different areas of the rough endoplasmic reticulum and the perinuclear space, as the main loci of immunoglobulin synthesis in different stages of B-cell development (Avrameas and Bouteille 1968; Leduc et al. 1968). By immunoelectron-microscopy it could be shown that different parts of immunoglobulin molecules are synthesized in different areas of individual cells (Newell et al. 1982). The possibility, technically, of tracing immunoglobulin production loci at the ultrastructural level has been of considerable significance for the understanding of the cytogenesis of various B-cell lymphomas (for literature see Mimura et al. 1986).

In addition to the immunoglobulin structures, cell-specific reagents have been valuable in the investigation of B cells. An illustrative example is presented in Fig. 1, which shows an immunoelectron-microscopic view of four lymphocytes immunostained with the mAb Ki-B5 reacting with B lymphocytes (Gralla et al., 1989; Hansmann et al., submitted). The small lymphocytes show rounded to slightly irregularly shaped nuclei, a coarse heterochromatin, and a small to medium-sized cytoplasm containing a few organelles such as monoribosomes and lysosomes as well as mitochondria. Due to the small amount of rough endoplasmic reticulum these cells are hardly identifiable as B lymphocytes at the ultrastructural level. This can be demonstrated using the mAb Ki-B5. The immunoreaction is confined to the outer cell

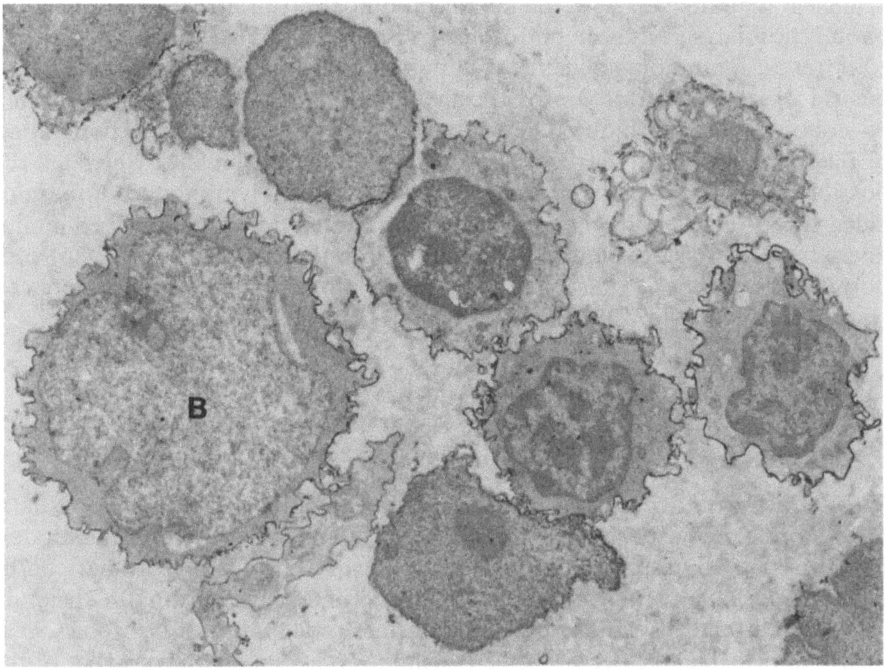

Fig. 1. Four lymphocytes and one blast cell (*B*) showing a positive immunoreaction on the cell membrane with the mAb Ki-B5, directed against B cells. In addition, five fragments of damaged cells. Immunoperoxidase reaction, cell suspension, ×7500

surface membrane, a conclusion also drawn from light-microscopic studies. In addition, on the left side in Fig. 1, a large blast is shown. This cell exhibits a large nucleus which is irregularly shaped and has sparsely distributed heterochromatin. The cytoplasm is narrow to medium-sized and contains densely packed ribosomes as well as a few ergastoplasmic profiles. Without additional immunohistochemical information, reliable classification of this blastic cell would not be feasible. Its positivity with the mAb Ki-B5, however, identifies it as being of B-cell line. Also in this case the Ki-B5 positivity is restricted to the outer plasma membrane surface: the reactivity is continuous along the membrane surrounding the cytoplasm, whereas intracytoplasmic organelles and the nucleus remain nonreactive. In addition to its reaction with B cells, Ki-B5 has been shown to coreact with about 20% of T8 lymphocytes (Gralla et al., 1989).

Comparable immunoreactivity at the ultrastructural level was demonstrated for the B-cell mAb Ki-B3 (Hansmann et al. 1986; Fellbaum et al. 1988). As with Ki-B5, Ki-B3 could be localized on the outer cell membrane of B cells, especially that of follicle mantle lymphocytes. In contrast to Ki-B5, Ki-B3 detects a smaller subpopulation of B lymphocytes. A detailed investigation of human germinal centers using a panel of monoclonal antibodies directed against B lymphocytes with the aid of immunoelectron-microscopy and morphometric analysis has been performed by SAID et al. (1986). They demonstrated different immunohistochemical staining patterns of gold particles at various stages of transformation of B cells in germinal centers using the protein A–colloidal gold technique. They were able to characterize a small population of B lymphocytes with markedly irregular or convoluted nuclei, which are the possible precursors for the development of rare B-cell lymphomas of multilobated type. Additionally, the findings which resulted from the combined immunoelectron-microscopy and morphometric techniques (SAID et al. 1986) supported the hypothesis that small lymphocytes invading germinal centers can transform directly to centroblasts.

3 T Cells

Viewed by means of conventional electron-microscopy, T lymphocytes usually have more irregularly shaped nuclei than B lymphocytes. Within the moderately broad cytoplasm a small number of focally arranged lysosomes can be detected. Despite certain ultrastructural criteria such as chromatin structure and amount and distribution of endoplasmic reticulum and lysosomes, it is nearly impossible to discern T and B lymphocytes reliably. This is one of the major advantages of the lineage-specific monoclonal antibodies.

Excellent examples of this line, in the case of T lymphocytes, are the T-cell antigen-specific receptor-related monoclonal Leu-4 (CD3) antibody and others with specificities to T-cell subsets, such as CD4 and CD8. As shown in Fig. 2, in immunoelectron-microscopic studies T lymphocytes represent medium-sized cells with a somewhat irregularly shaped nucleus. The condensed heterochromatin shows clear margination. The cytoplasmic rim, with a few organelles, remains nonreactive with all the above-mentioned T-cell-specific monoclonal antibodies. All three mAbs immunostain the external surface of T-cell cytoplasmic membrane. The reaction pattern is somewhat linear and continuous. Preferential accumulations do not regularly occur. There is good agreement between the results obtained in cell suspensions and those achieved with tissue sections. In cell suspensions the immunocytochemical staining pattern is more distinct. In tissue sections there is the important advantage of the possibility of surveying intercellular structural relations.

Using normal peripheral blood lymphocytes as well as leukemic lymphocytes and immunoelectron-microscopy, especially immunogold staining techniques, it was possible to identify and characterize T-cell subsets at the ultrastructural level (MATUTES et al. 1983), although features such as nucleo-cytoplasmic ratio, largeness of the Golgi field, number and arrangement of lysosomes, and the occurrence of parallel tubular structures were useful parameters of differentiation and typing of T cells and T-cell subsets. None of the criteria listed above turned out to be specific for a special type or an immunohistochemical marker constellation of these cells.

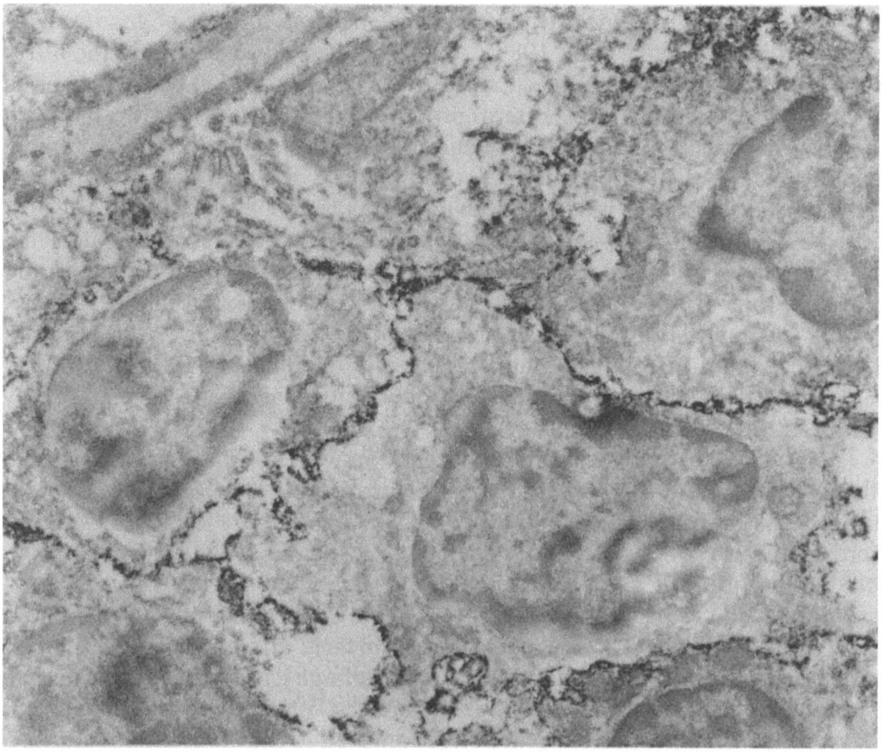

Fig. 2. Lymphocytes with slightly irregularly shaped nuclei and a medium-sized cytoplasm. Positive immunoreaction on the surface membrane with the anti-CD4 mAb. Immunoperoxidase reaction, ×12 500

4 Macrophages and Interdigitating Reticulum Cells

The human lymph node is equipped with a wide range of functional subtypes of macrophages and related cells. Some are found in sinuses while others populate perisinusoidal pulp cords or thymus-dependent paracortical areas, and scattered phagocytic cells occur within the B-cell follicles. Variations in light-microscopic and ultrastructural properties and major differences in antigen profile indicate their functional diversity. The conventional electron-microscopic findings of macrophages (for literature see CARR 1973) and interdigitating reticulum cells (KAISERLING and LENNERT 1974; for literature see VELDMAN and KAISERLING 1980) have been extensively recorded. In the following review we describe major immunoelectron-microscopic findings only. For the visualization of macrophages the pan-macrophage reagent Ki-M1 was utilized to reveal an example of the surface membrane-bound antigens (HANSMANN et al. 1984; RADZUN et al. 1984, 1988). In addition, the monoclonal antibody

Ki-M7 was applied to demonstrate the ultrastructural findings of an intracytoplasmic antigen (Kreipe et al. 1987). A similar immunoreactivity at the ultrastructural level is shown by the mAbs Ki-M6 (Parwaresch et al. 1986) and Ki-M8 (Radzun et al. 1987). Interdigitating reticulum cells, known as T-cell accessories in functional terms, are believed to be restricted to the thymus-dependent areas of the lymph node. It could be demonstrated at the ultrastructural level that these cells react with the mAb CD1a and with antibodies against the protein S-100 (Takahashi et al. 1981). The S-100 protein could be detected at the ultrastructural level in interdigitating reticulum cells in non-specific and dermatopathic lymphadenitis, the latter characteristically showing large amounts of interdigitating reticulum cells in the T zones. The S-100 protein was localized in the irregularly shaped nuclei, in the nuclear membrane, and in the broad, pale-looking cytoplasm in conventional electron microscopy (Takahashi et al. 1981).

The mAb Ki-M1 shows an immunoreaction with interdigitating reticulum cells in addition to different subtypes of macrophage. The immunoreaction is confined to the outer cell membrane, which forms more or less developed interdigitations (Hansmann et al. 1984; Radzun et al. 1984). The cytoplasm, including its organelles, and the nucleus are not reactive with this mAb.

Figure 3 shows a macrophage with an irregularly shaped nucleus and a large nucleolus located at the nuclear membrane. The chromatin is mainly condensed at the nuclear envelope. The macrophage has broad cytoplasm rich in organelles which exhibit vesicular structures often showing an electron-transparent area. The immunoreaction is confined to the outer cell membrane, which reveals many processes that contact the lymphocytes in the vicinity of the macrophage cell. Typical phagolysosomes are not visible in this section.

Ki-M1, as a pan-monocyte/macrophage monoclonal antibody, also detects a special variant of monocyte cell which is called an epithelioid cell. It is characterized by a mostly round to oval nucleus, a broad cytoplasm with a multicentric Golgi field, and many processes of the outer cell membrane. These epithelioid cells can be found under various reactive and neoplastic conditions. Furthermore, they show, as demonstrated in Fig. 4, a typical immunostaining of the outer cell membrane which is characteristic for all monocyte/macrophage cells detected by Ki-M1. Surrounding lymphocytes (Fig. 4), most of which are probably T cells, often show slightly irregularly shaped nuclei and a small to medium-sized cytoplasm. The lymphoid cells are negative with Ki-M1. Light microscopy revealed Piringer's lymphadenitis in this patient, which is characteristic mainly for toxoplasmosis infection.

Figure 5 shows a macrophage with a slightly irregularly shaped nucleus and a broad cytoplasm. Numerous vesicular structures can be seen in the cytoplasm. Many of these, and also membranous structures, show positive staining with the mAb Ki-M7, which is known to detect intracytoplasmic antigens mainly localized in lysosomal granules and membrane structures (Kreipe et al. 1987). This antibody typically shows a strong reaction in so-called stimulated macrophages and in multinucleated giant cells (Kreipe et al. 1988).

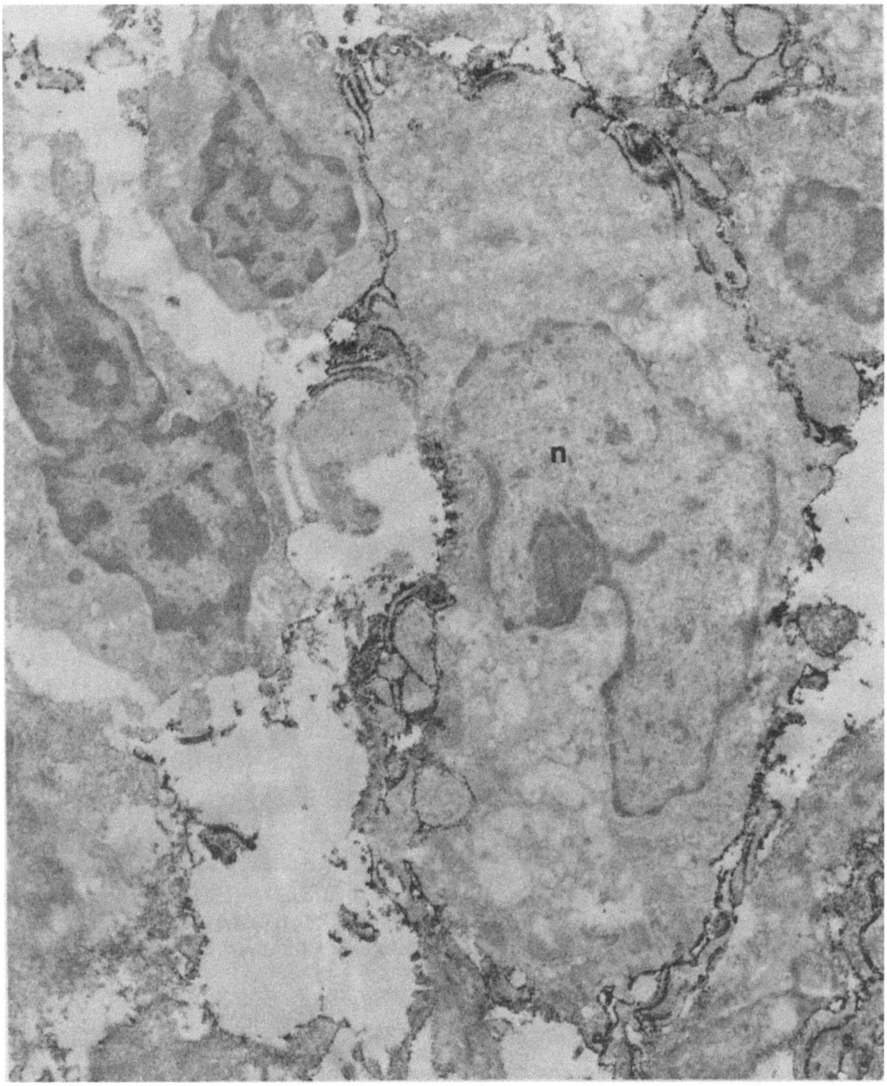

Fig. 3. Large monocyte/macrophage cell characterized by the mAb Ki-M1. The cell shows an irregularly shaped nucleus (*n*), a large nucleolus, and cytoplasmic processes with a positive immunoreaction. Immunoperoxidase, ×9000

5 Follicular Dendritic (Reticulum) Cells

Primary and secondary lymphoid follicles contain a varying number of cells that are designated follicular dendritic (reticulum) cells (FDCs). The original description was by MAXIMOW (1927), who noted the reticular or arachnoid

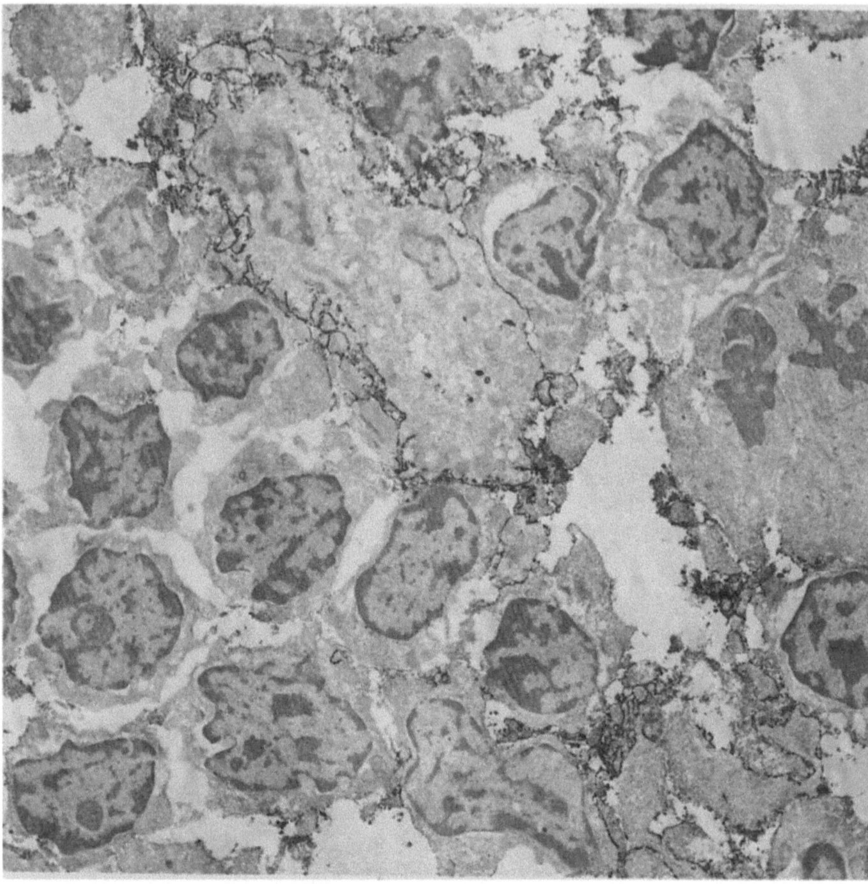

Fig. 4. Nonlymphoid cells with features of an epithelioid cell (*top*) showing immunoreaction of the outer cell membrane with the mAb Ki-M1. Positively stained cell processes are present at the *bottom right*. Surrounding lymphocytes are negative with this mAb. On the *right* of the figure a dividing cell is seen. Immunoperoxidase reaction, ×5700

morphology and nonphagocytosing nature of these cells. Later investigations by MITCHELL and ABBOTT (1965) disclosed the considerable functional significance of FDCs. In conventional ultrastructural studies FDCs build up a dense network, intercommunicating with their long (stretched) cytoplasmic projections, engulfing a large number of adjacent lymphoid cells. FDCs contain a medium-sized nucleus with a distinct nuclear membrane. Irrespective of the narrow rim of marginally condensed chromatin, a major part of the area of the nucleus is of low electron density. In the central part a small but distinct nucleolus is often encountered. The perinuclear part of the cytoplasm is poorly defined and is approximately as wide as adjacent lymphoid cells. Within this area of the cytoplasm a limited number of organelles, mainly comprising mitochondria and short profiles of ergastoplasm, are detectable. Phagosomes,

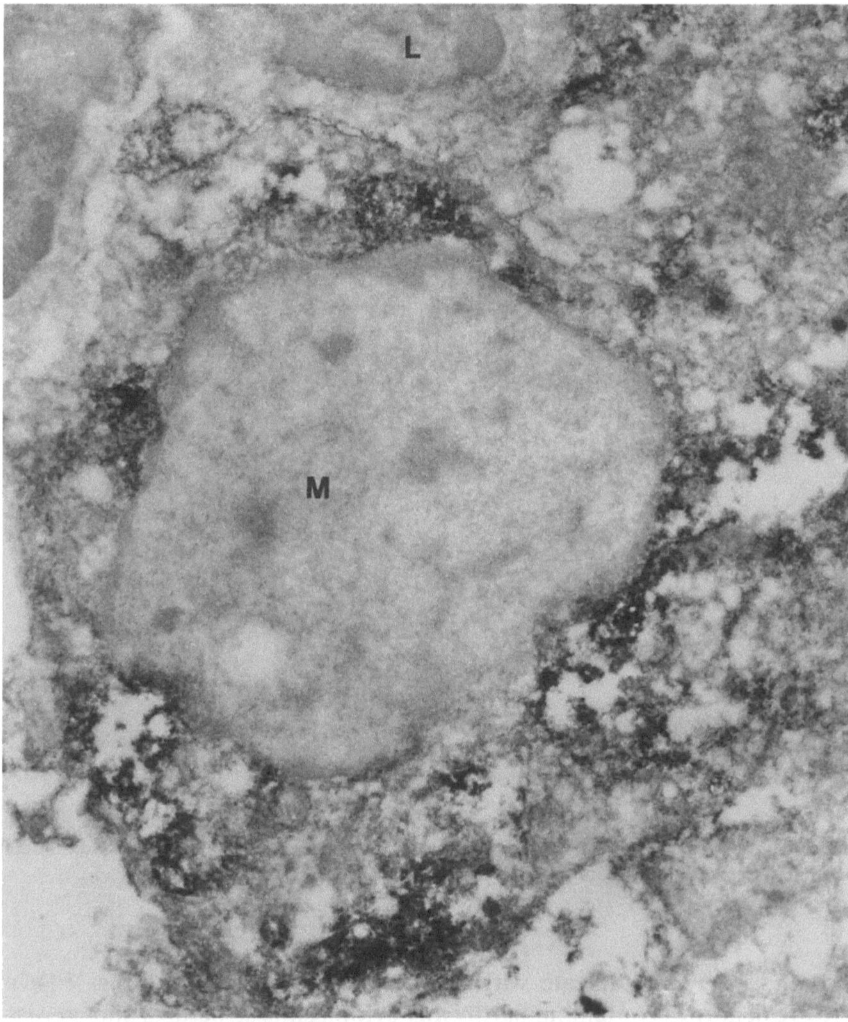

Fig. 5. Immunoelectron-microscopic picture of a macrophage (*M*) and a lymphocyte (*L*). The macrophage shows a broad cytoplasm with many vesicular and membranous structures positively stained with the mAb Ki-M7. Immunoperoxidase, ×7500

especially peroxidase-positive vesicular structures or vacuoles, are absent or inconspicuous. In some of the cells a narrow strand of microfilaments or parallel fibrillar structures occur. Peripherally the cytoplasm narrows increasingly into long cytoplasmic processes of varying width and length. Some of the FDCs show a wealth of narrow dendrites radiating around the central part of the nucleus. Such dendrites have been referred to as "villiform" by SZAKAL et al. (1985). Other dendrites show a beaded outline and are about 0.4 μm in width. Some of the dendrites are very long, reaching more than 300 μm in

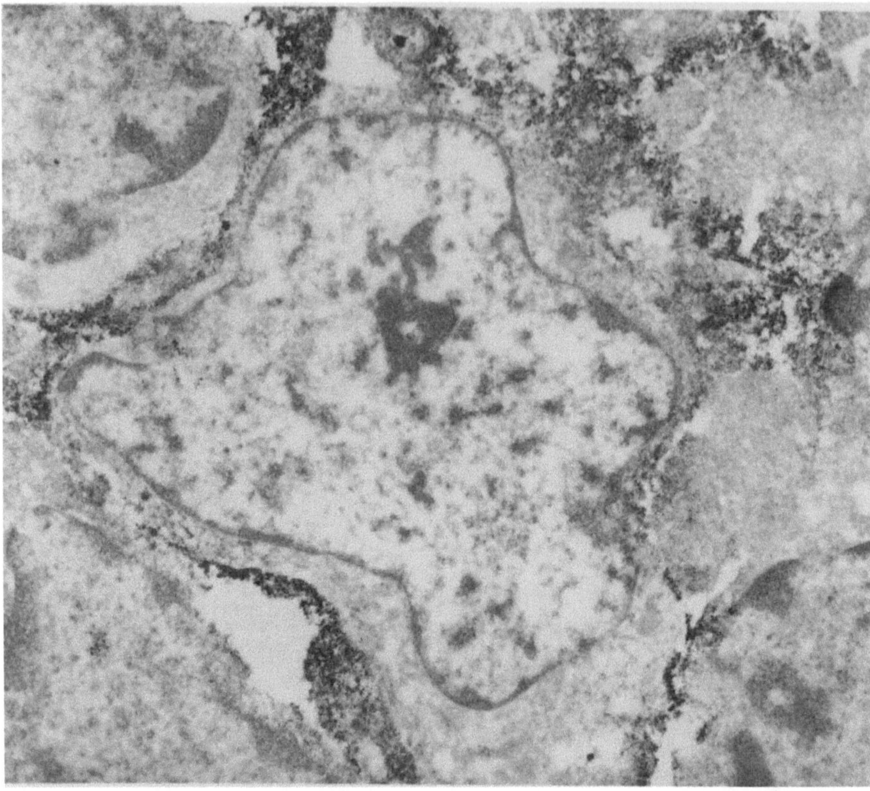

Fig. 6. Immunoelectron-microscopic picture of FDCs of a florid germinal center. The nucleus shows a medium-sized nucleolus. The dark immunoreaction product is localized mainly on the cell surface and its processes. Immunoperoxidase, Ki-M4, ×13 500

length and intercommunicate with adjacent lymphocytes and other FDCs. There are dendrites containing hardly any cytoplasmic structures and consisting of a double membrane duplicature. Others contain a number of scattered organelles and vesicular structures. In broader areas desmosomes are detectable on the membrane.

Immunoelectron microscopy has been a considerable aid in understanding various functional aspects of these cells. It is employed, among other purposes, for the substructural localization of immune complexes or antibodies (SZAKAL et al. 1988). The aim of various groups has also been to demonstrate selectively the complicated outline of FDCs by means of various cell-specific mAbs, among which R4/23 (STEIN et al. 1982), Ki-M4 (PARWARESCH et al. 1983 a, b), and Ki-M4R (WACKER et al. 1987) have been widely used. In this context we have been applying Ki-M4 and a new mAb, Ki-FDCp, both of which allow selective visualization of FDCs in the human system. Using these antibodies, an even immunostaining of the cell membrane is possible. The electron density

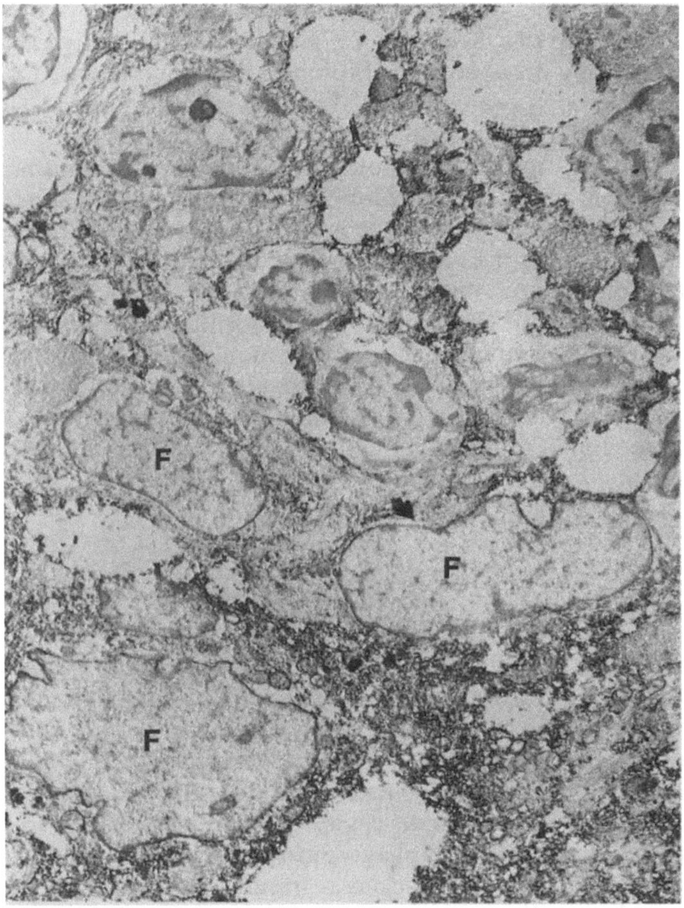

Fig. 7. Follicular dendritic cells (*F*) with positive immunostaining mainly on the cell surface, including the fine cell processes. Immunoperoxidase, Ki-FDCp, × 6000

of the immune complexes is localized more on the outer surface of the cytoplasm (Fig. 6). No considerable difference in the intensity of the electron density and the width of the antibody deposition is encountered along the length of stretched cytoplasmic dendrites. Almost no antibody deposition is detectable in the inner part of the cytoplasm, especially in the central area engulfing the nucleus. This also applies to the remote parts of the dendrites still containing narrow cytoplasmic bridges. Ki-M4 and Ki-FDCp show a comparable immunostaining at the ultrastructural level. In contrast to Ki-M4, Ki-FDCp occasionally shows an immunoreaction with the cell surface of follicle mantle lymphocytes. In Fig. 7 three FDCs are shown exhibiting an immunoreaction with Ki-FDCp. The positively stained processes surround germinal center cells and form a large network. It is difficult to determine whether the entire immunoreaction is part of the immunostaining of FDCs or whether some of the germinal center cells react with this mAb. Ki-FDCp works not only on frozen sections but also on routinely processed deparaffinized paraffin sections.

Immunoelectron microscopy has contributed considerably to the understanding of the morphofunctional relationships of various cell systems residing in lymph nodes. This applies especially to protein synthesis and mechanisms involved in the subcellular events of immunoglobulin secretion in plasma cells. With regard to lymphocytes, most light-microscopic findings could be critically evaluated and substantiated at the ultrastructural level. With no other cell type has the ultrastructural immunohistochemistry provided such an abundance of new information as with FDCs and other dendritic cell types. The majority of these cells serve as immune accessory cells modulating the diverse multitude of antigens into a form legible to lymphocytes with a specificially rearranged antigen receptor. The possibility of immunoelectron-microscopic tracing and specific detection of such structures opens up a wide range of new possibilities.

6 Sinus-Lining Cells

Sinus-lining cells have been the subject of occasional electron-microscopic studies (MORI and LENNERT 1969; SZAKAL et al. 1983). Their main feature is the large number of cytoplasmic projections which intercommunicate with each other. Sinus-lining cells are closely associated with multidirectional bundles of collagen fibers. Such fibers provide a certain static support enabling sinus-lining cells to be fixed within the sinus cavity. A small number of cytoplasmic organelles are detectable, whereas phagosomes or vacuoles containing foreign matter are extremely rare. The nucleus is irregularly shaped and is distinguished by a low chromatin content and a most often centrally located nucleolus. In contrast, in adjacent lymphocytes the nuclear form is irregular.

Immunoelectron-microscopic studies have rarely been extended to sinus-lining cells. This is mainly because the majority of immune reagents fail to react with sinus-lining cells. This is true of the majority of the endothelial antibodies and lectins. Using highly sensitive immunohistochemical methods it was maintained that antibodies specific to FDCs such as Ki-M4 or Ki-M4R (WACKER et al. 1987) reveal a positive subpopulation of sinus-lining cells. Recently developed reagents of high cellular specificity to FDCs, such as Ki-FDCp (TABRIZCHI, in press), or to sinus-lining cells, such as Ki-M9 or Ki-M9R (publication in preparation), render the other cell type positive, though with a considerably weaker intensity. Immunoelectron-microscopic features of sinus-lining cells correspond to those of other dendritic (reticulum) cells. The irregularly shaped, medium-sized nucleus is surrounded by a rim of cytoplasm which contains only a few organelles such as mitochondria or a short profile of ergastoplasm. The antibodies referred to above fail to immunostain intracytoplasmic structures and remain mostly confined to the

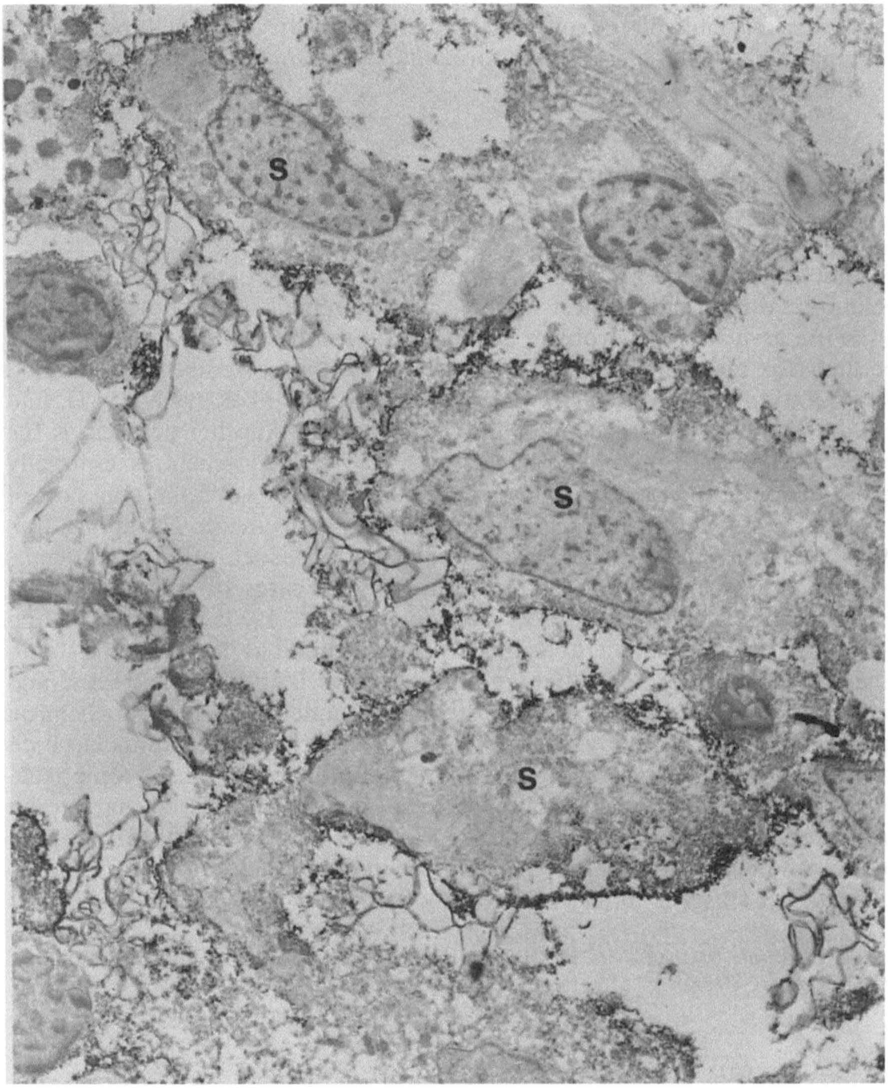

Fig. 8. Sinus of a lymph node in chronic nonspecific lymphadenitis. The sinus-lining cells (*S*) and their processes show a membrane-bound immunoreaction with the mAb Ki-M9. The lymphocytes are negative with this mAb. Immunoperoxidase, Ki-M9, × 6000

outer surface of the plasma membrane (Fig. 8). The linear deposition of the immune reagent lines up along the bizarre contour of the cytoplasm with a large number of cytoplasmic projections and dendrite-like cytoplasmic elongations. The electron density of the immunostaining shows only minor variations, lacking foci of accumulations or areas of complete absence of the immune precipitates. At low magnifications the arachnoid cellular form is clearly detectable, especially in the cells within the sinus cavity. Those cells populating marginal areas assume a long fusiform shape similar to that of the adjacent myofibroblasts.

7 Conclusions

Considering the achievements in immunoelectron microscopy, the available techniques do not nearly meet the present requirements. A major problem is tissue preservation; this problem is only partly resolved by the preembedding method (for literature see STERNBERGER 1979), the postembedding method (KAWARAI and NAKANE 1970), and ultracryosection (TOKUYASU 1983), and additional radical improvements are thus required. Another problem is the predictability of the acquired electron density of various structures, especially nuclear compartments. The basic recommendation remains the omission of contrast agents such as the various metal salts generally in use. The application of gold particles in combination with proteins for visualization of antigenic sites has found broad application, especially in cases of preservation by postembedding and in ultracryosections (ROTH 1982; BENDAYAN and ZOLLINGER 1983). Such methods have been recognized as useful for the simultaneous visualization of different antigens (for literature see HOLM and NESLAND 1988). The anticipated shortcoming, namely immunohistochemical agents and diluted antibody solutions lacking in efficient penetration, has been compensated for using combinations of immunoelectron-microscopic techniques, and additionally, by the application of many antibodies to characterize intracytoplasmic or even intranuclear antigens. This aspect of modern immunoelectron microscopy is of great assistance in the ultrastructural localization of the target antigens to an ever-growing number of monoclonal reagents.

Acknowledgements. We thank Mrs. M. Dirks for her technical assistance and Mrs. H. Brütting and Mrs. I. Karlberg-Stannik for preparation of the manuscript.

References

Avrameas S, Bouteille M (1968) Ultrastructural localization of antibody by antigen label with peroxidase. Exp Cell Res 53:166–176

Bendayan M, Zollinger M (1983) Ultrastructural localization of antigenic sites on osmium-fixed tissues applying the protein A-gold technique. J Histochem Cytochem 31:101–109

Carr J (1973) The macrophage. A review of ultrastructure and function. Academic, New York

Dobashi M, Terashima K, Imai Y (1982) Electron microscopic study of differentiation of antibody-producing cells in mouse lymph nodes after immunization with horseradish peroxidase. J Histochem Cytochem 30:67–74

Fellbaum C, Hansmann ML, Parwaresch MR, Lennert K (1988) Monoclonal antibodies Ki-B3 and LeuM1 discriminate giant cells of infectious mononucleosis and of Hodgkin's disease. Hum Pathol 19:1168–1173

Gralla J, Hansmann ML, Lumbeck H et al. (1989) Ki-B5, ein neuer monoklonaler Antikörper, der reaktive und neoplastische B-Zellen in konventionellen Paraffinschnitten erkennt. Verh Dtsch Ges Pathol 73:691

Hansmann ML, Radzun HJ, Kaiserling E, Parwaresch MR (1984) Immunoelectron microscopic demonstration of tissue antigens with monoclonal antibodies. Virchows Arch [B] 46:1–12

Hansmann ML, Wacker HH, Radzun HJ (1986) Paragranuloma is a variant of Hodgkin's disease with predominance of B cells. Virchows Arch [A] 409:171–181

Hansmann ML, Wacker HH, Gralla J, Lumbeck H, Kossmahl M, Heidebrecht HJ, Radzun HJ, Parwaresch MR (1990) Ki-B5: A monoclonal antibody unrelated to CD45 recognizes normal and neoplastic human B-cells in routine paraffin sections. Submitted

Holm R, Nesland JM (1988) Double-staining methods at the ultrastructural level applying colloidal gold conjugates. Ultrastruct Pathol 12:279–290

Kaiserling E, Lennert K (1974) Die interdigitierende Retikulumzelle im menschlichen Lymphknoten. Eine spezifische Zelle der thymusabhängigen Region. Virchows Arch [B] 16:51–61

Kawarai Y, Nakane PK (1970) Localization of tissue antigens in the ultrathin sections with peroxidase-labeled antibody method. J Histochem Cytochem 18:161–166

Köhler G, Milstein C (1975) Continuous cultures of fused cells secreting antibody of predefined specificity. Nature 256:495–497

Kreipe H, Radzun HJ, Parwaresch MR, Haislip A, Hansmann ML (1987) Ki-M7 monoclonal antibody specific for myelomonocytic cell lineage and macrophages in human. J Histochem Cytochem 35:1117–1126

Kreipe H, Radzun HJ, Rudolph P, Barth J, Hansmann ML, Heidorn K, Parwaresch MR (1988) Multinucleated giant cells generated in vitro. Terminally differentiated macrophages with down-regulated c-fms expression. Am J Pathol 130:232–243

Leduc EH, Avrameas S, Bouteille M (1968) Ultrastructural localization of antibody in differentiating plasma cells. J Exp Med 127:109–118

Matutes E, Crockard AD, Catovsky D (1983) The ultrastructural morphology of T lymphocytes in B-chronic lymphocytic leukaemia: a study with monoclonal antibodies and the immunogold technique. Br J Haematol 55:273–283

Maximow A (1927) Bindegewebe und blutbildende Gewebe. In: Möllendorf V (ed) Handbuch der mikroskopischen Anatomie des Menschen, vol 2/I. Springer, Berlin Heidelberg New York, pp 232–583

Mimura R, Hansmann ML, Lennert K (1986) Immunoelectron microscopic localization of immunoglobulin in B cell lymphomas. Virchows Arch [B] 52:207–220

Mitchell J, Abbott A (1965) Ultrastructure of the antigen-retaining reticulum of lymph node follicles as shown by high-resolution autoradiography. Nature 208:500–502

Mori Y, Lennert K (1969) Electron microscopic atlas of lymph node cytology and pathology. Springer, Berlin Heidelberg New York

Müller-Hermelink HK, Lennert K (1978) The cytologic histologic, and functional bases for a modern classification of lymphomas. In: Lennert K in collaboration with Stein H, Mohri N, Kaiserling E, Müller-Hermelink HK (eds) Malignant lymphomas others than Hodgkin's disease. Springer, Berlin Heidelberg New York, p 1–71

Newell DG, Hannam-Harris A, Karpas A, Smith JL (1982) The differential ultrastructural localization of immunoglobulin heavy and light chains in human haematopoietic cell lines. Br J Haematol 50:445–459

Parwaresch MR, Radzun HJ, Feller AC, Peters KP, Hansmann ML (1983a) Peroxidase-positive mononuclear leukocytes as possible precursors of human dendritic reticulum cells. J Immunol 131:2719–2725

Parwaresch MR, Radzun HJ, Hansmann ML, Peters KP (1983b) Monoclonal antibody Ki-M4 specifically recognizes human dendritic reticulum cells (follicular dendritic cells) and their possible precursor in blood. Blood 62:585–590

Parwaresch MR, Radzun HJ, Kreipe H, Hansmann ML, Barth J (1986) Monocyte/macrophage-reactive monoclonal antibody Ki-M6 recognizes an intracytoplasmic antigen. Am J Pathol 124:141–151

Peters JPJ, Rademakers LHPM, De Boer RJ, van Unnik JAM (1987) Cellular composition of follicles of follicle centre cell lymphomas in relation to germinal centres of reactive lymph nodes. A morphometrical electronmicroscopical study. J Pathol 153:233–244

Radzun HJ, Parwaresch MR, Feller AC, Hansmann ML (1984) Monocyte/macrophage specific monoclonal antibody Ki-M1 recognizes interdigitating reticulum cells. Am J Pathol 117:441–450

Radzun HJ, Kreipe H, Bödewadt S, Hansmann ML, Barth J, Parwaresch MR (1987) Ki-M8 monoclonal antibody reactive with an intracytoplasmic antigen of monocyte/macrophage lineage. Blood 69:1320–1327

Radzun HJ, Kreipe H, Zavazava N, Hansmann ML, Parwaresch MR (1988) Diversity of the human monocyte/macrophage system as detected by monoclonal antibodies. J Leukocyte Biol 43:41–50

Roth J (1982) The preparation of protein A-gold complexes with 3 nm and 15 nm gold particles and their use in labelling multiple antigens on ultra-thin sections. Histochemical J 14:791–801

Said JW, Sassoon AF, Chien K, Shintaku P, Pinkus GS (1986) Immunoultrastructural and morphometric analysis of B lymphocytes in human germinal centers. Evidence for alternate pathways of follicular transformation. Am J Pathol 123:390–397

Stansfeld AG, Diebold J, Kapanci Y et al. (1988) Updated Kiel classification for lymphomas. Lancet I:292–293, 603

Stein H, Gerdes J, Mason DY (1982) The normal and malignant germinal centre. Clin Haematol 11:531–559

Sternberger LA (1979) Immunocytochemistry, 2nd edn. John Wiley, New York

Szakal AK, Holmes KL, Tew JG (1983) Transport of immune complexes from the subcapsular sinus to lymph node follicles on the surface of nonphagocytic cells, including cells with dendritic morphology. J Immunol 131:1714–1727

Szakal AK, Gieringer RL, Kosco MH, Tew JG (1985) Isolated follicular dendritic cells: cytochemical antigen localization, Nomarski, SEM, and TEM morphology. J Immunol 134:1349–1359

Szakal AK, Kosco MH, Tew JG (1988) A novel in vivo follicular dendritic cell-dependent iccosome-mediated mechanism for delivery of antigen to antigen-processing cells. J Immunol 140:341–353

Tabrizchi H, Hansmann ML, Parwaresch MR, Lennert K (1990) Distribution pattern of follicular-dendritic cells in low-grade B-cell lymphomas of the gastrointestinal tract immunostained by Ki-FDCp, a new paraffin-resistant monoclonal antibody. Modern Pathology (in press)

Takahashi K, Yamaguchi H, Ishizeki J, Nakajima T, Nakazato Y (1981) Immunohistochemical and immunoelectron microscopic localization of S-100 protein in the interdigitating reticulum cells of the human lymph node. Virchows Arch [B] 37:125–135

Tokuyasu KT (1983) Present state of immunocryoultramicrotomy. J Histochem Cytochem 31:164–167

Tsunoda R, Terashima K, Takahashi K, Kojima M (1978) An ultrastructural study with enzyme-labeled antibody technique on immunoglobulin-containing cells in human tonsils, especially in germinal centers. Acta Pathol Jpn 28:53–75

Veldman JE, Kaiserling E (1980) Interdigitating cells. In: Carr I, Daems WT (eds) The reticuloendothelial system. A comprehensive treatise, vol 1: Morphology. Plenum, New York, pp 381–416

Wacker H-H, Radzun HJ, Mielke V, Parwaresch MR (1987) Selective recognition of rat follicular dendritic cells (dendritic reticulum cells) by a new monoclonal antibody Ki-M4R in vitro and in vivo. J Leukocyte Biol 41:70–77

Subject Index

Contents of Companion Volume 84/2

Index of Volumes 80–83 Current Topics in Pathology

Volume 80: Biological Characterization of Bone Tumors.
Edited by A. ROESSNER

Volume 81: Gastrointestinal Pathology. Edited by G. T. WILLIAMS

J. M. SLOAN, D. C. ALLEN, P. W. HAMILTON, P. C. H. WATT, The Place of Quantitation in Diagnostic Gastrointestinal Pathology
W. V. BOGOMOLETZ, Collagenous Colitis
A. B. PRICE, Ischaemic Colitis
P. S. TEGLBJÆRG, Intestinal Spirochaetosis
PH. U. HEITZ, P. KOMMINOTH, Biopsy Diagnosis of Hirschsprung's Disease and Related Disorders
P. HERMANEK, Malignant Polyps – Pathological Factors Governing Clinical Management
J. R. JASS, Prognostic Factors in Colorectal Cancer
N. A. SHEPHERD, H. J. R. BUSSEY, Polyposis Syndromes – An Update

Volume 82: Pathology of the Nucleus. Edited by J. C. E. UNDERWOOD

J. C. E. UNDERWOOD, Nuclear Morphology and Grading in Tumours
H. M. H. KAMEL, J. KIRK, P. G. TONER, Ultrastructural Pathology of the Nucleus
J. CROCKER, Nucleolar Organiser Regions
T. J. STEPHENSON, Quantitation of the Nucleus
P. QUIRKE, Flow Cytometry in the Quantitation of DNA Aneuploidy and Cell Proliferation in Human Disease
P. DAL CIN, A. A. SANDBERG, Karyotypic Analysis of Solid Tumors
G. TERENGHI, R. A. FALLON, Techniques and Applications of In Situ Hybridisation

Volume 83: Cell Receptors. Edited by G. SEIFERT

P. KARLSON, Historical Development of the Receptor Concept
R. D. HESCH, Classification of Cell Receptors
H. JÜPPNER, R. D. HESCH, Biochemical Characterization of Cellular Hormone Receptors
M. DIETEL, Morphological Characterization of Cell Receptors
D. RICHTER, W. MEYERHOF, F. BUCK, S. D. MORLEY, Molecular Biology of Receptors for Neuropeptide Hormones
J. LLOYD, R. TIBOLT, G. V. CHILDS, Peptide Hormone Receptors
I. DAMJANOV, Growth Factor Receptors
A. NIENDORF, U. BEISIEGEL, Low Density Lipoprotein Receptors
A. PROBST, G. MENGOD, J. M. PALACIOS, Neurotransmitter Receptors in Human Brain Diseases
M. VIERBUCHEN, Lectin Receptors
E. V. JENSEN, Steroid Hormone Receptors
H. HÖFLER, Oncogene and Receptor Expression
H.-E. STEGNER, W. JONAT, Breast Carcinoma
N. WERNERT, G. SEITZ, Prostatic Cancer – Immunohistochemistry of Steroid Hormone Receptors
M. R. PARWARESCH, H. KREIPE, H. J. RADZUN, G. GRIESSER, Malignant Lymphomas – Lineage Specific Receptors in the Diagnosis of Malignant Lymphomas and Myelomonocytic Neoplasias

MIX
Papier aus verantwortungsvollen Quellen
Paper from responsible sources
FSC® C105338

FSC
www.fsc.org

If you have any concerns about our products,
you can contact us on
ProductSafety@springernature.com

In case Publisher is established outside the EU,
the EU authorized representative is:
Springer Nature Customer Service Center GmbH
Europaplatz 3, 69115 Heidelberg, Germany

Printed by Libri Plureos GmbH
in Hamburg, Germany